£19 20

THE PHYSIOLOGICAL BASIS OF MEMORY

CONTRIBUTORS

D. A. Booth

Georges Chapouthier

Clifford N. Christian

Ronald G. Dawson

J. Anthony Deutsch

C. R. Gallistel

Susan D. Iversen

Arnold L. Leiman

James L. McGaugh

Donald A. Norman

Allen M. Schneider

Elizabeth K. Warrington

L. Weiskrantz

THE PHYSIOLOGICAL BASIS
OF MEMORY

Edited by

J. ANTHONY DEUTSCH

Department of Psychology
University of California, San Diego
La Jolla, California

ACADEMIC PRESS   *1973*   *New York and London*

ACADEMIC PRESS, INC.
111 Fifth Avenue, New York, New York 10003

26772

United Kingdom Edition published by
ACADEMIC PRESS, INC. (LONDON) LTD.
24/28 Oval Road, London NW1

LIBRARY OF CONGRESS CATALOG CARD NUMBER: 72-77336

PRINTED IN THE UNITED STATES OF AMERICA

CONTENTS

Chapter 8. Spreading Depression: A Behavioral Analysis
Allen M. Schneider

Chapter 9. Brain Lesions and Memory in Animals
Susan D. Iversen

**Chapter 10. An Analysis of Short-Term and Long-Term
Memory Defects in Man**
Elizabeth K. Warrington and L. Weiskrantz

**Chapter 11. What Have the Animal Experiments Taught
Us About Human Memory?**
Donald A. Norman

LIST OF CONTRIBUTORS

Numbers in parentheses indicate the pages on which the authors contributions begin

D. A. BOOTH (27), *Laboratory of Experimental Psychology, School of Biological Sciences, University of Sussex, Brighton, England*

GEORGES CHAPOUTHIER (1), *Laboratoire de Psychophysiologie, Universite Louis Pasteur, Strasbourg, France*

CLIFFORD N. CHRISTIAN (125), *Department of Psychology, University of California, Berkeley, California*

RONALD G. DAWSON (77), *Department of Psychology, University of Western Australia, Nedlands, Australia*

J. ANTHONY DEUTSCH (59, 113), *Department of Psychology, University of California, San Diego, La Jolla, California.*

C. R. GALLISTEL (175), *Psychology Department, University of Pennsylvania, Philadelphia, Pennsylvania*

SUSAN D. IVERSEN (305), *Department of Experimental Psychology, Cambridge, England*

ARNOLD L. LEIMAN (125), *Department of Psychology, University of California, Berkeley, California*

JAMES L. MC GAUGH (77), *Department of Psychobiology, University of California, Irvine, California*

DONALD A. NORMAN (397), *Department of Psychology, University of California, San Diego, La Jolla, California.*

ALLEN M. SCHNEIDER (269), *Department of Psychology, University College of Arts and Science, New York University, New York, New York*

ELIZABETH K. WARRINGTON (365), *National Hospital, Queen Square, London, W. C.*

L. WEISKRANTZ (365), *Department of Experimental Psychology, University of Oxford, Oxford, England*

PREFACE

This volume represents an attempt to collate in one source important information concerning the physiological substrate of memory and learning. The book should be useful to researchers and interested students alike. It has been written to be comprehended by an attentive reader even if he lacks previous background in the subject. The contributors have not merely been content to catalogue a series of facts. Findings and theories are critically evaluated so that the reader is given a realistic appraisal of the status of the field.

After the early, somewhat uncritical enthusiasm which ushered in the vast spate of work on the physical basis of memory, intense skepticism, disappointment, and disillusionment set in among many. However, a careful reading of the book will reveal that continuous progress is being made in the field and that the mood of self-doubt has actually produced a needed increase in sophistication. This heightening of intellectual refinement is necessary though perhaps not yet adequate to solve one of nature's most difficult and intriguing problems.

CHAPTER

1

BEHAVIORAL STUDIES OF THE MOLECULAR BASIS OF MEMORY[1]

GEORGES CHAPOUTHIER

I. INTRODUCTION

The achievement of molecular genetics has produced considerable evidence that hereditary information is stored in a chemical code, the DNA molecule. Because innate information can be stored in chemical form, many authors since

[1]We wish to thank Mr. G. Radcliffe, Jr. and Miss S. Greenfield for their counsel.

1

Monné (1948) and Katz and Halstead (1950) have postulated that acquired information might also be stored chemically.

The problem of acquisition of information by the brain brings us to a preliminary discussion of the concepts of learning and memory. There is no general agreement among psychologists about a definition of these terms. It does not seem necessary here, however, to discuss these definitions in depth, and in the context of the study of the molecular approach which follows, we could simply define these concepts by the use of the term information. In this sense, learning could appear as "acquisition and retention of information" by the nervous system (Ungar, 1970c), and memory, as the sum of all the information stored in the brain.

Only a few types of molecule have an information content high enough to code all the information required for the rather complex processes of learning and memory. The most likely to be involved in such a role are nucleic acids and proteins. Investigations of this hypothesis have been undertaken in recent years, and I should like to summarize the most important of them.

All the studies described in this chapter attempt to find a correlation between behavioral modifications occurring during learning and molecular changes. They can be divided into three main areas of investigation: (1) the study of chemical changes associated with learning, (2) the study of the effect of inhibitors of RNA and protein synthesis on learning, and (3) the bioassay methods for chemical correlates of learning.

II. CHEMICAL CHANGES ASSOCIATED WITH LEARNING

The simplest method for investigating the role of nucleic acids and proteins in learning and memory is to look for the quantitative or qualitative changes in these substances in the nervous system following learning. The principle is simple, but its application is not always easy. It is probable that only a comparatively small number of neurons are activated by a given learning situation and the resulting chemical changes are sometimes difficult to distinguish from the metabolic processes correlated with the activity of the nervous system.

Since another chapter of this volume explains in detail the neurochemical changes correlated with learning, and since that approach is not primarily a behavioral one, I should like merely to discuss the interpretation of the principal results.

First, it is extremely difficult to draw a general conclusion from the results obtained in this field for, in the various experiments, too many conditions vary widely. The animals used were either the usual laboratory animals or, in some cases, unusual ones, like chickens (Bateson, Horn, & Rose, 1969), pigeons (Bogoch, 1968), goldfish (Shashoua, 1968), or planarians (Corning & Freed, 1968; Crawford, King, & Siebert, 1965). The animals were trained in the following tasks: motor learning (Hydén & Lange, 1965, 1968; Shashoua, 1968), discrimination (Bowman & Strobel, 1969; Bogoch, 1968), avoidance (Altschuler, Kleban, Gold, Lawton, & Miller, 1969; Beach, Emmens, Kimble, & Lichey, 1969; Glassman, 1969; Gold, Altschuler, Kleban, Lawton, & Miller, 1969), or classical conditioning (Corning & Freed, 1968; Crawford et al., 1965). Numerous differences also exist in the chemical methods which can be carried out on nucleic acids and proteins, either directly on these substances after learning (Bogoch, 1968; Hydén, 1959, 1967, 1969) or by a more indirect way like the study of the incorporation of a nucleotide or its precursor (Bowman & Strobel, 1969; Glassman, 1969; Shashoua, 1968), or an amino acid (Beach et al., 1969; Bateson et al., 1969). And this chemical analysis itself may be done on various quantities of nervous tissue, from a single neuron (Hydén, 1959; Hydén & Egyhazi, 1962) to parts of the brain (Beach et al., 1969; Bowman & Strobel, 1969; Glassman, 1969; Hydén & Lange, 1968), or to the whole brain (Bogoch, 1968; Shashoua, 1968).

A second difficulty in the interpretation of this type of experiment is that it is not easy to distinguish between the chemical changes occurring in the brain after learning and the ones occurring after stimulation without learning (Ungar, 1970c). Increase in RNA and protein synthesis and even changes in RNA base ratio have been shown to occur in the brain after various types of stimulation without learning (Debold, Firschein, Carrier, & Leaf, 1967; Grampp & Edström, 1963; Rappoport & Daginawala, 1968). In this last study, the authors tried various olfactory stimuli on the isolated head of the catfish. Some stimuli, certainly new to the fish (like morpholine or amylacetate), caused changes in the RNA base ratio, but similar effects were caused by extracts of shrimp, certainly familiar to the animal. Moreover, some other new stimuli, like camphor, had no effect. It is possible that, even in the experiments including a control group of animals submitted to stimulation without learning, chemical changes following learning could result from quantitative differences rather than from qualitative ones. This could mean that a stimulation followed by retention needs a more active metabolism than a stimulation without retention (Ungar, 1970c).

Among the methods used to date, only two could prove the existence of qualitative changes during learning: DNA-RNA hybridization (Machlus & Gaito, 1969) and production of specific antibodies (Jankovic, Rakic, Veskov, & Horvat, 1969; Mihailovic & Jankovic, 1961; Rosenblatt, 1970). These methods, however, are still at a very early stage.

III. EFFECTS OF INHIBITORS OF RNA
AND PROTEIN SYNTHESIS ON LEARNING

Numerous drugs are known to have an effect—either facilitating or decreasing—on learning. A general review of this question has been written by McGaugh and Petrinovitch (1965). Interesting results were obtained on the effect on learning of drugs acting on synaptic transmission; this question is reviewed by Deutsch in another chapter of this volume. I should like to summarize here only the action of drugs which affect learning and memory by impairing RNA and protein synthesis.

Among the drugs used, the principal ones are 8-azaguanine and actinomycin D (which inhibit the transcription of DNA into RNA), puromycin (which blocks the peptide chain elongation in the ribosomes), and cycloheximide and acetoxycycloheximide (which block the amino acid transfer by t-RNA).

A. 8-Azaguanine and Actinomycin D

The first experiment in this field, the well-known study of Dingman and Sporn (1961), was done with 8-azaguanine. The authors trained rats to escape from mazes filled with water. Using 8-azaguanine, Dingman and Sporn showed that this substance can impair learning when injected before training, but has no effect when injected after. Although, in the authors' opinion (Dingman & Sporn, 1964), this experiment was not conclusive in itself, it can be considered the first attempt to affect learning by a substance acting on RNA synthesis.

A few attempts have been made using actinomycin D in mice (Barondes & Jarvik, 1964; Cohen & Barondes, 1966). It was shown that in a passive avoidance task (Barondes & Jarvik, 1964) and in a maze learning task (Cohen & Barondes, 1966), this drug affects neither the learning nor the retention in a test four hours later. Long-term studies were difficult because of the high toxicity of the substance.

More recently, Agranoff, Davis, Casola, and Lim (1967) found that intracerebral actinomycin D could impair memory consolidation in the goldfish, but did not affect long-term memory. These results are similar to those obtained by Agranoff's group with puromycin in the goldfish (Section III, B). Oshima, Gorbman, and Shimada (1969) injected homing salmon with actinomycin D. This treatment was able to inhibit olfactory discrimination by the animals between home water and other types of natural water. It was suggested by Oshima's experiments that inhibition of RNA synthesis could interfere with long-term olfactory memory in the homing salmon.

Evidence was produced by Glassman, Henderson, Cordle, Moon, and Wilson (1970) of the effects of actinomycin D in impairing the learning ability of headless cockroaches. The learning task for the animals was to keep their legs raised to avoid an electric shock (Horridge, 1962). It has been shown by Glassman's team that actinomycin D can impair the acquisition of this avoidance behavior. The mechanism of this action remains, however, unclear, and further work is still needed.

B. Puromycin

Studies on the effects of puromycin were undertaken using mice, goldfish, and homing salmon as experimental animals. The first results in this field were obtained in Flexner's laboratory with mice. The task used was a right-left discrimination in a Y-maze involving an avoidance criterion; the animals had to choose the correct arm within a few seconds. They were trained to a criterion of 9/10 correct choices. The injection of puromycin was intracerebral, since sub-cutaneous injections have been shown not to inhibit protein synthesis suffi-ciently to impair memory. Temporal injections of 90 μg each of puromycin impaired memory in animals trained 24 hours previously (Flexner, Flexner, & Stellar, 1963; Flexner, Flexner, Roberts, & De la Haba, 1964). This was cor-related with a marked inhibition of protein synthesis in the temporal area. If the injections are given 3 to 6 days after training, temporal injections alone are ineffective. To affect memory at this time, it is necessary to use six injections in various parts of the cerebral cortex (2 temporal, 2 ventricular, 2 frontal injec-tions). Flexner thinks that during 3 to 6 days there is a kind of short-term memory localized in the temporal region, but, after this time, there appears a longer term memory having no precise localization in the cortex. Deutsch (1969), however, pointed out that other explanations of this effect were pos-sible, especially differences in the dose necessary to suppress memory either 24 hours or several days after learning; the small dose present in the cortex after temporal injections could be sufficient to suppress recently acquired memory, but a higher dose, requiring several injections, would be necessary to erase many-day-old memory.

Flexner, Flexner, and Roberts (1967) have made interesting observations with this preparation: puromycin was without effect on overtrained animals and successive injections of puromycin became rapidly ineffective. The reasons for this are not clear. Flexner explains the second point by a more rapid elimination of puromycin from the brain, perhaps due to vascular changes.

Flexner and Flexner (1967) found that intracerebral injection of isotonic NaCl solution was able to suppress the amnesic effect of a prior injection of puromycin. This effect of saline injections was interpreted to be due to a washing off by saline of the abnormal peptides produced by puromycin. More recently Flexner and Flexner (1969) found that not only NaCl, but also other chlorides, an ultrafiltrate of blood serum, or even water alone could produce the same effect and restore memory after puromycin injection. The question re-mains whether this effect can really be interpreted as a washing off of abnormal peptides, or if a more indirect mechanism, such as the action of ions on cerebral electrical activity (Cohen, Ervin, & Barondes, 1966) could not partially interfere with the memory process.

Barondes' group trained mice in the same right-left discrimination. Their results are in agreement with Flexner's, but throw a new light on some aspects of the work. According to Barondes, puromycin does not impair the early stage of retention, but is highly effective a few hours after injection (Barondes & Cohen, 1966). This is, however, related to a strong impairment of electrical cerebral activity (Cohen et al., 1966). Barondes and his colleagues questioned whether some other action of puromycin besides its inhibition of protein synthesis might explain the amnesic effect.

While these results were obtained with a maze learning task with negative reinforcement, Ungerer (1969a) tried puromycin in mice trained in an instrumental learning situation with positive reinforcement. She was able to prove that puromycin injected in the brain in the same quantity and in the same places as were used to erase a maze learning is completely ineffective in an instrumental situation. Along with Flexner's results on overtained animals (Flexner *et al.*, 1967), this observation can suggest that puromycin is without effect on strongly consolidated learning. More experiments are still needed, however, to test this hypothesis.

Agranoff and Klinger (1964) devised in goldfish a conditioned avoidance to light in a shuttle tank. When learning is achieved in a session of twenty trials in one day, the score of the animal in a session 3 days later can be used as a measure of retention of learning. Puromycin, injected intracranially in doses from 90 to 210 μg during the 30 minutes which follow the first session, can impair retention, but there is no effect if the puromycin is injected more than 60 minutes after the first session (Agranoff, Davis, & Brink, 1965, 1966). If puromycin is injected before training, it does not affect it, but the retention shows impairment 3 days later. Agranoff's conclusion is that puromycin does not affect immediate memory during learning or long-term memory (60 minutes after learning), but that the drug can inhibit consolidation. Similar results seem to have been obtained by action of electroconvulsive shock immediately after learning (Davis, Bright, & Agranoff, 1965).

The effect of puromycin in the goldfish was confirmed by Potts and Bitterman (1967). These authors emphasized the fact that puromycin seems to suppress specifically conditioned fear; in an experiment with positive reinforcement, puromycin was without effect. It can be pointed out, however, that since the appetitive situation and the conditioned avoidance situation differ by many parameters, other explanations of the difference of effect of puromycin could be possible. As suggested by Deutsch (1969), a strongly consolidated training (as a task with positive reinforcement could be) would show less susceptibility to puromycin. In this aspect, the work of Potts and Bitterman with goldfish could be compared with the study of Ungerer (1969a) with mice.

More recently, evidence was produced by Oshima *et al.* (1969) of the ability of puromycin to inhibit olfactory discrimination of the homing salmon. This result is similar to the one obtained by the same authors with actinomycin D (Section III, A).

C. Cycloheximide and Acetoxycycloheximide

Acetoxycycloheximide was used by Flexner's group in mice trained in the same right-left discrimination as was used for the puromycin experiments. According to these authors, although acetoxycycloheximide produces a strong inhibition of protein synthesis, it seems to be without effect on either short-term or long-term memory. Moreover, simultaneous injections of acetoxycyclohex-imide and puromycin are also without effect on memory. Acetoxycyclohex-imide seems to "protect" memory from the action of puromycin (Flexner & Flexner, 1966). One of the many hypotheses attempting to explain this phenom-enon postulates that the action of puromycin is due to the synthesis of abnormal peptides which could interfere with memory; the formation of these peptides could be suppressed by acetoxycycloheximide (Flexner & Flexner, 1967; Flexner & Flexner, 1968). Reinis (1969) claimed to have shown the presence of such peptides by their effect on behavior, while Ungerer, Spitz, and Chapouthier (1969), using the same learning situation as Flexner, were unable to find them.

Barondes & Cohen (1967a) considered Flexner's criterion of nine correct responses out of ten was too severe and might mask the effect. To test this hypothesis, they submitted one group of mice to a prolonged training (criterion 9/10), another to a short training (criterion 3/4). Intracerebral injections of acetoxycycloheximide were able to impair memory for 3 hours to 7 days after injection in the animals submitted to short training, but not in the animals submitted to prolonged training. The criterion of 9/10 correct responses in such an easy learning task as left-right discrimination creates a kind of "overtraining" in the animals, which becomes resistant to acetoxycycloheximide.

In other experiments (Barondes & Cohen, 1968), it was shown that acetoxycycloheximide is able to suppress memory even in mice trained to the 9/10 correct response criterion in the case of a light-dark discrimination. Baron-des' group assumed that, since light-dark discrimination is a more difficult and less "natural" task for mice, there could be "less active stimulation of protein synthesis in the appropriate neural pathways" on each exposure to the cues, thus preventing the "overtraining" effect found with a 9/10 criterion in a left-right discrimination task.

Barondes and Cohen (1967b) have shown that simultaneous injections of cycloheximide and puromycin are without effect on memory. This result is similar to Flexner's results on the action on memory of acetoxycycloheximide-puromycin mixture (Flexner & Flexner, 1966).

Agranoff et al. (1966) found that acetoxycycloheximide, like puromycin (Section III, B), was able to inhibit the consolidation of a conditioned avoidance response when injected into goldfish after training. Similar results to those obtained with actinomycin D and puromycin (Section III, A and B) were obtained by Oshima et al. for the homing salmon. In insects, Brown and Noble (1967) and Glassman et al. (1970) were able to impair with cycloheximide the learning ability of headless cockroaches. These results are similar to those obtained by Glassman et al. (1970) with actinomycin D (Section III, A).

D. Effects of RNase

RNase is not an inhibitor of RNA or protein synthesis but an enzyme catalyzing the degradation of RNA. It is, however, interesting to compare the results obtained with antibiotics to some results obtained with RNase. This enzyme was used by Corning and John (1961) to suppress retention after regeneration in planarians (Section IV,A,2). More recently, Jaffard and Cardo (1968, 1969) have shown that RNase injected into the brain was able to suppress some retention, but not when learning was strongly consolidated. This observation could explain the negative results obtained with RNase by Stevens and Tapp (1966) in a pattern discrimination task; in such a difficult learning task, where the consolidation requires a large number of trials, RNase appears to be without effect once the animal has reached criterion. These results are similar to those obtained by Flexner et al. (1967) and Ungerer (1969a) with puromycin.

E. Discussion

It is difficult to draw general conclusions from all of these studies; I shall try, however, to do it for those works which use the mouse or the goldfish as the experimental animal. It is possible that Agranoff's "long-term" memory, on which the antibiotics are ineffective, could be compared to the overtraining situation in Flexner and Barondes' studies and to the strongly consolidated situation of Ungerer's experiments. It could be possible to delimit three stages in retention: first, immediate memory, on which the antibiotics were without effect, second, a stage of memory consolidation during which the antibiotics were effective, and, third, an "overtraining" situation insensitive to antibiotics. Many points remain unclear, however, and some authors, like Deutsch (1969), point out that antibiotics could eventually act on retention in a more indirect way, for example, by acting on a transmitter, than by direct inhibition of protein synthesis.

Whatever the interpretation of these results, whether the action is direct or indirect, the principal problem remains that the effects of antibiotics, like the analysis of chemical correlates of learning, do not prove that proteins have a specific role in learning and memory, but, rather, that learning and retention increase the general metabolism of the nervous system.

However, results of experiments on improvement of learning by drugs facilitating protein synthesis are less convincing. The effects on learning of tricyanoaminopropene (Egyhazi & Hydén, 1961; Chamberlain, Rothschild, & Gerard, 1963; McNutt, 1967) and of magnesium pemoline (Beach & Kimble, 1967) still remain controversial.

For more detailed information on this question, the reader is referred to the reviews by Glassman (1969), Ungerer (1969b), and Cohen (1970).

IV. BIOASSAY METHODS FOR THE CHEMICAL CORRELATES OF LEARNING

The principle of biological assay is to detect, not by biochemical means, but by biological effects, the chemical modifications that occur in animals. In the particular bioassay to be discussed below, "donor" animals are submitted to a certain type of training, then an extract of their nervous system is prepared and injected by various routes to "recipient" animals. The performance of these recipients in the task learned by the donors is then tested and compared with the performance given in the same task by control recipients (usually injected with an extract of "naive" nervous system). This method has the advantage of demonstrating the possibility of specific transfer of information, but like all bioassays it is a delicate technique, often a source of many artifacts (Gaddum, 1953). Because the test of the recipients is behavioral, the variability of responses is often even larger and the probability of error even greater than for ordinary bioassays. Compared with the procedures discussed in the two preceding sections: (1) the probability of error is much greater than in the direct analysis of chemical changes associated with learning because of the variability of the behavioral test, and (2) the possibility of artifacts is much greater than in the study of the effect on learning of a known single substance, such as an antibiotic drug, because the bioassay is used to test unknown and impure substances in the presence of several others. Therefore, this method involves the use of a large number of animals and the experiments must be replicated many times under different conditions.

A. Experiments on Planarians

The first experiments of this type were done on planarians in McConnell's laboratory. Because of the importance this category of experiments subsequently acquired, I should like to describe the principal results obtained in this field. The work of McConnell and his colleagues can be studied at three levels: the possibility of learning in planarians, the retention of learning after regeneration, and the "memory transfer through cannibalism" effect. This work was criticized at all three levels of the phenomena that McConnell claimed to have demonstrated.

1. Learning in Planarians

Before McConnell's results appeared, some authors had already observed phenomena resembling learning in planarians. Thompson and McConnell (1955) devised a method of "classical conditioning" of these animals. It is known that planarians are sensitive to light. After determination of the level of responses by planarians to light, the method consisted in the association of a light (conditioned stimulus) and electric shock (unconditioned stimulus). Thompson and McConnell showed that, after training, the experimental animals responded more to light than did the controls. Their conclusion was that the animals had been able to associate light to electric shock, that is, to be conditioned. Some authors (Halas, James, & Knutson, 1962; Bennett & Calvin, 1964) were unable to replicate this classical conditioning of planarians. Halas *et al.* showed that, in the planarian *Dugesia tigrina*, it was difficult to find a significant difference between the animals submitted to paired light and shock and some of the control groups. They concluded that McConnell's results did not show learning phenomena, but rather a general sensitization to light caused by some kind of manipulation of the animals. More recently, attempts have been made to demonstrate classical conditioning in two European species; the results were that only one of them showed an effect resembling classical conditioning (Chapouthier, Legrain, & Spitz, 1969). According to McConnell (1967), it is possible that some species, and even some strains in the same species, are refractory to classical conditioning.

The possibility of discrimination learning was shown in planarians by several authors. Best and Rubinstein (1962), Chapouthier, Pallaud, and Ungerer (1968), and Corning (1964) showed that it was possible to induce in planarians an elementary right-left discrimination. Other types of discrimination were used by Humphries (1961), Griffard and Pierce (1964), and by Block and McConnell (1967). Discrimination learning by planarians leads to an important problem: following the learning phase (during which the animal begins to choose significantly the "correct" arm of the maze and to avoid the arm where it receives punishment), a phase of rejection occurs (during which the animals paradoxically choose the "wrong" arm of the maze) (Best & Rubinstein, 1962; Chapouthier et al., 1968; Corning, 1964).

Some authors have reported positive results in complex operant conditioning in planarians (Lee, 1963; Seydoux, Girardier, Perrin, Ruphi, & Posternak, 1967), but these experiments are of such importance that much more replication in a number of laboratories is needed.

2. Retention of Learning after Regeneration

When cut in two, planarians are able to regenerate into two complete individuals. This peculiarity was used by McConnell, Jacobson, and Kimble (1959), who proved that, after regeneration, both sections of the animal show equal retention of classical conditioning. The same effect was observed by McConnell, Jacobson, and Maynard (1959) in the second generation of regenerated planarians. All these experiments caused McConnell to postulate, according to Hyden's work, that memory could have a molecular basis, possibly RNA. Experiments involving the action of RNase (Section III, D) seemed to confirm this hypothesis.

This observation was criticized by Brown, Dustman, and Beck (1966a,b). These authors claimed that the greater responsiveness to light of regenerated worms comes from the fact that the regenerated animals are smaller than the original ones, and it has been proved that smaller animals tend to be more responsive to light. This criticism, however, does not explain the fact that, in McConnell's experiments, the control group (regenerated and therefore smaller animals) responded significantly less than did the experimental animals.

The interpretation of Brown *et al.* can explain a comparison with animals before regeneration, but not with controls after regeneration. Moreover, many authors have shown different kinds of retention after regeneration. Westerman (1963) showed a retention of habituation and Ernhardt and Sherrick (1959) and Corning (1966) a retention of discrimination after regeneration.

3. *"Transfer of Memory through Cannibalism"*

When hungry, planarians are capable of cannibalizing other individuals of the same species cut up into suitably sized pieces. McConnell fed trained planarians to naive ones; this method was the equivalent of a crude injection of the supposed information-carrying molecule. The ability of the recipients of trained animals to respond to light was then tested and compared to the responses of recipients of naive animals in the same situation. The results of this experiment were positive, and McConnell (1962) claimed to have obtained a "transfer of memory through cannibalism." An experiment of the same type using purified RNA instead of fragments of planarians was carried out by Jacobson, Fried, and Horowitz (1966b); their results were also positive: the classical conditioning paradigm seemed able to be transferred by injection of trained RNA into the digestive cavity of naive animals.

The interpretation of this type of experiment remains difficult, because it must be postulated that RNA is not degraded by planarians. Moreover, although believing that classical conditioning can occur in planarians, some authors were not able to show a specific transfer of memory by cannibalism in these animals. Hartry, Keith-Lee, and Morton (1964) showed that not only cannibals of trained animals showed a greater ability to respond to light, but cannibals of some control groups also showed the same ability. Their interpretation is that experimental conditions in trained and in some control groups produce in the cannibalized animals the appearance of a general activating factor which makes the cannibals more sensitive to light. More recently I have shown that some physiological conditions like hunger can increase the response level of planarians to light (Chapouthier, 1967a). For the "transfer of memory by cannibalism" itself, I found that cannibals of some control groups (animals submitted to light alone) exhibited an increased responsiveness to light intermediate between that of the cannibals of naive planarians and the cannibals of trained planarians (Chapouthier *et al.*, 1969a). In such a situation, it was difficult to choose experimentally between the hypothesis of "transfer of memory through cannibalism" (McConnell) and the hypothesis of "activating substance [Hartry *et al.*]."

To answer this type of objection, McConnell (1966) tried to transfer discrimination learning. His results were positive and he claimed to have clearly demonstrated the specificity of the effect. Negative results, however, were obtained by Picket, Jennings, and Wells (1964), and Chapouthier (unpublished results).

In summary, there are apparently phenomena resembling learning in planarians and some retention after regeneration. The results of the bioassay methods, however, mostly using classical conditioning situations, are not sufficiently clear. The only proof of specific transfer of information in planarians would be the transfer of learned discrimination. These experiments will have to resolve the problem of the rejection phase (Section IV, A, 1). Such an important question needs more evidence produced by experiments from various laboratories. For more detailed information, the reader is referred to the reviews by Chapouthier *et al.* (1969a), Corning and Riccio (1970), and McConnell and Shelby (1970). The experiments on planarians have recently been extended by more clear-cut studies in vertebrates.

B. Experiments on Vertebrates

The first experiments in this field were published in 1965, almost simultaneously, by four groups of workers (Reinis; Fjerdingstad, Nissen, and Røigaard-Petersen; Ungar and Oceguera-Navarro; Babich, Jacobson, Bubash, and Jacobson). They were followed by a great controversy and many publications, some of them reporting negative results, some of them positive ones. Since then considerable evidence has been accumulated on the validity of the findings and at least twenty-two different laboratories have published positive results. Most of the negative results, obtained largely in the early stages of research in the field, can be explained in the light of the positive findings.

It is not possible here to review separately all the relevant publications. Systematic discussions have been published by Rosenblatt (1970), Ungar (1970b), and Ungar and Chapouthier (1971). I would like, however, to discuss a few aspects of this question, especially (1) the possible reasons for failure to replicate some positive results, (2) the type of training situation used, (3) the problem of the specificity of the bioassay, and (4) the question of the chemical identification of the responsible factors and of the molecular code of memory.

1. Reasons for Failure to Replicate the Bioassays

a. Chemical Composition. The first probable reason for inability to reproduce the positive experiments is the chemical composition of the extract used. Among the four original groups of workers, two (Fjerdingstad *et al.*, 1965; Babich *et al.*, 1965b) claimed to have obtained their results with an RNA preparation. Since it is now known (Ungar & Fjerdingstad, 1971) that the active factors are linked with RNA, but are not RNA, it can be understood how some investigators, using crude RNA preparations, have been able to obtain positive results while others, using more purified RNA, were unable to replicate them. Most of the negative results were obtained with RNA preparations, while the authors using crude extracts obtained positive results more easily (see Ungar & Chapouthier, 1971).

b. Dose. The clearest results were obtained with a high dose of extracts (Ungar & Irwin, 1967; Ungar, 1967a,b; Chapouthier & Ungerer, 1969). In these experiments each recipient received the equivalent of many times his brain weight. Moos, Levan, Mason, Mason, and Hebron (1969), and Rosenblatt (1969), however, obtained positive results with very small doses. Their results could perhaps be caused, in Moos' experiment, by a peculiar type of training situation (acquired aversion to saccharine) and, in Rosenblatt's case, to a different route of administration of the extracts (intravenous).

c. Interval between Injection and Testing of the Recipients. Most of the positive results were obtained when a sufficient interval was allowed between injection and testing of the recipients. The effect often only appears a few days after the injection. In many of the negative publications (Byrne and 22 others, 1966; Gross & Carey, 1965; Gordon, Deanin, Leonhardt, & Gwynn, 1966; Lambert & Saurat, 1967; Luttges, Johnson, Buck, Holland, & McGaugh, 1966), all the tests were done within 24 hours after the injection, which was too soon. It can be pointed out that the positive experiments which have used such a schedule were extremely difficult to replicate (Babich, Jacobson, & Bubash, 1965a; Babich, Jacobson, Bubash, & Jacobson, 1965b).

d. Duration of Donor Training. It is necessary not only to bring the donors to a certain criterion of training, but also to keep them at criterion for several days, probably to allow sufficient time for the active material to accumulate (Ungar, 1967a,b; Chapouthier & Ungerer, 1969). In some cases, however, an excess of training can decrease the effect (Ungar, 1967a).

e. Other Factors. There are many other factors which can interfere with the assay and many are interrelated. For example, the route of injection (which can be intraperitoneal, intravenous, or intracerebral) does not seem to be of considerable importance, but it is possible that intraperitoneal administration requires higher doses than other types of injection. As for the known factors, keeping the extracts at low temperature remains an elementary precaution. Animals which are either too young or too old do not seem to produce any effect when used as recipients (Adam & Faiszt, 1967). Food deprivation of recipients seems, according to Reinis (1965) to be important when donors are trained under the same conditions. More recently, Golub, Masiarz, Villars, and McConnell (1970) found that rest periods interposed during training of the donors increase significantly the performance of the recipients. There remain, of course, unknown parameters and there is no general rule guaranteeing a positive effect. The best way is to explore each situation by trial and error to determine the critical factors.

2. Types of Training in Positive Experiments

Many types of learning situations have been attempted with positive results. The principal ones are as follows.

Habituation to sound (Ungar & Oceguera-Navarro, 1965).

Habituation to a sound producing audiogenic seizure (Daliers & Rigaux-Motquin, 1968).

Habituation to air puffs (Ungar, 1967b).

Avoidance (Albert, 1966; Kleban, Altschuler, Lawton, Parris, & Lords, 1968).

Escape in a water maze (Essman & Lehrer, 1966).

Dark avoidance (Gay & Raphelson, 1967; Ungar, Galvan, & Clark, 1968; Fjerdingstad, 1969a; Golub, Epstein, & McConnell, 1969; Wolthuis, 1969).

Conditioned avoidance (Rosenblatt & Miller, 1966; Adam & Faiszt, 1967; Ungar, 1967a,b; Faiszt & Adam, 1968; Chapouthier, Pallaud, & Ungerer, 1969b; Chapouthier & Ungerer, 1969; Fjerdingstad, 1969c; Cohen, 1969).

Left-right discrimination (Rosenblatt & Miller, 1966; Essman & Lehrer, 1967; Ungar, 1967a,b; Ungar & Irwin, 1967; Krylov, Kalyuzhnaya, & Tongur, 1969).

Discrimination between two compartments (Jacobson, Babich, Bubash, & Goren, 1966a; Rosenblatt, 1969).

Choice of the lighted alley in a maze (Fjerdingstad et al., 1965; Ungar, 1967a,b; Ungar & Irwin, 1967; Gibby, Crough, & Thios, 1968; Rødigaard-Petersen, Nissen, & Fjerdingstad, 1968; Wolthuis, Anthoni, & Stevens, 1968).

Acquired avoidance of saccharine (Revusky & DeVenuto, 1967; Moos, Levan, Mason, Mason, & Hebron, 1969).

Conditioned avoidance of drinking (Weiss, 1970).

Learning of a detour by chicks (Rosenthal & Sparber, 1968).

Wire climbing (Gibby & Crough, 1967).

Color discrimination in goldfish (Zippel & Domagk, 1969).

Black and white discrimination (Dyal & Golub, 1967).

Alimentary conditioned reflexes (Reinis, 1965, 1968).

Instrumental learning in a Skinner box (Rosenblatt & Miller, 1966; Rosenblatt, Farrow, & Herblin, 1966a; Rosenblatt, Farrow, & Rhine, 1966b; Byrne & Samuel, 1966; Byrne & Hughes, 1967; Dyal, Golub, & Marrone, 1967; Dyal & Golub, 1968; Golub & McConnell, 1968; McConnell, Shigehisha, & Salive, 1968; Chapouthier et al., 1969b; Golub et al., 1970).

Alternation in a Skinner box (Fjerdingstad, 1969b).

Conditioned approach (Babich et al., 1965a,b; Jacobson, Babich, Bubash, & Jacobson, 1965; McConnell et al., 1968).

Fixation of postural asymmetry (Giurgea, Daliers, & Mouravieff, 1969).

It should be noted that some situations are evidently nontransferable. This seems to be the case in the choice of the dark alley of a maze (Luttges et al., 1966; Ungar, 1967a; Ungar & Irwin, 1967; Chapouthier & Ungerer, 1968, 1969).

Most of the publications cited above report experiments done in rodents (rats or mice). One (Rosenthal & Sparber, 1968) used chicks, and a few (Zippel

& Domagk, 1969; Fjerdingstad, 1969c) used goldfish. Experiments with other animal groups would be useful.

Recently Braud (1970) showed in goldfish that even extinction could be transferred by brain extracts. In his experiment, recipients were injected with brain extracts prepared from donors that had acquired and then extinguished a conditioned avoidance response in a shuttle tank; the recipients extinguished the response significantly faster than the controls. These results, if they are confirmed, would suggest the possibility that both acquisition and extinction are active processes, correlated with the synthesis of molecules. This had already been suggested in a different situation by some experiments of Jacobson et al. in planarians (1966b). In their experiments, however, there was no transfer of extinction, but, on the contrary, extracts prepared from extinguished planarians produced a positive transfer effect; this would suggest that in the extinguished donors the "positive" molecules remain present, but are inhibited by some other substance. Chapouthier (1967b) showed that, taking into account this similarity of active mechanisms, it could be possible to construct a mathematical theory explaining many peculiarities of learning phenomena. More experimental work is still needed in the field, for such a new conception of extinction needs much more proof than is supplied in these two studies.

For more detailed information relating to the entire problem the reader is referred to reviews by Rosenblatt (1970), Ungar (1970b), and Ungar and Chapouthier (1971).

3. Specificity of the Bioassay

The question of the specificity of the bioassay and of the limits of this specificity is certainly one of the most important questions in this field. Among the several authors claiming positive results, most have used a procedure of testing the recipients with reinforcement. In this case, the only thing they can prove is a facilitation of learning in the animals injected with trained brain extract, but not a specific transfer of information.

The best arguments in favor of a relative specificity of the extracts are the results published by Ungar (1967a,b), who has performed "cross transfer" experiments between habituation to two different stimuli and between two types of avoidance tasks. The negative results of these "cross transfer" experiments suggest that the extract of donor brains trained in a certain situation has a specific effect on recipients tested in the same situation. More recently, Zippel & Domagk (1969) were able to transfer color discrimination in the goldfish, showing specificity within the same sensory modality. These experiments have been replicated in Ungar's laboratory (Ungar, Galvan, & Chapouthier, in preparation) with an attempt to find out how narrow a difference between the wavelengths can be used while still maintaining a transfer effect. But the question of the limits of specificity of the bioassay still remains an important one and more experiments are needed to determine these limits precisely.

4. Chemical Identification of the Active Material; the Possibility of a Molecular Code of Memory

Because of the influence of Hyden's and McConnell's experiments, many authors have thought, as already stated, that the substance responsible for transfer effects was RNA. This idea is at the origin of many negative results. Others, with no preconceived ideas, began with crude extracts and proposed the hypothesis that small molecules, probably peptides, were responsible for the effects (Ungar & Oceguera-Navarro, 1965; Rosenblatt *et al.*, 1966; Chapouthier, 1968; Fjerdingstad, 1969a; Giurgea *et al.*, 1969). It has recently been proved by Ungar and Fjerdingstad (1971) that the RNA preparations were active because of the presence of peptides linked to RNA. This complex can be dissociated at low pH and, after separation from the active peptide, the RNA has no transfer activity.

The first active peptide, isolated from brains of rats trained to avoid a dark box (Ungar *et al.*, 1968), has been completely purified and identified (Ungar, Ho, Galvan, & Desiderio, 1970). It was found that it was a peptide composed of 15 amino acids having the following sequence: Ser-Asp-Asn-Asn-Glu-Glu-Gly-Lys-Ser-Ala-Glu-Gln-Gly-Gly-Tyr-NH$_2$.

The isolation of other active substances is a function of the limits of the specificity of the bioassay. Using enzymic digestions, Ungar (1970a) was able to show chemical differences in four extracts eliciting different behaviors. Further studies of purification and isolation of new peptides are presently being done in Ungar's laboratory, but it would certainly be useful if other laboratories began experiments of this type.

If Ungar's hypothesis is correct, that a great number of such peptides are synthesized in the brain in various situations and are able to elicit various types of behavior when injected into recipients, it could be possible to identify a large number of these substances. Since these substances would represent a chemical translation of the behavioral information, it could then be possible to decipher the code of this translation (Ungar, 1969; Ungar & Chapouthier, 1971).

A few speculations have already been made on the possible mechanisms of such a coding in the brain, trying to take into account all the experimental data described earlier. The most convincing theories at the moment postulate that molecules could direct the traffic of nerve impulses along neural pathways through an appropriate chemical coding of the synapses (Szilard, 1964; Rosenblatt, 1967; Ungar, 1968; Best, 1968). In these theories, therefore, the chemical code is understood as a complement to the structural and electrical codes of the nervous system. A general review of the theories of information processing in the nervous system has been written by Ungar (1970c).

Although the hypotheses of chemical coding of neural pathways are in agreement with most of the results known at present, our knowledge of this problem still remains extremely incomplete and a great deal of experiments are still needed to confirm the present results and to increase our understanding of the nervous system.

V. CONCLUSIONS

The principal results obtained up to now concerning the role of nucleic acids and proteins in learning and memory bring us to the following conclusions:

1. It is possible to show by chemical methods that there are quantitative and qualitative differences in the RNA and protein contents of the brain in naive and trained animals. It is difficult, however, to determine whether these changes result from the learning itself or from a nonspecific increase in brain metabolism.

2. RNA and protein synthesis play a role in the early stage of memory consolidation. This phenomenon can be altered by various inhibitors of RNA and protein synthesis, whose mechanism of action has not yet been clearly defined.

3. Bioassay methods show that during learning there is a formation of peptides in the trained brain. These peptides are able to alter the behavior of recipient animals when injected into them in sufficient doses. At least in the case of vertebrates, these products seem to show a specificity to the learned situation, the extent of which must be determined more precisely. In a question of such importance, much more work is still necessary; it is hoped that many laboratories will undertake studies which can lead to knowledge of a molecular code of memory.

REFERENCES

Adam, G. & Faiszt, J. Conditions for successful transfer effects. *Nature*, 1967, Vol. 216, 198-200.

Agranoff, B. W., Davis, R. E., & Brink, J. J. Memory fixation in goldfish. *Proceedings National Academy of Sciences USA*, 1965, Vol. 54, 788-793.

Agranoff, B. W., Davis, R. E., & Brink, J. J. Chemical studies on memory fixation in goldfish. *Brain Research*, 1966, Vol. 1, 303-309.

Agranoff, B. W., Davis, R. E., Casola, L., & Lim, R. Actinomycin D blocks formation of memory of shock avoidance in goldfish. *Science*, 1967, Vol. 158, 1600-1601.

Agranoff, B. W., & Klinger, P. D. Puromycin effect on memory fixation in the goldfish. *Science*, 1964, Vol. 146, 952-953.

Albert, D. J. Memory in mammals: evidence for a system involving nuclear ribonucleic acid. *Neuropsychologia*, 1966, Vol. 4, 79-92.

Altschuler, H., Kleban, M. H., Gold, M., Lawton, M. P., & Miller, M. Neurochemical changes in the brains of albino rats as related to aversive training. *Journal of Biological Psychology*, 1969, Vol. 11(2), 33-38.

Babich, F. R., Jacobson, A. L., & Bubash, S. Cross-species transfer of learning: effect of ribonucleic acid from hamsters on rat behavior. *Proceedings of the National Academy of Sciences USA*, 1965, Vol 54, 1299-1302. (a)

Babich, F. R., Jacobson, A. L., Bubash, S., & Jacobson, A. Transfer of a response to naive rats by injection of ribonucleic acid extracted from trained rats. *Science*, 1965, Vol. 149, 656-657. (b)

Barondes, S. H., & Cohen, H. D. Puromycin effect on successive phases of memory storage. *Science*, 1966, Vol. 151, 594-595.

Barondes, S. H., & Cohen, H. D. Delayed and sustained effect of acetoxycycloheximide on memory in mice. *Proceedings of the National Academy of Sciences USA*, 1967, Vol. 58, 157-164. (a)

Barondes, S. H., & Cohen, H. D. Comparative effects of cycloheximide and puromycin on cerebral protein synthesis and consolidation of memory in mice. *Brain Research*, 1967, Vol. 4, 44-51. (b)

Barondes, S. H. & Cohen, H. D. Effect of acetoxycycloheximide on learning and memory of a light-dark discrimination. *Nature*, 1968, Vol. 218, 271-273.

Barondes, S. H. & Jarvik, M. E. The influence of actinomycin D on brain RNA synthesis and on memory. *Journal of Neurochemistry*, 1964, Vol. 11, 187-195.

Bateson, P. P. G., Horn, G., & Rose, S. P. R. Effects of an imprinting procedure on regional incorporation of tritiated lysine into protein of chick brain. *Nature*, 1969, Vol. 223, 534-535.

Beach, G., Emmens, M., Kimble, D. P., & Lickey, M. Autoradiographic demonstration of biochemical changes in the limbic system during avoidance training. *Proceedings of the National Academy of Sciences USA*, 1969, Vol. 62, 692-696.

Beach, G., & Kimble, D. P. Activity and responsivity in rats after magnesium pemoline injections. *Science*, 1967, Vol. 155, 698-701.

Bennett, E. L., & Calvin, M. Failure to train planarians reliably. *Neurosciences Research Program Bulletin*, 1964, Vol. 2, 3-24.

Best, J. B., & Rubinstein, I. Maze learning and associated behavior in planaria. *Journal of Comparative & Physiological Psychology*, 1962, Vol. 55, 560-566.

Best, R. M. Encoding of memory in the neuron. *Psychological Reports*, 1968, Vol. 22, 107-115.

Block, R. A. & McConnell, J. V. Classically conditioned discrimination in the planaria *Dugesia dorotocephala*. *Nature*, 1967, Vol. 215, 1465-1466.

Bogoch, S. *The biochemistry of memory*. London & New York: Oxford University Press, 1968.

Bowman, R. E., & Strobel, D. A. Brain RNA metabolism in the rat during learning. *Journal of Comparative & Physiological Psychology*, 1969, Vol. 67, 448-456.

Braud, W. G. Extinction in goldfish:facilitation by intracranial injection of RNA from brains of extinguished donors. *Science*, 1970, Vol. 168, 1234-1236.

Brown, B. M., & Noble, E. P. Cycloheximide and learning in the isolated cockroach ganglion. *Brain Research*, 1967, Vol. 6, 363-366.

Brown, H. M., Dustman, R. E., & Beck, E. C. Experimental procedures that modify light response frequency of regenerated planaria. *Physiology and Behavior*, 1966, Vol. 1, 245-249. (a)

Brown, H. M., Dustman, R. E., & Beck, E. C. Sensitization in planarian. *Physiology and Behavior*, 1966, Vol. 1, 305-308. (b)

Byrne, W. L. & Hughes, A. Behavioral modification by injection of brain extract from trained donors. *Federation Proceedings*, 1967, Vol. 26, 676.

Byrne, W. L. & Samuel, D. Behavioral modification by injection of brain extract prepared from a trained donor. *Science*, 1966, Vol. 154, 418.

Byrne, W. L., Samuel, D., Bennett, E. L., Rosenzweig, M. R., Wasserman, E., Wagner, A. R., Gardner, R., Galambos, R., Berger, B. D., Margules, D. L., Fenichel, R. L., Stein, L., Corson, J. A., Enesco, H. E., Chorover, S. L., Holt, C. E., III, Schiller, P. H., Chiappetta, L., Jarvik, M. E., Leaf, R. C., Dutcher, J. D., Horovitz, Z. P., & Carlson, P. L. Memory transfer. *Science*, 1966, Vol. 153, 658-659.

Chamberlain, T. J., Rothschild, G. H., & Gerard, R. W. Drugs affecting RNA and learning. *Proceedings of the National Academy of Sciences USA*, 1963, Vol. 49, 918-924.

Chapouthier, G. Taux de reponse à la lumière en relation avec le cannibalisme chez la planaire *Dugesia lugubris*. *Comptes Rendus Academie Sciences Serie D.*, 1967, Vol. 265, 2047-2050. (a)

Chapouthier, G. Esquisse d'une théorie moléculaire de la mémoire et de l'oubli. *Revue du Comportement Animal*, 1967, Vol. 4, 1-9. (b)

Chapouthier, G. Le transfert de molecules de mémoire chez les vertébrés. *L'Année Biologique*, 1968, Vol. 7, 275-285.

Chapouthier, G., Legrain, D., & Spitz, S. La planaire en tant qu'animal de laboratoire dans les recherches psychophysiologiques. *Expérimentation Animale*, 1969, Vol. 1, 269-280. (a)

Chapouthier, G., Pallaud, B., & Ungerer, A. Relations entre deux reactions des planaires face à une discrimination droite-gauche. *Comptes Rendus Academie Sciences Serie D.*, 1968, Vol. 266, 905-907.

Chapouthier, G., Pallaud, B., & Ungerer, A. Note préliminaire concernant l'effet sur l'apprentissage des broyats de cerveau conditionné. *Revue du Comportement Animal*, 1969, Vol. 3, 55-63. (b)

Chapouthier, G., & Ungerer, A. Effet de l'injection d'extraits de cerveau conditionné sur l'apprentissage. *Comptes Rendus Academie Sciences Serie D.*, 1968, Vol. 267, 769-771.

Chapouthier, G. & Ungerer, A. Sur l'effet de certains extraits de cerveau conditionné sur l'apprentissage. *Revue du Comportement Animal*, 1969, Vol. 3, 64-71.

Cohen, A. Effects of whole brain homogenate on transfer of information in rats. *Journal of Biological Psychology*, 1969, Vol. 9(2), 27-29.

Cohen, H. D. Learning, memory, and metabolic inhibitors. In G. Ungar (Ed.), *Molecular mechanisms in memory and learning*. New York: Plenum Press, 1970. Pp. 59-70.

Cohen, H. D., & Barondes, S. H. Further studies of learning and memory after intracerebral actinomycin D. *Journal of Neurochemistry*, 1966, Vol. 13, 207-211.

Cohen, H. D., Ervin, F., & Barondes, S. H. Puromycin and cycloheximide: Different effects on hippocampal electrical activity. *Science*, 1966, Vol. 154, 1557-1558.

Corning, W. C. Evidence of a right-left discrimination in planarians. *Journal of Psychology*, 1964, Vol. 58, 131-139.

Corning, W. C. Retention of a position discrimination after regeneration in planarians. *Psychonomic Science*, 1966, Vol. 5, 17-18.

Corning, W. C., & Freed, S. Planarian behavior and biochemistry. *Nature*, 1968, Vol. 219, 1227-1229.

Corning, W. C., & John, E. R. Effect of ribonuclease on retention of conditioned response in regenerated planarians. *Science*, 1961, Vol. 134, 1363-1365.

Corning, W. C., & Riccio, D. The planarian controversy. In W. L. Byrne (Ed.), *Molecular approaches to learning and memory*. New York: Academic Press, 1970. Pp. 107-149.

Crawford, T., King, F., & Siebert, L. Amino acid analysis of planarians following conditioning. *Psychonomic Science*, 1965, Vol. 2, 49-50.

Daliers, J., & Rigaux-Motquin, M. L. Transfer of learned behaviour by brain extracts. 1. Audiogenic seizure. *Archives International Pharmacodynamics*, 1968, Vol. 176, 461-463.

Davis, R. E., Bright, P. J., & Agranoff, B. W. Effect of ECS and puromycin on memory in fish. *Journal of Comparative & Physiological Psychology*, 1965, Vol. 60, 162-166.

Debold, R. C., Firshein, W., Carrier, S. C., III, & Leaf, R. C. Changes in RNA in the occipital cortex of rats as a function of light and dark during rearing. *Psychonomic Science*, 1967, Vol. 7, 379-380.

Deutsch, J. A. The physiological basis of memory. *Annual Review of Psychology*, 1969, Vol. 20, 85-104.

Dingman, W., & Sporn, M. B. The incorporation of 8-azaguanine into rat brain RNA and its effects on maze learning by the rat: an inquiry into the chemical basis of memory. *Journal of Psychiatry Research*, 1961, Vol. 1, 1-11.

Dingman, W., & Sporn, M. B. Molecular theories of memory. *Science*, 1964, Vol. 144, 26-29.

Dyal, J. A., & Golub, A. M. An attempt to obtain shifts in brightness preference as a function of injection of brain homogenates. *Journal of Biological Psychology*, 1967, Vol. 9(2), 29-33.

Dyal, J. A., & Golub, A. M. Further positive transfer effects obtained by intraperitoneal injections of brain homogenates. *Psychonomic Science*, 1968, Vol. 11, 13-14.

Dyal, J. A., Golub, A. M., & Marrone, R. L. Transfer effects of intraperitoneal injection of brain homogenates. *Nature*, 1967, Vol. 214, 720-721.

Egyhazi, E., & Hydén, H. Experimentally induced changes in the base composition of the ribonucleic acids of isolated nerve cells and their oligodendroglial cells. *Journal of Biophysics & Biochemistry Cytology*, 1961, Vol. 10, 403-410.

Ernhardt, E. N., & Sherrick, C. Retention of a maze habit following regeneration in planaria *(D. maculata)*. Paper presented at the Midwestern Psychological Association, St. Louis, Missouri, 1959.

Essman, W. B., & Lehrer, G. M. Is there a chemical transfer of learning? *Federation Proceedings*, 1966, Vol. 25, 208.

Essman, W. B. & Lehrer, G. M. Facilitation of maze performance by "RNA extracts" from maze-trained mice. *Federation Proceedings*, 1967, Vol. 26, 263.

Faiszt, J., and Adam, G. Role of different RNA fractions from the brain in transfer effect. *Nature*, 1968, Vol. 220, 367-368.

Fjerdingstad, E. J. Chemical transfer of learned preference. *Nature*, 1969, Vol. 222, 1079-1080. (a)

Fjerdingstad, E. J. Chemical transfer of alternation training in the Skinner box. *Scandinavian Journal of Psychology*, 1969, Vol. 10, 220-224. (b)

Fjerdingstad, E. J. Memory transfer in goldfish. *Journal of Biological Psychology*, 1969, Vol. 11(2), 20-25. (c)

Fjerdingstad, E. J., Nissen, T., & Røigaard-Petersen, H. H. Effect of ribonucleic acid (RNA) extracted from the brain of trained animals on learning in rats. *Scandinavian Journal of Psychology*, 1965, Vol. 6, 1-5.

Flexner, J. B., & Flexner, L. B. Restoration of memory lost after treatment with puromycin. *Proceedings of the National Academy of Sciences USA*, 1967, Vol. 57, 1651-1654.

Flexner, J. B., & Flexner, L. B. Further observations on restoration of memory lost after treatment with puromycin. *Yale Journal of Biology and Medicine*, 1969, Vol. 42, 235-240.

Flexner, J. B., Flexner, L. B., & Stellar, E. Memory in mice as affected by intracerebral puromycin. *Science*, 1963, Vol. 141, 57-59.

Flexner, L. B., & Flexner, J. B. Effect of acetoxycycloheximide and acetoxycycloheximide-puromycin mixture on cerebral protein synthesis and memory in mice. *Proceedings of the National Academy of Sciences USA*, 1966, Vol. 55, 369-374.

Flexner, L. B., & Flexner, J. B. Studies on memory: the long survival of peptidyl-puromycin in mouse brain. *Proceedings of the National Academy of Sciences USA*, 1968, Vol. 60, 923-927.

Flexner, L. B., Flexner, J. B., & Roberts, R. B. Memory in mice analyzed with antibiotics. *Science*, 1967, Vol. 155, 1377-1383.

Flexner, L. B., Flexner, J. B., Roberts, R. B., & De la Haba, G. Loss of recent memory in mice as related to regional inhibition of cerebral protein synthesis. *Proceedings of the National Academy of Sciences USA*, 1964, Vol. 52, 1165-1169.

Gaddum, J. H. Bioassays and mathematics. *Pharmacological Reviews*, 1953, Vol. 5, 87-134.

Gay, R., & Raphelson, A. "Transfer of learning" by injection of brain RNA: a replication. *Psychonomic Science*, 1967, Vol. 8, 369-370.

Gibby, R. G., & Crough, D. G. RNA-induced enhancement of wire climbing in the rat. *Psychonomic Science*, 1967, Vol. 9, 413-414.

Gibby, R. G., Crough, D. G., & Thios, S. J. RNA-enhancement of a single discrimination task. *Psychonomic Science*, 1968, Vol. 12, 295-296.

Giurgea, C., Daliers, J., & Mouravieff, F. Pharmacological studies on an elementary model of learning: the fixation of an experience at spinal level. *Abstracts, fourth international congress on pharmacology*. Basel, Switzerland: Schwabe, 1969. Pp. 291-292.

Glassman, E. The biochemistry of learning: an evaluation of the role of RNA and protein. *Annual Review of Biochemistry*, 1969, Vol. 38, 605-646.

Glassman, E., Henderson, A., Cordle, M., Moon, H. M., & Wilson, J. E. Effect of cycloheximide and actinomycin D on the behaviour of the headless cockroach. *Nature*, 1970, Vol. 225, 967-968.

Gold, M., Altschuler, H., Kleban, M. H., Lawton, M. P., & Miller, M. Chemical changes in the rat brain following escape training. *Psychonomic Science*, 1969, Vol. 17, 37-38.

Golub, A. M., Epstein, L., & McConnell, J. V. The effect of peptides, RNA extracts, and whole brain homogenates on avoidance behavior in rats. *Journal of Biological Psychology*, 1969, Vol. 11(1), 44-49.

Golub, A. M., Masiarz, F. R., Villars, T., & McConnell, J. V. Incubation effects in behavior induction in rats. *Science*, 1970, Vol. 168, 392-394.

Golub, A. M., & McConnell, J. V. Transfer of a response bias by injection of brain homogenates: a replication. *Psychonomic Science*, 1968, Vol. 11, 1-2.

Gordon, M. W., Deanin, G. G., Leonhardt, H. L., & Gwynn, R. H. RNA and memory: a negative experiment. *American Journal of Psychiatry*, 1966, Vol. 122, 1174-1178.

Grampp, W., & Edström, J. E. The effect of nervous activity on ribonucleic acid of the crustacean receptor neuron. *Journal of Neurochemistry*, 1963, Vol. 10, 725-731.

Griffard, C. D., & Pierce, J. T. Conditioned discrimination in the planarian. *Science*, 1964, Vol. 144, 1472-1473.

Gross, C. G., & Carey, F. M. Transfer of learned response by RNA injection: failure of attempts to replicate. *Science*, 1965, Vol. 150, 1749.

Halas, E. S., James, R. L., & Knutson, C. S. An attempt at classical conditioning in the planarian. *Journal of Comparative & Physiological Psychology*, 1962, Vol. 55, 969.

Hartry, A. L., Keith-Lee, P., & Morton, W. D. Planaria: memory transfer through cannibalism reexamined. *Science*, 1964, Vol. 146, 274-275.

Horridge, G. A. Learning of a leg position by the ventral nerve cord in headless insects. *Proceedings of the Royal Society*, 1962, Vol. 157, 33-52.

Humphries, B. Maze learning in planaria. *Worm Runner's Digest*, 1961, Vol. 3(2), 114-116.

Hydén, H. Biochemical changes in glial cells and nerve cells at varying activity. *Biochemistry of the central nervous system*. Vol. 3. New York and London: Pergamon Press, 1959. Pp. 64-89.

Hydén, H. Behavior, neural function and RNA. *Progress Nucleic Acid Research*, 1967, Vol. 6, 187-218.

Hydén, H. Trends in brain research on learning and memory. In S. Bogoch (Ed.), *The future of the brain sciences*. New York: Plenum Press, 1969. Pp. 265-279.

Hydén, H., & Egyhazi, E. Nuclear RNA changes in nerve cells during a learning experiment in rats. *Proceedings of the National Academy of Sciences USA*, 1962, Vol. 48, 1366-1372.

Hydén, H., & Lange, P. W. A differentiation in RNA response in neurons early and late in learning. *Proceedings of the National Academy of Sciences USA*, 1965, Vol. 53, 946-952.

Hydén, H., & Lange, P. W. Protein synthesis in the hippocampal pyramidal cells of rats during a behavioral test. *Science*, 1968, Vol. 159, 1370-1373.

Jacobson, A. L., Babich, F. R., Bubash, S., & Jacobson, A. Differential-approach tendencies produced by injection of RNA from trained rats. *Science*, 1965, Vol. 150, 636-637.

Jacobson, A. L., Babich, F. R., Bubash, S., & Goren, C. Maze preferences in naive rats produced by injection of ribonucleic acid from trained rats. *Psychonomic Science,* 1966, Vol. 4, 3-4. (a)

Jacobson, A. L., Fried, C., & Horowitz, S. D. Planarians and memory, *Nature*, 1966, Vol. 209, 599-601. (b)

Jaffard, R. & Cardo, B. Influence de l'injection intracorticale de ribonucléase sur l'acquisition et la rétention d'un apprentissage alimentaire chez le rat. *Journal de Physiologie, Paris*, 1968, Vol. 60 (Supplement 2), 470.

Jaffard, R., & Cardo, B. Influence de l'injection intracorticale de ribonucléase sur l'apprentissage d'une discrimination visuelle chez le rat. *Journal de Physiologie, Paris*, 1969, Vol. 61 (Supplement 2), 322-323.

Jankovic, B. D., Rakic, L., Veskov, R., & Horvat, J. Effect of intraventricular injection of anti-brain antibody on defensive conditioning reflexes. *Nature*, 1968, Vol. 218, 270-271.

Katz, J. J., & Halstead, W. D. Protein organizations and mental function. *Psychology Monographs*, 1950, Vol. 20, 1-38.

Kleban, M. H., Altshuler, H., Lawton, M. P., Parris, J. L., & Lords, C. A. Influence of donor-recipient brain transfers on avoidance learning. *Psychological Reports*, 1968, Vol. 23, 51-56.

Krylov, O. A., Kalyuzhnaya, P. I., & Tongur, V. S. Possible conveyance of conditioned connection by means of a biochemical substrate. *Zhurnal Vysshei Nervnoi Deyatel'nosti imeni Pavlova*, 1969, Vol. 19, 286.

Lambert, R., & Saurat, M. RNA et transfert d'apprentissage: une réplique d'expérience. *Bulletin CERP*, 1967, Vol. 16, 435-438.

Lee, R. M. Conditioning of a free operant response in planaria. *Science*, 1963, Vol. 139, 1048-1049.

Luttges, M., Johnson, T., Buck, C., Holland, J., & McGaugh, J. An examination of "transfer of learning" by nucleic acid. *Science*, 1966, Vol. 151, 834-837.

Machlus, B., & Gaito, J. Successive competition hybridization to detect RNA species in a shock avoidance task. *Nature*, 1969, Vol. 222, 573-574.

McConnell, J. V. Memory transfer through cannibalism in planarians. *Journal of Neuropsychiatry*, 1962, 3 (Supplement 1), 42-48.

McConnell, J. V. New evidence for "transfer of training" effect in planarians. Symposium on the biological bases of memory traces, XVIII International Congress of Psychology, Moscow, 1966.

McConnell, J. V. Specific factors influencing planarian behavior. In W. C. Corning & E. C. Ratner (Eds.), *Chemistry of learning; invertebrate research*. New York: Plenum Press, 1967. Pp. 217-233.

McConnell, J. V., Jacobson, A. L., & Kimble, D. P. The effects of regeneration upon retention of a conditioned response in the planarian. *Journal of Comparative & Physiological Psychology*, 1959, Vol. 52, 1-5.

McConnell, J. V., Jacobson, R., & Maynard, D. M. Apparent retention of a conditioned response following total regeneration in the planarian. *American Psychologist Abstracts*, 1959, Vol. 14, 410.

McConnell, J. V., & Shelby, J. M. Memory transfer experiments in invertebrates. In G. Ungar (Ed.), *Molecular mechanisms in memory and learning.* New York: Plenum Press, 1970. Pp. 71-101.

McConnell, J. V., Shigehisha, T., & Salive, H. Attempts to transfer approach and avoidance responses by RNA injections in rats. *Journal of Biological Psychology*, 1968, Vol. 10 (2), 32-50.

McGaugh, J. L., & Petrinovitch, L. Effects of drugs on learning and memory. *International Review of Neurobiology*, 1965, Vol. 8, 139-196.

McNutt, L. 1,1,3-tricyano-2-amino-1-propene: a pharmacological attempt to enhance learning ability. *Proceedings of the American Psychological Association*, 1967, Vol. 2, 77-78.

Mihailovic, L., & Jankovic, B. D. Effect of intraventricularly injected anti-n. caudatus antibody on the electrical activity of the cat brain. *Nature*, 1961, Vol. 192, 665-666.

Monné, L. Functioning of the cytoplasm. In F. F. Nord (Ed.), *Advances in enzymology.* Vol. 8. New York: Wiley (Interscience), 1948.

Moos, W. S., Levan, H., Mason, B. T., Mason, H. C., & Hebron, D. L. Radiation induced avoidance behavior transfer by brain extracts of mice. *Experientia*, 1969, Vol. 25, 1215-1219.

Oshima, K., Gorbman, A., & Shimada, H. Memory-blocking agents: effects on olfactory discrimination in homing salmon. *Science*, 1969, Vol. 165, 86-88.

Picket, J. B. E., III, Jennings, L. B., & Wells, P. H. Influence of RNA and victim training on maze learning by cannibal planarians. *American Zoologist*, 1964, Vol. 4, 411-412.

Potts, A., & Bitterman, M. E. Puromycin and retention in the goldfish. *Science*, 1967, Vol. 158, 1594-1596.

Rappoport, D. A. & Daginawala, H. F. Changes in nuclear RNA of brain induced by olfaction in catfish. *Journal of Neurochemistry*, 1968, Vol. 15, 991-1006.

Reinis, S. The formation of conditioned reflexes in rats after the parenteral administration of brain homogenate. *Activitas Nervosa Superior*, 1965, Vol. 7, 167-168.

Reinis, S. Block of "memory transfer" by actinomycin D. *Nature*, 1968, Vol. 200, 177-178.

Reinis, S. Indirect effect of puromycin on memory. *Psychonomic Science*, 1969, Vol. 14, 44-45.

Revusky, S. H., & Devenuto, F. Attempt to transfer aversion to saccharine solution by injection of RNA from trained to naive rats. *Journal of Biological Psychology*, 1967, Vol. 9 (2), 18-22.

Røigaard-Petersen, H. H., Nissen, T., & Fjerdingstad, E. J. Effect of ribonucleic acid (RNA) extracted from the brain of trained animals on learning in rats. III. Results obtained with an improved procedure, *Scandinavian Journal of Psychology*, 1968, Vol. 9, 1-16.

Rosenblatt, F. Recent work on theoretical models of biological memory. In J. Tou (Ed.), *Computer and information sciences*. Vol. 2, New York: Academic Press, 1967. Pp. 33-56.

Rosenblatt, F. Behavior induction by brain extracts: a comparison of two procedures. *Proceedings of the National Academy of Sciences USA*, 1969, Vol. 64, 661-668.

Rosenblatt, F. Induction of specific behavior by mammalian brain extracts. In G. Ungar, (Ed.), *Molecular mechanisms in memory and learning*. New York:Plenum Press, 1970. Pp. 103-147.

Rosenblatt, F., Farrow, J. T., & Herblin, W. F. Transfer of conditioned responses from trained rats to untrained rats by means of a brain extract, *Nature*, 1966, Vol. 209, 46-48.   (a)

Rosenblatt, F., Farrow, J. T., & Rhine, S. The transfer of learned behavior from trained to untrained rats by means of brain extracts, I and II. *Proceedings of the National Academy of Sciences USA*, 1966, Vol. 55, 548-555, 787-792.   (b)

Rosenblatt, F., & Miller, R. G. Behavioral assay procedures for transfer of learned behavior by brain extracts, Parts I and II. *Proceedings of the National Academy of Sciences USA*, 1966, Vol. 56, 1423-1430, 1683-1688.

Rosenthal, E., & Sparber, S. B. Transfer of a learned response by chick brain homogenate fed to naive donors. *The Pharmacologist*, 1968, Vol. 10, 168.

Seydoux, J., Girardier, L., Perrin, M. C., Ruphi, M., & Posternak, J. M. Essai de mise en evidence d'un conditionnement de type operant chez la planaire *Dugesia lugubris*. *Helvetica Physiologica & Pharmacologica Acta*, 1967, Vol. 25, 436-438.

Shashoua, V. E. RNA changes in goldfish brain during learning. *Nature*, 1968, Vol. 217, 238-240.

Stevens, D. A., & Tapp, J. T. Effect of ventricular injections of ribonuclease on learned discrimination and avoidance tasks in the rat. *Psychological Reports*, 1966, Vol. 18, 286.

Szilard, L. On memory and recall. *Proceedings of the National Academy of Sciences USA*, 1964, Vol. 51, 1092-1099.

Thompson, R., & McConnell, J. V. Classical conditioning in the planarian, *Dugesia dorotocephala*. *Journal of Comparative & Physiological Psychology*, 1955, Vol. 48, 65-68.

Ungar, G. Transfer of learned behavior by brain extracts. *Journal of Biological Psychology*, 1967, Vol. 9 (1), 12-27.   (a)

Ungar, G. Chemical transfer of acquired information. *Proceedings of the Vth International Congress of the Collegium Internationale Neuropsychopharmacologicum*. Amsterdam: Excerpta Medica, 1967. Pp. 169-175.   (b)

Ungar, G. Molecular mechanisms in learning. *Perspectives Biological Medicine*, 1968, Vol. 11, 217-232.

Ungar, G. Molecular neurobiology: reflections on the first ten years of a new science. *Journal of Biological Psychology*, 1969, Vol. 11 (2), 6-9.

Ungar, G. Role of proteins and peptides in learning and memory. In G. Ungar (Ed.), *Molecular mechanisms in memory and learning*. New York: Plenum Press, 1970. Pp. 149-175.   (a)

Ungar, G. Chemical transfer of acquired information. In A. Schwartz (Ed.), *Methods in pharmacology*, Volume 1. New York: Appleton-Century-Croft, 1971. P. 479. (b)

Ungar, G. Molecular mechanisms in information processing. *International Review of Neurobiology*, 1970, Vol. 13, 223-253.   (c)

Ungar, G., & Chapouthier, G. Mécanismes moléculaires de l'utilisation de l'information par le cerveau. *L'Année Psychologique*, 1971, Vol. 1, 153-183.

Ungar, G., & Fjerdingstad, E. J. Chemical nature of the transfer factors; RNA or protein? Proceedings of the symposium on biology of memory (Tihany, Hungary, September 1-4, 1969). In G. Adam (Ed.), *Biology of Memory*. New York, Plenum Press, 1971. Pp. 137-143.

Ungar, G., Galvan, L., & Chapouthier, G. Possible chemical coding of color discrimination in goldfish brain. In preparation.

Ungar, G., Galvan, L., & Clark, R. H. Chemical transfer of learned fear. *Nature*, 1968, Vol. 217, 1259-1261.

Ungar, G., Ho, I. K., Galvan, L., & Desiderio, D. M. Isolation and identification of a specific behavior-inducing peptide extracted from brain. *Proceedings Western Pharmacology Society*, 1970, in press.

Ungar, G., & Irwin, L. N. Transfer of acquired information by brain extracts. *Nature*, 1967, Vol. 214, 453-455.

Ungar, G., & Oceguera-Navarro, C. Transfer of habituation by material extracted from brain. *Nature*, 1965, Vol. 207, 301-302.

Ungerer, A. Effets comparés de la puromycine et de *Datura stramonium* sur la rétention d'un apprentissage instrumental chez la souris. *Comptes Rendus Academie Sciences Serie D.*, 1969, Vol. 269, 910-913. (a)

Ungerer, A. Antibiotiques et mémoire: rôle de l'ARN et de la synthèse protéique dans la fixation de la mémoire. *Revue du Comportement Animal*, 1969, Vol. 3, 72-80. (b)

Ungerer, A., Spitz, S., & Chapouthier, G. Sur les polypeptides toxiques impliqués par Flexner dans l'effacement de la memoire par la puromycine. *Comptes Rendus Academie Sciences Serie D.*, 1969, Vol. 268, 2472-2475.

Weiss, K. P. Measurement of the effects of brain extract on interorganism information transfer. In W. L. Byrne (Ed.), *Molecular approaches to learning and memory*. New York: Academic Press, 1970. Pp. 325-334.

Westerman, R. A. Somatic inheritance of habituation of responses to light in planarians. *Science*, 1963, Vol. 140, 676-677.

Wolthuis, O. L. Inter-animal information transfer by brain extracts. *Archives internationales de Pharmacodynamie*, 1969, Vol. 182, 439-442.

Wolthuis, O. L., Anthoni, J. F., & Stevens, W. F. Interanimal transfer of information by brain extracts. *Acta Physiologica & Pharmacologica Neerlandica*, 1968, Vol. 15, 93.

Zippel, H. P., & Domagk, G. F. Versuche zur chemischen Gedachtnisübertragung von farbdressierten Goldfischen auf undressierte Tiere. *Experientia*, 1969, Vol. 25, 938-940.

CHAPTER

2

PROTEIN SYNTHESIS AND MEMORY

D. A. BOOTH

1. POSSIBLE RELATIONSHIPS OF PROTEIN SYNTHESIS TO MEMORY

A. Memory as Part of the Biology of Proteins

Every living function depends on protein which the organism has synthesized for itself. The capacity to remember past experiences which the brain gives to higher organisms can be no exception.

Virtually all the covalent bond formation and destruction in a cell is catalyzed and controlled by enzymic protein. In addition, the spatiotemporal organization of the mature eukaryote cell largely depends on compartmentation by lipid membranes whose stability and transport operations are determined by enzymic and structural species of protein. As to protein origin, there are no general mechanisms for assigning protein from other organisms to its function within the cell of the feeding organism. Furthermore, unless they remain in a strongly hydrophobic environment, all endogenous proteins are subject to breakdown by proteolytic enzymes and must be replaced by new molecules having the same amino acid sequence. Thus, it would be surprising to find any biological function which could be maintained in the long term without continuing protein synthesis.

As is the case for many organs, half the dry weight of the brain is protein. Probably a substantial proportion of protein species in the brain are peculiar to the structures and substances involved in the movement of electrical events along and between neuronal membranes, and the maintenance of this specialized function of dendrites, somata, axons, and interneuronal clefts. It remains to be seen how much of the genetic load of higher organisms is the program for synthesizing these proteins and those controlling the interconnection of regions and neuron cell types during brain development: presumably more than the 2.4 percent of the genome which is active in adult rat brain (Stevenin, Samec, Jacob, & Mandel, 1968). A question which is central to the topic of this chapter is whether there are additional regulatory and structural genes which are involved only in memory: if there are, then how many, and, if hundreds rather than a few, by what biochemical mechanisms environmentally caused differences in brain activity select among them, and how the memory protein(s) coded in these structural genes influence the effects of environment on brain processes controlling behavior. If there are no memory genes, then there remains the question of what sort of neuronal differentiation or growth it is which functions in this context as well as others, if protein synthesis is in fact crucial to memory retention.

B. Must Each Memory Trace Be New Protein?

Some gross brain functions persist for many hours, perhaps days, when synthesis of new protein has been drastically inhibited.

Electrical transmission in an invertebrate preparation continues for 12 hours in the presence of puromycin (Toschi & Giacobini, 1965), as indeed it also does (Huneeus-Cox, Fernandez & Smith, 1966) when the axon cytosol is extruded, eliminating the axonal membrane's supply of protein from the perikaryon and whatever small amount of protein-synthesizing machinery the axon itself may contain. Some preexisting protein attached to the axon membrane is necessary (Rojas, 1965).

Apparently much of the behavioral capacity of vertebrates such as a teleost (Agranoff, Davis, & Brink, 1966) and a rodent (Barondes & Cohen, 1967) survives during and after hours of massive inhibition of protein synthesis.

Such findings are readily understandable when we discover that many brain proteins have a half-life of 2–3 weeks (Lajtha & Toth, 1966). All the same, neuronal malfunction and death must eventually ensue if new protein is lacking indefinitely, and of course with it would go memory. (There is, however, no evidence that the lethal effects of the DNA transcription inhibitor actinomycin D are attributable to neuronal lack of protein: the cause of death is likely to be accumulation of toxic products because of liver damage.)

Nevertheless, protein synthesis might be expected to be more critical to remembering than to some other brain functions, because the retention of a given aspect of environmental information is not an innate or invariant capacity, but one with a birth time of its own. At the physiological level, the establishment of a particular memory must involve a change in state of the transfer function of some variable stage of neuronal transmission (assuming that all behavior is specified by physical brain processes). Most hypotheses as to the mechanism of this flip in transmission properties—ranging from synaptic growth to coding of electrical discharge patterns into macromolecular structures—seem to presuppose creation of new protein especially to comprise the trace, and in some cases continued augmentation of protein synthesis to maintain it. Yet there is no valid a priori argument that a change in protein synthesis must be crucial to long-term retention of memory. There are as yet very few examples of changes in function in neural tissue which have been demonstrated to depend on production of new protein. The available analogies are the adrenergic induction of the enzyme controlling pineal melatonin synthesis (Axelrod, Schein, & Wurtman, 1969) and adaptive enzyme changes in starvation ketosis (Smith, Satterthwaite, & Sokoloff, 1969).

1. Alternative Possibilities

Any number of transmissivity modulation mechanisms could be irreversible and persist indefinitely and yet involve only existing proteins and no change in their replacement mechanism. The change in transmission properties could be maintained by cooperative phenomena, such as crystalline growth in the case of a conformational change in a membrane, autocatalysis or allosteric positive feedback in the case of a change in activity of an existing enzyme, and intercellular binding or other interaction in the case of a topological crisis. If, for example, synapses were formed as a consequence of coincidence of electrical activity in an axon terminal and a dendrite during the period they happen to be in contact because of random outgrowth on the part of either, materials to stabilize the synapse could be accumulated from axonal and dendritic transport, rather than being broken down as would occur otherwise. To give another example (one which it is not fashionable to invoke as a memory mechanism), some myelin probably lasts a lifetime, undoubtedly because of the stability of the membrane structure once formed in that environment (Vandendeuval, 1966), and increased myelination might introduce sufficient changes in spatial summation to be an effective information-holding mechanism.

2. High Brain Protein Synthesis Rate

The rates of protein formation and destruction in the brain are of the same order as in the liver, many of whose known functions involve replacing proteins and rapidly adjusting their concentration. It has sometimes been argued that the average rate of protein synthesis in the brain is too high to be accounted for by known cellular needs and, so, is likely to be involved in memory. However, neurons are really secretory cells. Furthermore some of the secretions are peptide hormones and probably peptide transmitters or synaptic modulators. Even though very little of this protein leaves the brain, that which remains is unlikely to be taken up intact into cells, rather than broken down and resynthesized from amino acids. Neurons may well be continuously growing cells, with high protein turnover as axonal and dendritic processes enlarge and retract. Whatever its functions, large amounts of material are now known to be transported at various speeds down (and some material up) axons (Sjöstrand, 1969). Unless there is precise control of distalward transport by some upward signal, excess material must be transported and broken down at the nerve ending if not needed. The breakdown products could be used for energy or to control activity. Axonal consumption of protein may therefore account for a large proportion of the turnover of brain proteins.

Brain tissue is also unusual in its use of endogenous substrates as immediate sources for the synthesis of energy-yielding compounds. The brain uses glucose alone as exogenous energy source (not lipid in addition, as do other organs), but much of the glucose on which brain metabolism is ultimately dependent is incorporated into amino acids and thence protein, and also into lipid and glycogen. The brain uses these polymeric molecules as energy sources. The existence of this macromolecular calorie buffer is no doubt adaptive as it makes the brain tissue among the least affected by short-term changes in concentrations of circulating metabolites. As the brain produces one-fifth of the total body heat (from 3 percent of body weight), use of protein for energy probably accounts for a good deal of the high synthetic rate.

3. Large Information Capacity of Protein Structure

In the early phases of the expansion of interest in the biochemistry of memory which has taken place in the last decade, a lot of the psychological literature focused on the suggestion that large repetitive molecules like proteins and nucleic acids must contain all the behavior-specifying information of memory in their sequential structure. Most people familiar with neuroanatomy or with the biochemistry of protein synthesis have always regarded this as a most implausible argument. Even the analogy of antibody recognition of an unlimited range of antigens has not weakened this evaluation. Indeed, the analogy has come to strengthen the evaluation, as those workers on antibody synthesis who believed in "instructive" mechanisms have accepted the now virtually universal belief in a "selective" mechanism of some sort.

It is false to suppose that we cannot explain the ability of the brain to model the environment in ways that bear no relation to the phylogenetic past (nor indeed any specifiable future) unless we assume that electrical activity in the brain instructs the synthetic mechanisms which sequence of amino acids or nucleotides to make.

In the first place, neuronal interconnections seem amply sufficient to carry a lifetime's memories. The approximate figures commonly accepted are 10^3 for the average number of neurons connected to a mammalian central neuron and 10^{10} for the number of neurons in the human brain. Taking the high estimate of the maximum rate of information processing in man of 10^2 bits per second, a lifetime of waking hours spent processing at that rate would pass about 10^{11} bits. Now we know that nothing like this rate is maintained continuously—it is approached only during relatively brief bouts of highly skilled performance. Furthermore, it is doubtful whether most of the information transmitted is also retained indefinitely. Above all, that which is retained is far more economically coded than in a series of binary choices. So if only one in 10^4 neuronal interconnections has irreversibly modifiable conductivity, there would be ample representational capacity, even if the interconnections changed conductivity merely in yes/no fashion and were all in parallel. In fact, interneuronal connections are in series through a network, and conductivity changes may be graded, giving much higher capacity.

Second, even if one does postulate that variations in the structure of the biochemical substance comprising the memory trace do contribute to specification of the spatiotemporal distribution of electrical activity in the recall process, this does not solve the coding problem. Indeed, the postulate complicates the explanation, for the brain processes involved in the registration of memory still have to select that chemical which has the appropriate effect during recall. Hypotheses involving some arbitrary electrical or chemical modification of DNA or RNA structure, even when they do not ignore the determinateness with which the mechanism of protein synthesis is known to be regulated, usually do nothing to solve the central problem—how registration specifies just those chemical changes, which in turn specify the appropriate electrical activity for retrieval. However, this is not to go to the conceptual extreme that some have, and to say that Locke was wrong to suppose that experience instructs the brain and Plato was right to suppose that mental experiences merely select reminiscences. Both were wrong. The mind is instructed by experience and this instruction is variations in brain transmission states being selected. Even in the description of mechanisms of protein synthesis, "instruction" versus "selection" is merely a matter of conceptual level of the analysis: the messenger RNA instructs the ribosome which protein to make and yet the messenger-ribosome complex selects each amino acid in turn during the construction of a protein molecule (Jerne,1955).

If one expects the memory code to be in the spatiotemporal properties of the nerve net, rather than in molecular structure, once again there is no need to assume that selection has to operate among innately meaningful neuronal connections. Much information could, in fact, be represented by a selection of interneuronal conductivity changes which is meaningful only in virtue of the organism's pervious history of selection of functional connections within the random aspects of the innate broad pattern of interconnections. Indeed, now that statistical model networks have been shown to be capable of building their own representations of input regularities, the problem is no longer to explain how any mechanism can learn, but, rather, to explain the limits on the learning capacity of biological brains, given that they do contain elements having irreversibly variable transmission states.

C. Mechanisms which Change the Rate of Protein Synthesis

Even though we do not have to assume that memory is coded in protein structure, nor even that a unitary biochemical mechanism of neuronal plasticity involves creation of new protein molecules especially for it during consolidation, many of the changes in cellular function of whose mechanism we have gained some idea do involve changes in the rate of synthesis of protein molecules. We are beginning to appreciate the variety in the mechanisms by which cells vary protein synthesis, and if memory is a change of neuronal function of this type, we must examine the whole range of possible mechanisms.

1. Known Range of Mechanisms

a. Gene Activation. If the establishment, and, perhaps, the maintenance, of the trace does, as a matter of fact, require extra new protein, the requirement of long-term stability does not imply that the mechanism goes right back to a change in gene activity. Appearance of a new enzyme and increase in cell size or activity often involves changes in DNA transcription, but newly expressed genes can become repressed again and new growth can regress when the change-initiating conditions are removed. Stability is introduced by more specific mechanisms. A new growth could be maintained long after a transient burst of synthesis had passed if it brought into contact two cells whose background activities were sufficient to keep them touching. A newly activated structural gene would continue to be transcribed as messenger RNA if the protein formed on the RNA template maintained an interaction between a regulator gene and the rest of the cell such that the structural gene remains unrepressed. A very large proportion of the genes in metazoan cells are regulatory and must be involved in mechanisms of selective activation of the minute fraction of the genome that is active at any given time in any given cell—mechanisms likely to be far more complex than the selective repression mechanisms that exist for a minority of genes in bacteria.

Only about 2 percent of the DNA in rat brain seems to be active in the synthesis of RNA (Stevenin *et al.*, 1968), though it should be noted that this is sufficient for many tens, even hundreds, of thousands of proteins. Usually a good deal of different DNA is active in different tissues in the mammal, and the DNA in use changes markedly during differentiation of a cell. The inactive parts of the genome are repressed by proteins which do not seem to have any selectivity for any part of it: lysine-rich histones keep the DNA tightly coiled until they are acetylated; arginine-rich histones keep RNA polymerase inactive; nucleophosphoprotein may be phosphorylated to take histone off either. The derepressors must therefore be selective as the repressors are in bacteria. The bacterial repressor substances isolated thus far are protein (Gilbert and Müller-Hill, 1966; Ptashne, 1967). However, some or all of the metazoan activators may be in the very rapidly turning over, high molecular weight nuclear RNA fraction; this never leaves the nucleus and may not act as a template for protein synthesis at all, but rather serves as a highly selective, rapidly responsive expression of the regulatory genes acting on the structural genes which do make templates from protein synthesis. There is, however, no evidence that this aspect of protein synthesis control by RNA synthesis is crucial for memory (Section IV).

b. Cell Division. In contrast to the immunocompetent cell in the secondary phase of elaboration of antibody-producing cells, the stability of the trace is not in all probability achieved by DNA replication and cell division. There is no appreciable neuronal multiplication in adult mammalian brain. Enriched experience has been reported to cause glial multiplication (Diamond, Krech, & Rosenzweig, 1964; Altman & Das, 1964). Altman has raised a question as to the identity of these cells, whether they have been adequately distinguished from undifferentiated cells which are migrating and will develop into microneurons (Altman, 1967). Even transformations from one type to the other on a small scale has not been excluded: dedifferentiation readily occurs in cultures of dispersed neurons; pigment cells in the salamander retina can redifferentiate into neurons (Stone, 1950). However, in all these cases there is no conclusive evidence of postnatal cell multiplication, as opposed to differentiation or redifferentiation of existing cells with a full chromosomal DNA content, (although perhaps replicating DNA for nucleoli and mitochondria). Furthermore, disruption of DNA synthesis seems to have no effect on learning in goldfish (Casola, Lim, Davis, & Agranoff, 1968). DNA incorporation may relate to memory in the rat, nevertheless (Gaito, 1971).

c. Varied Translation Rates. Now, further, there is no need to suppose that transcription of new RNA has to occur immediately before new proteins, or greatly increased amounts of existing proteins, are synthesized. Some forms of messenger RNA are extremely stable in mammalian and other metazoan systems, compared with bacterial templates which generally have half-lives of only a few minutes. Although metazoan gene expression can be activated as quickly as bacterial (Kidson, 1965), even the fastest decaying gene products have half-lives of the order of an hour or more (Trakatellis, Axelrod, & Montjar, 1964). Some vertebrate messenger RNA may last for weeks or even the lifetime of the animal. Lens crystallin (Papaconstantinou, 1967), erythrocyte hemoglobin (Marks, Burka, & Schlessinger, 1962) and feather keratin (Humphreys, Penman, & Bell, 1964) are all proteins which can be synthesized for days independently of nuclei to maintain RNA concentrations. This order of stability is not peculiar to cells which are going to lose their nuclei, as it has been found in muscle (Yaffe & Feldman, 1964) and pancreas (Wessells & Wilt, 1965). However, these cases do involve cells which have stopped dividing, and also specialized protein. If the consolidation of the memory trace does turn out to depend on protein synthesis on a stable template in mature neurons, it would not be surprising, therefore, if the protein were unique to neurons, and even to memory retention.

Mechanisms regulating the rate of messenger translation (e.g., in the action of some hormones) are currently under intensive study. Active messenger may be used with varying efficiency. It is not certain how inactive messenger is protected from ribonuclease in the mammalian cell. At least in amphibian and invertebrate eggs and embryos, a protein coat seems to be involved: messenger, sometimes separate from ribosomes, sometimes in inactive polysomes, can be made both active and sensitive to ribonuclease by treatment with a proteolytic enzyme (Monroy, Maggio & Rinaldi, 1965; Spirin, 1966). In the case of plant seeds containing messenger RNA stable for a year or more (Dure & Waters, 1965)—even thousands of years in the case of the lotus!—presumably dehydration is important to the stabilization. Possibly the lipid in the membrane to which many metazoan ribosomes are bound, in vertebrate brain and other tissues, plays an important part in providing a hydrophobic environment for messenger RNA. Messenger that is available for use is translated at a rate which depends not only on a supply of energy and of all the necessary amino acids but also on specialized control factors, for example initiating and terminating the construction of a particular protein molecule.

d. Speculative Examples of Changes in Synaptic Protein. Whether or not long-lived messenger is used, an enormous variety of mechanisms involving protein synthesis could be imagined which could effect the change in neuronal transmission properties mediating memory retention. A presynaptic change is more likely to require stable template which has survived axonal transport from the nucleus in the perikaryon. However, the Golgi complex often visible subsynaptically may also contain long-lived messenger RNA which responds to a change in synaptic activity with synthesis of a protein which alters postsynaptic characteristics. The proportion of genome expressed, directly or indirectly, could be multicistronic and already active ("growth") or perhaps constitutes only a few new cistrons ("differentiation"). Recently some anatomical evidence has finally been obtained for changes in synaptic configuration in response to gross stimulation of the mammalian brain—changes in size (Cragg, 1967) or location (Raisman, 1969). However, the memory trace could well be invisible even under the electron microscope. To give an illustration: release of an unusually large amount of transmitter from an axon collateral synapsing with an inhibitory microneuron might increase the permeability of the postsynaptic membrane to such an extent that the transmitter, a breakdown product, or the usual ions pass through in quantities sufficient to trigger synthesis of transmitter receptor protein, either by acting on a local messenger, or perhaps by direct interaction with the nucleus which is close to the soma membrane in many central neurons and, indeed, is extracellular in virtue of channels from plasma membrane to nuclear membrane through the endoplasmic reticulum. The increased efficiency of transmission could be maintained, once triggered, by arrival of transmitter in more usual amounts. If the inhibitory neuron synapsed with a third neuron which has always been facilitated hitherto by direct synaptic contact from the first neuron, than a burst of firing in the first neuron will have triggered a decrease of conductivity between it and the third neuron—a negative feedback system, which Bliss, Burns, and Uttley (1968) suggest is a more likely memory mechanism than facilitation of synaptic conduction.

2. Investigation of Protein Synthesis

One does not have to be a molecular biologist to make some assessment of the biochemical validity of a report that protein synthesis correlates with learning or is necessary to memory retention. The remainder of this chapter surveys the common methods of studying protein synthesis, describing their principles, and some primary canons of interpretation of experimental reports. Some of the best examples to date of the use of each method in the study of the biochemistry of the memory trace are given as illustrations. Procedural details are not described: those not biochemically qualified who want to start work in this area should consult biochemist colleagues and the relevant handbooks of experimental methods. Also, the difficulties of behavioral interpretation of such work are not dealt with here; detailed critical reviews of that side of the problem have appeared quite recently (e.g., Booth, 1967, 1970; Cohen, 1970; Deutsch, 1969).

II. INCREASES IN AMOUNT OF PROTEIN

An acceleration in the rate of synthesis of a particular protein will be reflected in an increase in its concentration in those cells involved, unless protein breakdown accelerates equally or to a greater extent. If many species of protein are involved, as in outgrowth of a cell process, this acceleration might be detectable as a slight increase in total protein. It would be more likely to be detectable as an increased concentration of a species or group of proteins identified by their physical properties, chemical composition, or enzymic or other function.

A. Physical Fractionation of Proteins

The variations between species of protein in their molecular weights and conformation, their sequences of amino acids and their proportions of diamino and dicarboxylic amino acids cause them to vary in physical properties sufficiently to separate into distinct populations when passed through a porous medium, particularly under the influence of an electric field applied either across the medium (as in electrophoresis) or at the molecular level within the medium (as in ion exchange chromatography).

Virtually all the proteins in brain tissue can be dispersed using a detergent. This leaves lipids and polysaccharides in association with them, even after centrifugation at moderate power. Also, the dispersion contains small molecules and ions unless it is dialysed. Alternatively, the tissue (or a lipid-free sediment precipitated from it) can be dispersed in buffered solutions, which extract a selection of proteins which depends on the pH and ionic strength of the dispersion. The concentrated protein preparation is then placed at the starting point of a moderately polar wet medium, e.g., in a slot in a block of gel such as starch or polyacrylamide for electrophoresis, or on the top of a column of ion exchange cellulose for washing through with buffer solutions of increasing effectiveness at disrupting the association between protein and the exchange moiety on the cellulose. Amounts of protein in the various fractions can be measured by ultraviolet absorption or by photometry on the results of histochemical staining or colorimetric reactions (chemical or enzymic).

A single component on any one type of separation, even if it appears homogeneous on rechromatography, does not necessarily contain a single species of protein. The "S-100 protein"—a highly acidic protein band peculiar to brain tissue—has been resolved into more than three components (McEwen & Hydén, 1966). However, the persistence of a symmetrical peak through several widely different types of separative method would be good evidence that the peak is homogeneous. The problem then becomes the identification of its molecular weight, amino acid sequence and functional properties *in vitro*. The average mass of a protein species which exists in an approximately spherical conformation can be determined from its sedimentation rate in an analytical ultracentrifuge or by gel filtration mixed with proteins of known molecular weight—the smaller proteins being slowed during filtration by passing into the holes in the gel. Amino acid sequence determination is an exploding technology involving selective hydrolysis of the pure protein and larger peptides derived from it, followed by chromatography and determination of amino acid composition of the smaller peptides after complete hydrolysis. A picture of overlapping sequences can be built up by deduction, and checked by other techniques such as, in some cases, X-ray crystallography. If studies of memory mechanisms ever reach this stage, and the protein is nonenzymic or concentrated in nerve ending ghosts or some other membrane, such data are likely to be crucial because probably in that case there would be, in addition to the biochemistry of the trace, a biophysics of memory retention which may relate directly to the electrical membrane characteristics studies by neurophysiologists.

Many of these isolation and separation procedures are mild enough to allow enzymic activity to be measured, either on the support or in an eluate. Radioactive incorporation can be measured by scintillation or direct counting on a sheet support, in a preparation from an eluate, or by gas counting after combustion. Autoradiography on the gel or paper provides a much more sensitive measure, although it is not so easy to quantify. A reliable separation and assay method can be used to locate variation in concentration of the protein component between brain and other tissues, regions of brain, types of cell, and types of centrifugally separated subcellular fraction, such as membrane-bound ribosomes, synaptic vesicles, and emptied fragments of nerve endings (synaptosome ghosts).

Bogoch (1968) has achieved one of the most impressive fractionations of total brain protein to date which he has put to various uses. From an interest in the nature of the memory trace, Bogoch and collaborators have compared the pattern of chromatographic peaks from the brain of untrained pigeons with the pattern from brains of pigeons trained by one or other of two procedures to peck the left key for grain when a buzzer was off, and the right when it was on. Two or three fairly discrete and adequately identifiable peaks of more acidic protein were greater in size in trained animals, and the increase in amount roughly correlated in one group with the individual pigeon's speed of acquisition of the discrimination. These protein mixtures are rich in acidic sugar moieties, which should influence the role which the glycocalyx might play in interactions between neurons (Adey, 1967; Pease, 1966; Pappas & Purpura, 1966). It remains to be seen from further behavioral comparisons whether the change in concentration of these brain protein components is specific to establishment of a memory.

Hydén & Lange (1970a,b) have performed microelectrophoretic separations on solubilized dispersions of samples from the hippocampus of rats which had been given exercise at reaching for food pellets with their nonpreferred forepaw. Control animals used their preferred paw, and so were less frustrated and were not acquiring a new paw preference (although this was not measured). The increase in dexterity with specifically the nonpreferred paw was paralleled by increases in amounts of at least two brain-specific proteins, the antiserum to one of which interfered with dexterity or perhaps motivation. Haljamäe & Lange (1972) have reported that an apparently new fraction is in fact the S-100 brain-specific protein with a changed calcium content and partial unfolding of the protein chain. These acidic proteins and changes in their conformation may alter membrane permeability to cations, at least temporarily. A role in memory retention remains to be established, both for these proteins and for the hippocampus.

B. Enzymic Assay of Protein Concentration

The function of many species of protein molecule is to catalyze some limited class of chemical reaction. The rate at which this reaction proceeds in a solution of free enzyme molecules which contains a defined excess of reactants (substrate) and any necessary activating ions and cofactors is a function of the number of enzyme molecules present. Given that associated molecules are not keeping the enzyme at very low activity or with very poor access to substrate, even relatively impure preparations can be assayed for concentrations of specific proteins by their enzymic activity. The basic requirements are that the assay incubation by carried out under fixed conditions of duration, temperature, and incubation mixture composition, and the amount of measured reaction product (or disappearance of substrate) be a monotonic, preferably linear, rising function of the amount of standard enzyme preparation in the incubation mixture, over the range of amounts of enzyme to be measured. Subtler matters of interpretation are also vital. The method of measuring the product of enzyme action should not be sensitive to other materials which might arise by the action of other enzymes, or to contaminants in the tissue preparations which are being assayed for enzyme activity. The latter point is controlled by blanks containing various amounts of enzyme but no substrate. Most important of all for the theoretical implication of results, the specificity of the assay must be critically assessed. That is, the assay must distinguish between various known types of enzyme which may be able to catalyze the measured reaction. The most well-known example in the memory field is the distinction between acetyl-cholinesterase and the less specific enzyme cholinesterase (or pseudo-cholin-esterase). From their subcellular localizations, these enzymes seem to have very different functions: acetylcholinesterase being involved in lowering acetyl-choline concentration close to the postsynaptic receptors and pseudocholin-esterase at other sites in and out of cells where acetylcholine accumulations might have untoward effects. Enzymic breakdown of acetylcholine should not be attributed to the specific enzyme except in so far as the same tissue preparations fail to hydrolyze choline esters of longer chain acids, e.g., butyryl-choline.

It is also possible to deduce the effective activity of an enzyme *in vivo* from measurements of the tissue concentrations of the substrate and product. If all of the measured quantities of substrate and product can be assumed to be in rapid exchange with pools directly interacting with enzyme molecules, and if the tissue is in steady state with respect to this reaction (i.e., effective substrate and product concentrations are not changing), then the ratio of substrate and reactant concentrations is a measure of the concentration of active enzyme molecules.

Only enzyme assays on *in vitro* tissue preparations have been exploited thus far in connection with effects of experience on brain processes. These studies have involved massive and prolonged differences in environmental complexity, the behavioral consequences of which are ill-defined but almost certainly include changes in information processing and emotional capacity over and above the storage of usable information about past environmental contingencies. Assay of the enzymes which conceivably could be represented in the new protein which seems to be necessary for retention (Section V) has yet to be performed in work concerned particularly with the biochemistry of the trace, using specific training and retention tasks. Presumably, the possibilities which could be tested are so multitudinous that workers interested in protein synthetic correlates of learning wish first to obtain some partial purification of the protein concerned, and so get some pointers from its regional and subcellular distribution and perhaps its physical properties. Pharmacological disruption of memory can also be a guide to the enzymes most likely to be involved. For example, it would be interesting to see whether the changes in cholinergic transmission which seem necessary to retention or retrieval according to Deutsch and co-workers (Chapter 3) are correlated with changes in either cholineacetylase, cholinesterases or choline reuptake in synaptosome preparations. It would be surprising if a change in availability of acetylcholine at a synapse was not either caused by, or the cause of, a change in amount of one of these enzymes.

C. Bioassay

If the establishment of the trace involves increased amounts of a small soluble protein or peptide, it is conceivable that this could be detected in the brain of a trained animal by its behavioral effects on recipients to which it was administered by a suitable route. It might facilitate consolidation or disrupt learning or retention by confusion. Conceivably, a whole class of protein might be involved, which varied in structure with site in the brain because of a role in brain development—the protein at a given site may even have selective affinity for neurons related to that site. In that case, behavior might be biased selectively towards certain modes of sensitivity, reactivity, or action when the brain protein from animals trained in specific tasks is administered. Whatever the mechanism, brain preparations do seem capable of influencing behavior. The statistically most certain series of differences in effects on behavior between brain materials from trained and untrained animals have come from the laboratories of Rosenblatt (Rosenblatt, Farrow, & Rhine, 1966) and Ungar (1969). However, we await a demonstration of informational instruction of behavior by preparations from brain tissues: a logically watertight design involves at least two tasks and four groups of recipients (Booth, 1972). Material from donors trained in one task must facilitate recipients' performance in that task relative to the performance of another group of recipients in the other task, and, also, in the same experiment, material from donors trained in the second task must facilitate in the task relative to the first task. Whether or not all of the chemical transfers of training observed by these or other groups turn out to be strictly informational, it is relevant here to note that both Ungar and Rosenblatt have evidence that the materials necessary to transfer are susceptible to some protein hydrolyzing enzymes, but not to ribonuclease under the conditions tested. Albert (1966) has reported a neuroanatomically more localized transfer source of which the opposite was true. Low values for molecular weight of the active agent (as found by Rosenblatt) are important for the interpretation here because a protease could remove protection from RNA which is then broken down by endogenous RNase (see Section I,C,1). If replication or extension of Albert's paradigm can confirm his result, there is, of course, no reason why polynucleotides should not be able to bias behavior if proteins or peptides can. Some messenger RNA must program synthesis of the peptide. Indeed, Reiniš (1969) has reported that a chemical transfer effect can be blocked by treating the recipient with actino-mycin D. If this disruption of transfer is not because of a general disturbance of behavior by actinomycin, this suggests that transfer materials require new RNA to bias behavior; perhaps they act directly on the chromosomes, or an increase in their concentration at an extranuclear site triggers increased RNA and protein synthesis like some hormones do.

Even if we prove the possibility of chemical transfer of information, we will have to beware of confounding the bioassay used in the purification and characterization of the active material by behavioral changes of other sorts. For example, donors which have been trained in aversive tasks might have changed concentrations of adrenocorticotropin or its releasing factor in the hypothalamus. ACTH can have marked effects on avoidance learning and extinction, but these have recently been shown to be very probably attributable to effects of the peptide hormone on emotionality (Weiss, McEwen, Silva, & Kalkut, 1969), not to any cognitive biasing. Furthermore, behavioral and biochemical analysis will not be sufficient to elucidate the role of any biochemical substances which are implicated in the trace by this method. Physiological and anatomical factors will also have to be specified: for example, a correlation between chemical structure and behavioral information content would not be evidence for chemical coding of memory unless it was also shown that the chemical structure differences do not correlate with regional or cellular uptake or neurophysiological effectiveness of the material. Anatomically selective changes in vascular permeability (Chyatte, Mele, & Anderson, 1967) or neuronal uptake

(Lajtha, 1964) could well have selective effects on or within a sensory modality, on a motor pattern, or on the perception of or intention under a certain environmental contingency (Dyal, 1971).

III. RADIOISOTOPIC ESTIMATION OF PROTEIN SYNTHESIS.

A. Radioautography

The location and the number of radioactive atoms in a tissue preparation can be assessed by the effect of particles from radioisotope disintegration on an adjacent photographic emulsion. The picture that a section of brain tissue can give of the distribution of radioactivity over its surface is of greatest value as a wide anatomical survey, unprejudiced by the sampling procedures necessary to biochemical analysis of blocks of tissue or single cells. The method can resolve detail down to a few micra and has the sensitivity of a cumulative record of disintegrations during an exposure period many times longer than commonly used in scintillation counting. However, any claim that the radioautograph relates to variations in rates of protein synthesis within the tissue must be evaluated in terms of the experimental procedures described in the report.

1. General Interpretation of Autographs

In the first place, the general radioautographic control procedures should have been run. Nonradioactive experimental tissue should be exposed along with every batch of radioactive samples to ensure that chemical reactions between the slice and the emulsion have not created or suppressed a latent image (chemography). A chemographic image could reflect localized variations in tissue metabolism, but these need have nothing to do with the biochemical reactions involving the radioactive precursor which was used. Many known chemographs result from concentrations of histological stain or fixative. Chemography controls also ensure that the visual features assessed are grains and not structures in the tissue or the emulsion which may be difficult for the eye and impossible for a microphotometer to discriminate under bright field illumination except with extremely short depth of focus. Dark field microscopy is better as it exploits the distinctive scattered reflection of light by silver grains.

Microphotographs and even microphotometer readings must be supplemented by grain counts over structures or areas of tissue which have been selected by explicit operations. If structures such as neurons or large subcellular organelles (e.g., cell nuclei) are chosen and grain count differences of only 20 or 30 percent are found, the surrounding areas should be checked for a similar difference between conditions. In sections only a few micra thick, such variations could reflect merely molecular redistribution or conformational changes. Location of grains over cytosol organelles such as synaptic vesicles is highly dubious without sophisticated preparative and statistical techniques, because the size of the silver halide crystals in the finest grain emulsion limits resolution to far less than that of the electron microscope. The grain counting in each tissue sample should have been done without knowledge of the experimental condition being viewed, and, indeed, the autoradiographs of experimental and control conditions should also have been prepared "blind" and in parallel. If comparisons between slides are made (and the risk of artefacts requires that counts should not be restricted to one or two samples), either very many slides should be compared or the radioactive standards which should be on each slide should have shown negligible variations among slides.

2. Biochemical Interpretation of Grain Count Differences

Grain counts are biochemically meaningless without several controls. Isotopic measures follow atoms not molecules.

The radioactive precursor for radioautographic studies of protein synthesis should be a molecule which goes into proteins rather than other large molecules and rather than being catabolized for energy or to give fragments used in the synthesis of other substances. Since the precursor has to get into cells, this implies an amino acid, preferably an essential one, and histidine probably better than leucine, valine, or lysine, and certainly better than tryptophan or tyrosine. The longer between injection and tissue fixation, the more radioactivity will have passed into lipids, nucleic acids, and so on, both directly and by protein breakdown.

Even under optimum conditions, the radioactivity cannot be assumed to be primarily in protein unless the distributions of grains after various tissue treatments are appropriate. Soluble molecules may have been extracted from the tissue before it was coated with emulsion: amino acid catabolites, amino acyl RNA and peptides, for example, will have been lost at any aqueous treatment, and soluble proteins lost during any perfusion before fixation. Deliberate extraction of small molecules prior to exposure must be used to check whether they contribute appreciably to the radioautograph. Dry radioautography at low temperatures will be necessary to check that the label has not been misleadingly redistributed in the tissue before or during exposure if there is some interest in soluble proteins or an assessment of variations in protein precursors. In the case of most proteins, application of lipid solvents or of nucleases before exposure should not affect the picture, but incubation of tissue with one or more proteolytic enzymes should markedly reduce the grain count differences (while incubation for the same time in the medium used for enzyme incubation does not).

Even if the radioautograph by such criteria does show a differential distribution of radioactive proteins, this does not by any means indicate differences in synthesis rate. A radioautograph shows, at most, the pattern of isotope which has been and remains incorporated into protein by the time of tissue fixation. As discussed in more detail in the next subsection, this incorporation is an integral of the variation over time of radioisotope concentration in the immediate precursors out of which protein is made, and of radioactive protein breakdown rate relative to previously synthesized protein. More incorporation in one place than in another may result from faster transport of amino acid, slower breakdown by transamination, faster combination with transfer RNA, new protein containing species of greater than previous average concentration of the precursor amino acid, longer half-life of the new protein, or other factors—all quite distinct from an increased rate of protein synthesis, i.e., the production of greater numbers of any given species of protein molecule during the time sampled. Estimation of precursor pool radioactivity is not practicable by radio-autography. Pharmacological disruption specifically of ribosomal function cannot be used except in any rare case in which the control tissue shows no incorporation, for in other cases the baseline would be shifted and elimination of the incorporation difference would be uninterpretable.

Thus radioautography is best suited to a search for sites showing marked incorporation changes. Samples from these sites then have to be examined by other methods to see whether increases or decreases in rate of protein synthesis are involved.

3. Protein Incorporation during Learning

Altman and co-workers have looked for several years in circular areas of various brain regions for increases in grain density which might have been caused by engaging the rats in various activities for periods of hours after injection of tritiated leucine or glycine (Altman, Das, & Chang, 1966). They found increases relative only to controls which had been accommodated to the handling necessary for injection of isotope or to the activity required in the task. They did not test the possibility that the extent or distribuiton of increased incorporation could be related to the amount of information the rats had acquired. They attributed the differences entirely to an effect of unfamiliar handling or activity. This certainly may be a major factor, but Altman discusses only an acute stress reaction to the novel experience. Contributions from long-lasting conditioning and habituation effects have not been excluded. It is not unreasonable to suppose that dramatic involuntary experiences dominate the representational systems in the brain in a way that the adjustment of details of instrumental activities may not.

Altman's group have varied, to a fair extent, the dose of isotope and the interval between injection and tissue fixation, but intervals less than an hour do not appear to have been investigated, nor have variations in the time of injection before and after training. Their procedures are demonstrated to be capable of showing incorporation differences between certain behavioral conditions, but, unfortunately, negative results from even the most exhaustive study of the more interesting behavioral differences can carry little weight in the face of any positive results obtained by other techniques. We can hope for a combination of positive and negative results in future experiments, as that would narrow the range of interpretation of positive effects.

Rensch & Rahmann (1966) and these workers with Skrzipek (1968) report distinctive distributions of isotope incorporation over the tecta of teleosts which had been injected with radioactive histidine and then exposed for 10 minutes to a lighted spot, stripe, or pair of stripes. It remains to be seen whether the electrical activity which is evoked in the tectum by the visual patterns increases or decreases incorporation (or both). If protein incorporation has been increased in certain cells, the protein formed may not be particularly stable, as the radioautographic pattern disappears at between one and two days. It will be interesting to see whether a blockade of tectal protein synthesis can disrupt retention by the fish of discriminations based on these visual patterns.

Beach, Emmens, Kimble, & Lickey (1969) have found that grain counts over neuronal nuclei in a hippocampal region and in medial septum show up to 20 percent differences between rats trained in one-way active avoidance and both yoked and passive controls, all prehabituated and injected with leucine– ^{3}H. They have yet to establish that the differences are attributable to protein and also are not due to nuclear size changes. The differences were not found in septal regions, some subcortical sensory relays, or liver. Very appropriately, this work is being followed up using dissection, fractionation, and analysis procedures. If protein synthesis is increased in nuclei during learning, this could reflect changes in one of the classes of protein which probably influence DNA function.

B. Scintillation and Geiger Counting

Radioactive decay in a tissue sample can be monitored by measuring photons released by interaction of the emitted particles with a phosphor in solution with or around the sample. This counting technique has advantages and disadvantages relative to the use of combusted samples in a gas flow counter or dried samples under a Geiger counter window. Although these latter techniques are quite adequate for studies of protein synthesis, the present discussion will be restricted to the scintillation method because of its popularity.

Radioisotopes vary in the maximum of the energy range over which particles are emitted. Thus ^{14}C concentration in a sample can be estimated from the rate of events in a high energy range and ^{3}H (tritium) concentration in the same sample from the low energy counts per minute, less the low energy counts expected from the ^{14}C. Often three "windows" are available, allowing a third isotope such as ^{32}P to be counted, at the cost of some loss of reliability in practice. This facility makes double or triple isotope experiments possible. An

RNA precursor and a protein precursor labeled with different radioisotopes can be injected into the same animal, or, more important for memory experiments, samples from experimental and control animals, injected with the same precursor but different isotopes, can be combined for the isolation of protein and its analysis, eliminating effects of the marked variability in purification procedure on the sensitivity of the experiment.

1. General Interpretation of Counts

As with any other method of measuring radioactivity, the rate of recorded counts is not identical to the rate of disintegrations in the sample. First, local and cosmic radiation from outside the sample has to be subtracted. Also background-corrected counts from "blank" samples are often not negligible, because of slight cross-contamination between multiple samples. Under good conditions these corrections are less than 1 percent of total counts. When corrections are less than an order below total counts, a longer time should have been spent in counting each sample, and statistical questions should no longer be ignored, even though they often are. Every report should give typical examples of raw counts per minute and counting times, especially for samples of low activity. Presentation of derived data exclusively is acceptable only if every aspect is given a valid statistical evaluation.

Then, second, the ratio between corrected counts and actual disintegrations should have been assessed for each sample. The efficiency of the counter, phosphor, and sample geometry for the isotope used must be known to get absolute values of isotope concentration. This is often not needed but the variance in efficiency estimates could be important when efficiencies are low—50 percent or less. What is more crucial than general counting efficiency is the suppressing effect of the composition of each sample on the detectability of disintegrations in it (quenching); statistically reliable count differences between experimental samples, whether of high or low activity, need have no relation to differences in concentration of radioisotope. The counter used may have a radioactive source with which the quench of each sample is tested, but the validity of this external quench correction should be tested by measures of internal quenching—adding a known amount of radioisotope to a duplicate sample or to the original for recounting. Statement of the quenching correction procedure used is vital to the interpretation of studies involving the counting of crude protein preparations.

2. Biochemical Interpretation of Corrected Counts

For studies of protein synthesis, one must first be sure that the counts come from protein. Some of the arguments over the first reports claiming chemical transfer of training in rodents have had the benefit of emphasizing that chemical purity is a specifiable degree of approximation to an ideal. An "RNA preparation" or a "protein preparation" almost always has measurable amounts of other materials in it. A standard first step in preparation of protein samples in precipitation from the cold tissue dispersion by trichloracetic acid. This brings down virtually all the protein and large peptides, soluble and particulate, but even after several TCA washes, membrane protein will still have lipid attached; nucleoprotein, nucleic acids, and other materials will remain occluded. At least lipid, glycolipid, RNA, and DNA extraction procedures should be applied if the claim is that the counts are in protein. Either the procedures used should have been shown to be effective for brain tissue or some assay of the residium should demonstrate this (assaying samples of extracts for negligible extraction of radioactivity is a very insensitive test).

One may then have a valid measure of isotope incorporation into protein, as with radioautography. The next problem is to relate incorporation to synthesis, and here isolation procedures have the advantage. One could, in principle, isolate a sample of amino acyl-tRNA—even the transfer ester specifically of the injected radioactive amino acid. Given that initiation of protein chains on the ribosome is normally the rate-limiting step in translation from existing messenger RNA, the relation between isotope concentration in this precursor and in the protein population should exclude variations in amino acid transport and metabolism, which are very likely to follow from intensive neuronal activity. However, this amount of isotope in the protein has been incorporated over a time period during which isotope concentrations (as indicated by specific activity) in precursor species have been changing rapidly. Therefore, estimation of synthesis using only a correction from the protein presursor specific activity ratio at the time of protein isolation is highly dubious. There should at least be estimates of precursor specific activity at a few time intervals before the main measure. Now, also, it is not generally practicable, of course, to measure the specific activity of the immediate precursor of protein. Indeed it is also impossible to measure the specific activity in only the population of precursor molecules immediately available to the ribosomes. So the crudeness of the measure of total protein in the tissue sample has to be further compounded by a measure of total precursor activity, which even includes radioactive molecules which are not on the synthetic pathway from injected precursor to protein. Nevertheless, even a total soluble radioactivity measure at various times up to the time of the protein incorporation measure can give information about the contribution of variations in cellular uptake of amino acids and in reutilization of amino acids from protein breakdown. This recycling of amino acids is particularly important in the brain, which is the organ with the least net uptake response to changes in blood amino acid concentration (Lajtha, 1964).

The breakdown of old and new proteins could also significantly affect the interpretation of incorporation measures. Decreased breakdown of all protein or of only new protein, or increased breakdown of old protein, would increase incorporation. Such variations in breakdown rate are known to be important in the liver. This means that a hypothesis of changed protein synthesis is only justified if corrected incorporation data are supplemented by turnover data, that is, protein is labeled and then the effects of the learning experience on loss of radioactivity determined.

3. Protein Incorporation Correlates of Training

Gaito, Mottin, & Davison (1968) measured pool-corrected incorporations (relative specific activities) of protein preparations from various portions of brain, as well as concentrations of protein, RNA, and DNA, after injection of valine-^{14}C and 15 trials in 15 minutes of one-way active avoidance acquisition reinforced by a conventional 1.5 mA electric shock to the feet. Controls were placed in the avoidance chamber without shocks. Some brain regions showed consistent incorporation differences in two experiments. Cerebellum and medial ventral cerebral cortex samples showed greater protein relative specific activity in trained than control rats, and anterior dorsal cerebral cortex showed less. Protein/nucleic acid ratios generally followed the same pattern, supporting an interpretation in terms of changes in protein synthesis or breakdown. The optimist might hope that these regional changes reflect motor, emotional, and cognitive differences, respectively, between trained and control rats. Correlates in yoked rats, overtrained rats, and other behavioral controls will help indicate whether any of the differences could reflect establishment of a memory trace. Conceivably the decrease in dorsal cortex may be related to the depression of RNA incorporation in sensorimotor cortex observed by Zemp, Wilson, & Glassman (1967). Studies of amino acid incorporation into brain protein in nonlearning situations by no means always show increases with gross changes in electrical activity patterns; Rose (1967) found a phase of decreased incorporation after bringing dark-reared rats into the light, and Orrego and Lippman (1967) found only decreases on electrical stimulation of cerbral cortex slices *in vitro*.

The increases in protein and RNA incorporation are observed in these situations by Gaito's group and Glassman's group seem to be attributable mainly to the limbic system (although excluding the hippocampus). The possibility that some aspects of the trace lie in structures like the amygdala or the septum in rats cannot be exluded. Hydén and Lange (1968) have recently supplemented their studies of RNA composition of neocortex samples with an examination of amino acid incorporation into hippocampal protein. However, these results to date relate only to exercise of a paw, and not demonstrably to the acquisition of a motor skill or preference, although McEwen (1968) has reported a preliminary correlation which is suggestive in that respect. Incidentally, the Hydén and Lange study also illustrates the care needed in the interpretation of isotope results. They took the admirable precaution of carrying out a control experiment to check whether precursor specific activity was in fact linearly related to protein specific activity in the relevant hippocampal region over the range of protein specific activities observed in their main experiment. Their plot of precursor dose (Hydén & Lange, 1969) against specific activity shows very large scatter. They assume that a linear relation over the dose range underlies the scatter, but an asymptote of incorporation at medium doses seems quite possible from the data points they present. If this were the case, then high precursor concentrations would not necessarily give proportionately higher incorporations into protein, given a constant rate of protein synthesis. Hence, their observations of higher precursor radioactivity in the control group and similar protein radioactivity in control and exercised groups does not necessarily indicate that the rate of protein synthesis in the control conditions is lower than during exercise. Thus, the need for caution in interpreting pool-corrected incorporation values is very evident, especially in tissue samples which often are much larger than those used in Hydén's laboratory.

IV. CHANGES IN CONTROL OF PROTEIN SYNTHESIS

The sole known activity of nucleic acids is the regulation and specification of protein synthesis. So variation in type or amounts of DNA or RNA implies variation in their expression as new protein molecules.

A. Deoxyribonucleic Acid

At present there is no way of isolating the genetic material of the chromosomes, or the DNA recently discovered in mitochondria, in a form which reliably reflects its functional state in the cell. The materials (presumably histones and perhaps other proteins) which keep genes inactive are only held to the DNA by electrostatic and other noncovalent bonds, which are liable to be disrupted during isolation. Also new associations could easily be formed during disruption of the cell. We are dependent on analysis of RNA to determine what the DNA is doing.

Incipient cell division can be detected as synthesis of DNA. From what we know of the cells of adult mammalian brain, such increases in amount of DNA or appreciable incorporation of radioisotope into DNA can only reflect glial or perhaps mitochondrial multiplication. Although one cannot exclude a priori the possibility that glia might modulate neuronal transmission at or around synapses or by myelination, there is no evidence that establishment of a memory correlates with DNA synthesis. There is evidence that microneurons are formed in certain regions of mature brain. This possibly occurs more widely than has been hitherto suspected or proved and, if so, may even mediate the trace (Altman, 1967; see I,C,1,b above). However these neurons differentiate from preexisting cells, and probably no DNA synthesis is involved.

B. Ribonucleic Acid

Growth of a cell would probably depend on an increased number of ribosomes whether or not this required faster synthesis of messenger RNA. The extra RNA might have a different proportion of bases than the previous average, but it need not contain previously absent species of RNA. Differentiation, in any sense, down to a switch of activity of a single gene, involves the appearance of new species of messenger RNA.

Changes in average rate of creation or destruction of new RNA molecules of all types may be detectable by changes in total amount of RNA per cell (i.e., RNA/DNA ratio) or by isotopic methods similar in principle to those discussed above in connection with protein synthesis. A change in RNA polymerase activity may be seen.

Further information can be sought by preparing RNA-rich portions, either by extracting much of the RNA from a tissue dispersion, or by preparing a portion of the range of subcellular particles which is rich in ribosomes. The spectrum of molecular sizes in an RNA extract can be examined for changes with tissue status.

The profile of RNA fractions seen after centrifugation through a gradient of increasing sucrose concentration sometimes changes. This often represents no more than a change in the average number of ribosomes associated with messenger RNA molecules, not any change in rate of synthesis of an RNA type: however, the more polysomes and the heavier they are for a given number of ribosomes, the more protein is being produced under normal conditions. Sometimes a relative increase in messenger RNA can be detected. Nonetheless, a change in density gradient profile often does not accompany an increase in RNA synthesis rate and the consequent increase in new protein and, so, such changes should not be required as a condition of acceptance of an hypothesis of raised protein synthesis rate.

Appreciably increased amounts of messenger RNA should be reflected in increased rate of protein synthesis *in vitro* under conditions where messenger concentrations are limiting. With the aid of radioisotopes it might one day prove possible to demonstrate that messenger preparations from a given brain region containing a new memory trace synthesize a distinctive new fraction of protein. At present, evidence for a new messenger RNA species can more easily be obtained by hybridizing total RNA preparations with denatured DNA from the same animal species. Single-stranded DNA can be absorbed on to a solid support and will bind RNA molecules when base sequences in the RNA match those of unoccupied stretches of DNA. The RNA in the hybrid is not sensitive to ribonuclease under certain conditions and, so, the membrane can be cleared of unhybridized RNA. The hybridization is slow even at high temperatures and salt concentrations and, so, a high ratio of RNA to DNA is essential, although this introduces complications from RNA–RNA hybrids. The rate is very dependent on the frequency of exactly or approximately complementary sequences on the DNA, and, so, some species of RNA reach equilibrium between binding and release much earlier during incubation than others; indeed, it is doubtful whether asymptote is reached before appreciably RNA breakdown supervenes, especially in the case of mammalian preparations which contain a high proportion of very complex unique sequences. Some sequences are reiterated and will hybridize rapidly, but the bulk would take weeks to saturate. All the same, DNA which has been hybridized as efficiently as practicable with RNA from cells in one condition sometimes still binds RNA prepared from similar cells in another condition. When this happens it implies that some RNA species from the second condition readily find free complementary regions on the DNA, that is, they are present in far higher concentrations than in the RNA preparation from the first condition. This interpretation is reasonable only if the RNA preparations have been incubated with the DNA in two successive steps, to minimize complications arising from competition for sites on DNA. It also depends on the reverse sequence of incubations showing that RNA from the first condition is not bound by DNA hybridized with RNA from the second condition. Radioactive RNA is used for the second incubation as the extra RNA bound is usually very little, and, so, this control experiment requires reversed labeling procedures.

With mammalian preparations it is not really safe to conclude that an increase in concentration of a particular RNA species as indicated by hybridization experiments represents activity of a previously inactive gene. Faster transcription or slower breakdown of RNA from a whole group of nonreiterated genes could give the same result.

Some indication of a change in the relative concentrations of different RNA species in the tissue can also be obtained by determinations of the proportions of the four purine or pyrimidine bases in the total RNA. The RNA in the ribonucleoprotein of ribosomes dominates the RNA of cells having at least moderate-sized cytosol compartments. Thus a large rise in messenger production may produce a shift of average base compostition. If many genes are involved, this is likely to be in a direction towards the base composition complementary to the average for DNA, because the base ratios of the ribosome genes are often higher than average in cytosine and guanine.

Hydén and colleagues found changes in RNA concentration and composition in very small samples from the cerebral cortex of rats exercised in a way which should change their paw preference (Hydén & Egyházi, 1964; Hydén & Lange, 1965). Bowman & Stroebel (1969) have studied incorporation into RNA during reversal of T-maze approach learning. Avoidance tasks have also been used. Glassman's group have exploited radioautography (Zemp *et al.*, 1967) and sucrose density-gradient techniques (Adair, Wilson, Zemp, & Glassman, 1968; Adair, Wilson, & Glassman, 1968) in following up a change they observed in whole brain RNA incorporation during brief training of mice to jump to a shelf to avoid shock. Machlus & Gaito (1969) have used hybridization on whole brain preparations, having found evidence for localized RNA incorporation differences in a study of dissected rat brain samples taken after brief training in position-discriminated avoidance. However, the results were unsatisfactory because, as Clifford, Gaito, & Takai (1971) have recently noted, far from saturating amounts of RNA were used.

These studies vary greatly in the behavioral situations used and in the degree of anatomical localization of the biochemical correlates of training. The results of the different methods are generally consistent with there being a rise in net synthesis of RNA specific to the brain during and immediately after the activity involved in learning in the rat. This may be triggered or maintained by neuronal metabolic needs, although the evidence is that these can have the opposite effect (Prives & Quastel, 1969). Alternatively, perhaps the protein whose synthesis seems to be necessary to retention (see Section V, below) activates synthesis of RNA by enzymic or allosteric action. It is difficult to believe that this new RNA is necessary to the maintenance of memory in the early stages soon after its initial synthesis—for example, as template for the protein synthesis which is necessary—because gross disruption of transcription from DNA does not block retention of a discriminated task over 24 hours following acquisition (Barondes & Cohen, 1967). If many genes are involved, as the DNA-like base ratios and the wide spectrum of molecular weights suggest, the faster synthesis may reflect higher RNA polymerase activities. The resulting increased capacity for protein synthesis might conceivably be important for the long-term stabilization of the trace, rather than its initial establishment for which protein synthesis is necessary within hours of learning. However, the RNA synthesis may simply be involved in increasing the capacity of a transmission pathway for repeated use, without any modulation of the pathway's input-output relationships that would mediate new memory.

V. BIOCHEMICAL PHARMACOLOGY OF PROTEIN SYNTHESIS

If properly used, pharmacological methods can be powerful tools in the investigation of biochemical theories. The criteria as applied to behavioral studies are as follows: the drugs used should have well-understood biochemical effects which have been demonstrated to occur in the mammalian brain, not just in other tissues. A drug which is found to change behavior significantly should be shown to have the supposed effect in the strain of animal used at the dose and site at which its administration affects behavior. Chemically related drugs not having the biochemical effect of interest should be shown not to affect behavior in the same way. Even all this is not sufficient evidence that the biochemical effect being considered is involved in the behavior. The behavioral change could be caused by some other biochemical or biophysical action of the drug, known or unknown, however specific the drug is generally considered to be. (It has been well said that the specificity of a drug is inversely proportional to the extent to which its mechanism of action has been investigated.) Pharmacological studies only become definite biochemical evidence when the function being examined is affected by three or four or more drugs of widely differing structures—even of widely differing modes of action on the same biochemical system—which have only one known biochemical action in common. This criterion has yet to be met in studies of the effects of antibiotics on memory retention. Gartside's (1968) study of a long-term electrophysiological plasticity in rat cerebral cortex is an interesting and probably relevant example that does have this advantage. Several minutes' anodal polarization causes an increase in neuronal firing rate which lasts for several hours at least. Gartside found that protein synthesis inhibitors as different as cycloheximide, chloramphenicol, neomycin, and tetracycline all prevented the appearance of this aftereffect, without disrupting the increase in firing rate which normally occurred during polarization.

A knowledge of dose-response relationships is also necessary to an adequate evaluation of this sort of evidence. A study of the variation of the behavioral effect with the dose of drug administered is not an optional extra for those who find satisfaction in the collection of parametric data on otherwise well-established phenomena. A pharmacologist insists on such data because they are theoretically essential to any comparison of substances, routes, or conditions which involve an effect in one case and not in another. As Deutsch (1969) has pointed out, the deduction of delocalization of the trace from the need of multiple injections of antibiotic late after learning is not valid unless it is shown that dose-response relationships are the same soon and long after training. A negative result might depend on too low a dose, or, in certain cases, on too high a dose. When a concentrated solution of a chemically reactive drug is rapidly introduced locally in the brain, there is difficulty in justifying the supposition that it changes behavior by a mechanism for which the drug is specific at low concentration; the effect should also be seen when the same amount of drug is introduced in a more dilute solution or more slowly.

The report to date with the best behavioral indications of a disruption of memory retention by an antibiotic is by Barondes & Cohen (1967). They used a position discriminated escape task in those studies, and have another discriminated escape task in other work (Barondes & Cohen, 1968; Cohen & Barondes, 1968). They tested for state-dependent retrieval deficits. Also, they used a disruptor of ribosomal function, acetoxycycloheximide, which inhibits protein synthesis at very low concentrations, increasing the chances that its assumed specificity is real. Its mode of action is not as well understood as is that of puromycin, for example, but its action is not as likely to produce materials as deleterious as the incomplete proteins generated by puromycin. There exists a good selection of other inhibitors of protein synthesis which can penetrate mammalian cells and, so, there is every opportunity to establish definite biochemical implications by pharmacological studies. The behavioral problems of establishing that the psychological disruption is due to loss of the memory trace remain enormous, indeed, basically insoluble, for no behavioral test can exclude the possibility that an apparent retention deficit is actually only a blockade of retrieval mechanisms. This approach has therefore to be combined with a search for biochemical correlates specific to establishment of a new memory, that is, biochemical changes distinct from correlates merely of exercise of that memory in the same perceptual, motivational, and emotional situation, using the same pattern of actions and reactions as are involved in its registration.

VI. BIOCHEMISTRY AND MEMORY RESEARCH

Part of the purpose of this chapter has been to dispel the illusion that biochemical variables are more tangible or unambiguously measurable than behavioral variables—a biochemical result in relation to behavior is Real Science entering psychology! The substantive phenomena of metabolic biochemistry are as different from billiard balls, chairs, and tables as is the substance of psychology, namely the interpretations and intentions existing in the behavior of the animal or human subject. The biochemist has no more right to regard behavior as somehow too nebulous for him to handle than the psychologist has need to fool himself, or anyone else, that marks made by a pen recorder are what put objectivity into the theoretical analysis of behavior.

Even though some of the biochemists' measures do happen to be amounts of material stuffs, the comforts of a covertly materialist metaphysics are no guarantee of valid theoretical interpretation of the measures in terms of dynamic chemical physiology of the cell. The problems of alternative plausible conjectures and their investigation by further experiment are of the same form for both sciences. Therefore, of course, chemical characterization of the memory trace (like other areas of the biochemistry of behavior) has at least twice the problems of straight biochemistry or straight experimental psychology; and, so, at this early stage of the enterprise, it often has less than half the theoretical depth of the current unidisciplinary research in either field.

Nonetheless, there is progress in relating protein synthesis and other biochemical processes to long-term memory. Arguments over the data to hand have at least increased the general appreciation of the correct questions to ask. As the manpower working on the biochemistry of memory expands, it would be good if more effort went into developing experimental paradigms which are capable of answering the important questions than has been spent in some other areas of memory physiology, in which crucial experiments are done several years after they were identified, while most of the effort goes into multiple parametric replications of a prematurely standardized paradigm involving virtually unexplored behavioral and physiological mechanisms. We need joint application of pharmacological disruption and biochemical correlate approaches to the role of protein synthesis; for the learning tasks, we need modality-specific discriminations, movement-specific skills, and the like, and those examples of acquisition of these defined types of information which have some known neurophysiological and neuroanatomical basis.

A working hypothesis consistent with the data to hand is that retention of a memory normally depends on the creation of additional protein within some minutes of registration, and this new protein is, at a few hours after registration, more critical to the retention of information than new protein is to the use of older memories or of innate transmission pathways. The strongest support for this general hypothesis comes, at the moment, from the pharmacological approach. This, in the nature of the case, can never establish that retention is mediated by the chemical processes disrupted by the drugs, but some examples continue to survive the fiercest tests for retrieval deficits that have thus far been made. As yet we have no idea whatsoever of the nature of these molecules or the setting that enables the brain to use them in information retention; also, it remains a mystery at what stage the RNA which programs their synthesis is made.

It must be emphasized that these questions about the physical character of the trace are only a minute fraction of the problem of explaining memory. Other chapters in this book bring out the complexities of the neurophysiology and anatomy of memory mechanisms. The biochemical trace is a usable representation of the past in virtue of its context in the neuronal network and the organism's continuing environment. The physics of computer memories is a fairly minor aspect of computer technology! Investigation of the logic of the "machine codes" of memory neurophysiology and the "program languages" or memory experimental psychology constitutes the bulk of the challenge of the memory phenomenon to research into brain and behavior. However, identifying the biochemical principle of the state change to which all these processes give meaning is a genuine scientific problem relevant to body-mind relationships and conceivably of eventual clinical import. Also, it might lead us to some interesting neurochemistry, even if we should not pin our hopes on finding some mechanism previously unknown in all of molecular biology.

REFERENCES

Adair, L. B., Wilson, J. E. & Glassman, E. Brain function and macromolecules, IV. Uridine incorporation into polysomes of mouse brain during different behavioral experiences. *Proceedings of the National Academy of Sciences*, 1968, Vol 61, 917-922.

Adair, L. B., Wilson, J. E., Zemp, J. W., & Glassman, E. Brain function and macromolecules, III. Uridine incorporation into polysomes of mouse brain during short-term avoidance conditioning. *Proceedings of the National Academy of Sciences*, 1968, Vol. 61, 606-613.

Adey, W. R. Neurophysiological correlates of information transaction and storage in brain tissue. *Progress in Physiological Psychology*, 1967, Vol. 1, 1-42.

Agranoff, B. W., Davis, R. E., & Brink, J. J. Chemical studies on memory formation in goldfish. *Brain Research*, 1966, Vol. 1, 303-309.

Albert, D. J. Memory in mammals: Evidence for a system involving nuclear ribonucleic acid. *Neuropsychologia*, 1966, Vol. 4, 79-92.

Altman, J. Postnatal growth and differentiation of the mammalian brain, with implications for a morphological theory of memory. In G. C. Quarton, T. Melnechuk, & F. O. Schmitt (Eds.), *The Neurosciences*. New York: Rockefeller University Press, 1967. Pp. 723-743.

Altman, J., & Das, G. D. Autoradiographic examination of the effects of enriched environment on the rate of glial multiplication in adult rat brain. *Nature*, 1964, Vol. 204, 1161-1163.

Altman, J., Das, G. D., & Chang, J. Behavioral manipulations and protein metabolism of the brain: effects of visual training on the utilization of leucine-^{3}H. *Physiology and Behavior,* 1966, Vol. 1, 111-115.

Axelrod, J., Schein, H. M., & Wurtman, R. J. Stimulation of Δ^{14}C-melatonin synthesis from ^{14}C-tryptophan by noradrenaline in rat pineal in organ culture. *Proceedings of the National Academy of Sciences*, 1969, Vol. 62, 544-549.

Barondes, S. H., & Cohen, H. D. Delayed and sustained effect of acetoxycycloheximide on memory in mice. *Proceedings of the National Academy of Sciences*, 1967, Vol. 58, 157-164.

Barondes, S. H., & Cohen, H. D. Memory impairment after subcutaneous injection of acetoxycycloheximide. *Science*, 1968, Vol 160, 556-557.

Beach, G., Emmens, M., Kinble, D. P. & Lickey, M. Autoradiographic demonstration of biochemical changes in the limbic system during avoidance training. *Proceedings of the National Academy of Sciences*, 1969, Vol. 62, 692-696.

Bliss, T. V. P., Burns, B. D., & Uttley, A. M. Factors affecting the conductivity of pathways in cerebral cortex. *Journal of Physiology*, 1968, Vol. 195, 339-367.

Bogoch, S. *The Biochemistry of Memory*. New York: Oxford University Press, 1968.

Bowman, R. E., & Stroebel, D. A. Brain RNA metabolism in the rat during learning. *Journal of Comparative & Physiological Psychology*, 1969, Vol. 67, 448-456.

Booth, D. A. Vertebrate brain ribonucleic acids and memory retention. *Psychological Bulletin*, 1967, Vol. 68, 149-177.

Booth, D. A. Neurochemical changes correlated with learning and memory retention. In G. Ungar (Ed.), *Molecular Mechanisms in Memory and Learning*. New York: Plenum Press, 1970.

Booth, D. A. Review of E. J. Fjerdingstad (Ed.), *Chemical transfer of learned information. Quarterly Journal of Experimental Psychology*, 1972, Vol. 24, 116-117.

Casola, L., Lim, R., Davis, R. E., & Agranoff, B. W. Behavioral and biochemical effects of intracranial injection of cytosine arabinoside in goldfish. *Proceedings of the National Academy of Sciences*, 1968, Vol. 60, 1389-1395.

Chyatte, C., Mele, K. E. C., & Anderson, B. L. R. Brain blood-shift theory: verification of a predicted gradient in tactual-auditory rivalry. *International Journal of Neuropsychiatry*, 1967, Vol. 9, 360-364.

Clifford, J., Gaito, J., & Takai, M. RNA species during visual stimulation. *Nature*, 1971, Vol. 234, 90-91.

Cohen, H. D. Learning, memory and the metabolic inhibitors. In G. Ungar (Ed.), *Molecular Mechanisms in Memory and Learning*. New York: Plenum Press, 1970.

Cohen, H. D., & Barondes, S. H. Effect of acetoxycycloheximide on learning and memory of a light-dark discrimination. *Nature*, 1968, Vol. 218, 271-273.

Cragg, B. G. Effect of first exposure to light on synaptic dimensions in rat visual cortex. *Nature*, 1967, Vol. 215, 251-253.

Deutsch, J. A. The physiological basis of memory. *Annual Review of Psychology*, 1969, Vol. 20, 85-104.

Diamond, M. C., Krech, D., & Rosenzweig, M. R. The effects of enriched environment on the histology of the rat cerebral cortex. *Journal of Comparative Neurology*, 1964, Vol. 123, 111-119.

Dure, L., & Waters, L. Long-lived messenger RNA: Evidence from cotton seed germination. *Science*, 1965, Vol. 147, 410-412.

Dyal, J. A. Transfer of behavioral bias and learning enhancement: a critique of specificity experiments. In G. Ádám (Ed.), *Biology of Memory*. Budapest: Akadémiai Kiadó, 1971. Pp. 145-159.

Gaito, J. *DNA Complex and Adaptive Behavior*. Englewood Cliffs, New Jersey: Prentice-Hall, 1971.

Gaito, J., Mottin, J., & Davison, J. H. Chemical variation in the ventral hippocampus and other brain sites during conditioned avoidance. *Psychonomic Science*, 1968, Vol. 13, 259-260.

Gartside, I. B. Mechanisms of sustained increases of firing rate of neurones in the rat cerebral cortex after polarization: Role of protein synthesis. *Nature*, 1968, Vol. 220, 383-384.

Gilbert, W., & Müller-Hill, B. Isolation of the lac repressor. *Proceedings of the National Academy of Sciences*, 1966, Vol. 56, 1891-1898.

Haljamäe, H. & Lange, P. W. Calcium content and conformational changes of S-100 protein in the hippocampus during training. *Brain Research*, 1972, Vol. 38, 131-142.

Humphreys, T., Penman, S., & Bell, E. The appearance of stable polysomes during the development of chick down feathers. *Biochemical & Biophysical Research Communications,* 1964, Vol. 17, 618-623.

Huneeus-Cox, F., Fernandez, H. L., & Smith, B. H. Effects of redox and sulfhydryl reagents on the bioelectric properties of the giant axon of the squid. *Biophysics Journal*, 1966, Vol. 6, 675-689.

Hydén, H., & Egyházi, E. Changes in RNA content and base composition in cortical neurons of rats in a learning experiment involving transfer of handedness. *Proceedings of the National Academy of Sciences*, 1964, Vol. 52, 1030-1035.

Hydén, H., & Lange, P. W. A differentiation in RNA response in neurons early and late in learning. *Proceedings of the National Academy of Sciences*, 1965, Vol. 53, 946-952.

Hydén, H., & Lange, P. W. Protein synthesis in the hippocampal pyramidal cells of rats during a behavioral test. *Science*, 1968, Vol. 159, 1370-1373.

Hydén, H., & Lange, P. W. Protein synthesis during learning. *Science*, 1969, Vol. 164, 200-201.

Hydén, H. & Lange, P. W. Brain-cell protein synthesis specifically related to learning. *Proceedings of the National Academy of Sciences*, 1971, Vol. 65, 898-904.

Hydén, H. & Lange, P. W. S-100 brain protein: correlations with behavior. *Proceedings of the National Academy of Sciences*, 1971, Vol. 67, 1959-1966 (b).

Jerne, N. K. The natural-selection theory of antibody formation. *Proceedings of the National Academy of Sciences*, 1955, Vol. 41, 849-857.

Kidson, C. Kinetics of cortisol action on RNA synthesis. *Biochemistry & Biophysics Research Communications*, 1965, Vol. 21, 282-289.

Lajtha, A. Protein metabolism of the nervous system. *International Review of Neurobiology*, 1964, Vol. 6, 1-98.

Lajtha, A., & Toth, J. Instability of cerebral proteins. *Biochemical & Biophysical Research Communications*, 1966, Vol. 23, 294-298.

Machlus, B., & Gaito, J. Successive competition hybridization to detect RNA species in a shock avoidance task. *Nature*, 1969, Vol. 222, 573-574.

Marks, P., Burka, E. R., & Schlessinger, D. Protein synthesis in erythroid cells, I. *Proceedings of the National Academy of Sciences*, 1962, Vol. 48, 2163-2171.

McEwen, B. S. Cellular dynamics of brain proteins. In F. D. Carlson (Ed.), *Physiological and Biochemical Aspects of Nervous Integration*. Englewood Cliffs, New Jersey: Prentice-Hall, 1968. Pp. 361-381.

McEwen, B. S., & Hydén, H. A study of specific brain proteins on the semimicro scale. *Journal of Neurochemistry*, 1966, Vol. 13, 823-833.

Monroy, A., Maggio, R., & Rinaldi, A. M. Experimentally induced activation of the unfertilized sea urchin egg. *Proceedings of the National Academy of Sciences*, 1965, Vol. 54, 107-111.

Orrego, F., & Lipmann, F. Protein synthesis in brain slices. Effects of electrical stimulation and acidic amino acids. *Journal of Biological Chemistry*, 1967, Vol. 242, 685-671.

Papaconstantinou, J. Molecular aspects of lens cell differentiation. *Science*, 1967, Vol. 156, 338-346.

Pappas, G. D., & Purpura, D. P. Distribution of colloidal particles in extracellular space and synaptic cleft substance of mammalian cerebral cortex. *Nature*, 1966, Vol. 210, 1391-1392.

Pease, D. C. Polysaccharides associated with the exterior surface of epithelial cells: kidney, intestine, brain. *Journal of Ultrastructure Research*, 1966, Vol. 15, 555-588.

Prives, C., & Quastel, J. H. Effects of cerebral stimulation on the biosynthesis *in vitro* of nucleotides and RNA in brain. *Nature*, 1969, Vol. 221, 1053.

Ptashne, M. Isolation of the λ phage repressor. *Proceedings of the National Academy of Sciences*, 1967, Vol. 57, 306-313.

Raisman, G. Neuronal plasticity in the septal nuclei of the adult rat. *Brain Research*, 1969, Vol. 14, 25-48.

Reiniš, S. Block of "memory transfer" by actinomycin D. *Nature*, 1968, Vol. 220, 177-178.

Rensch, B., and Rahmann, H. Autoradiographische Untersuchungen über visuelle "Engramm"-Bildung bei Zahnkarpfen. *Pflügers Archiv*, 1966, Vol. 290, 158-166.

Rensch, B., Rahmann, H., & Skrzipek, K. H. Autoradiographische Untersuchungen über visuelle "Engramm"-Bildung bei Fischen (II). *Pflügers Archiv*, 1968, Vol. 304, 242-248.

Rojas, E. Membrane potentials, resistance and ion permeability in squid giant axons injected or perfused with proteases. *Proceedings of the National Academy of Sciences*, Vol. 53, 306-311.

Rose, S. P. R. Changes in incorporation of ^{3}H-lysine into protein in rat visual cortex following first exposure to light. *Nature*, 1967, Vol. 215, 253-255.

Rosenblatt, F., Farrow, J. T., & Rhine, S. The transfer of learned behavior from trained to untrained rats by means of brain extracts, II. *Proceedings of the National Academy of Sciences*, 1966, Vol. 55, 787-792.

Sjöstrand, J. Rapid axoplasmic transport of labelled proteins in the vagus and hypoglossal nerves of the rabbit. *Experimental Brain Research*, 1969, Vol. 8, 105-112.

Smith, A. L., Satterthwaite, H. S. & Sokoloff, L. Induction of brain D(–)–B– hydroxybutyrate dehydrogenase activity by fasting. *Science*, 1969, **163** 79-81.

Spirin, A. S. On "masked" forms of messenger RNA in early embryogenesis and other differentiating systems. *Current Topics in Developmental Biology,* 1966, Vol. 1, 1-28.

Stevenin, J., Samec, J., Jacob, M., & Mandel, P. Détermination de la fraction du génome codant pour les RNA ribosomiques et messangers dans le cerveau du rat adulte. *Journal of Molecular Biology*, 1968, Vol. 33, 777-793.

Stone, L. S. Neural retina degeneration followed by regeneration from surviving retinal pigment cells in grafted adult salamander eyes. *Anatomical Record*, 1950, Vol. 106, 89-108.

Toschi, G., & Giacobini, E. Puromycin and the impulse activity of crayfish stretch-receptor neuron. *Life Science*, 1965, Vol. 4, 1831-1834.

Trakatellis, A. C., Axelrod, A. E., & Montjar, M. Studies on liver messenger ribonucleic acid. *Journal of Biological Chemistry*, 1964, Vol. 239, 4237-4244.

Ungar, G. Chemical transfer of acquired information. In A. Schwartz (Ed.), *Methods in pharmacology*. New York: Appleton-Century-Crofts, 1969.

Vandenheuval, F. A. Lipid-protein interactions and cohesional forces in the lipoprotein systems of membranes. *Journal of the Americal Oil Chemical Society*, 1966, Vol. 43, 258-264.

Weiss, J. M., McEwen, B. S., Silva, M. T. A., & Kalkut, M. F. Pituitary-adrenal influences on fear responding. *Science*, 1969, Vol. 163, 197-199.

Wessells, N. K., & Wilt, F. H. Action of actinomycin D on exocrine pancreas cell differentiation. *Journal of Molecular Biology*, 1965, Vol. 13, 767-779.

Yaffe, D., and Feldman, M. The effect of actinomycin D on heart and thigh muscle cells grown *in vitro*. *Developmental Biology,* 1964, Vol. 9, 347-366.

Zemp, J. W., Wilson, J. E., & Glassman, E. Brain function and macromolecules, II. Site of increased labeling of RNA in brains of mice during a short-term training experience. *Proceedings of the National Academy of Sciences*, 1967, Vol. 58, 1120-1125.

CHAPTER

3

THE CHOLINERGIC SYNAPSE AND THE SITE OF MEMORY

J. ANTHONY DEUTSCH

I. INTRODUCTION

The idea that learning and memory are due to some form of change of synaptic conductance is very old, having been suggested by Tanzi in 1893. It is a simple idea and in many ways an obvious one. However, the evidence that learning is due to changes at the synapse has hitherto been meager.[1] Though changes do occur at a spinal synapse as a result of stimulation, there is no evidence that the changes are those utilized in the nervous system for informa-

---

[1] Eccles (1961, 1964) has attempted to supply such evidence by studying the effect of stimulation on transmission across a synapse at the spinal level. After repetitive stimulation, a stimulus produces a larger effect at the synapse than before stimulation. More recently, Spencer and Wigdor (1965) and Beswick and Conroy (1965) have also shown such an effect. On the other hand, Fentress and Doty (1966) have reported a depression of responsiveness at a synapse following stimulation.

tion storage. To use an analogy, if we pass large amounts of current across resistors in a computer, temporary increases in temperature and perhaps even permanent increases in resistance occur. However, such an experiment shows only that the computer could store information by using "poststimulation" alterations in its resistors, but not that this is the actual way in which the computer does store information. Furthermore, Sharpless (1964) has pointed out that learning is not due to simple use of stimulation of a pathway and he therefore questions whether the phenomena studied by Eccles (1961, 1964) have anything to do with learning as observed in the intact organism. Nevertheless, this does not mean that learning is not due to synaptic changes of some sort. It means only that a different experimental test of the possibility must be devised.

In designing our experimental approach to this problem, clues from human clinical evidence were used. After blows to the head sustained in accidents, events which occurred closest in time prior to the accident cannot be recalled (retrograde amnesia). Such patches of amnesia may cover days, or even weeks. The lost memories tend to return, with those most distant in time from the accident becoming available first (Russell & Nathan, 1946). In the Korsakoff syndrome (Talland, 1965), retrograde amnesia may gradually increase until it covers a span of many years. An elderly patient may end up remembering only his youth, while there is no useful memory of the more recent intervening years. From such evidence concerning human retrograde amnesia we may conclude that the changes that occur in the substrate of memory take a relatively long time and are measurable in hours, days, and even months. If we suppose from this that the substrate of memory is synaptic, and that it is slowly changing, then it may be possible to follow such synaptic changes using pharmacological methods. If the same dose of a synaptically acting drug has different effects on remembering, depending on the age of the memory (and this can be shown for a number of synaptically acting drugs), we may assume that there has been a synaptic alteration as a function of time since learning, and we may infer that such a synaptic change underlies memory.

Pharmacological agents are available which can either increase or decrease the effectiveness of neural transmitters (Goodman & Gilman, 1965). For instance, anticholinesterase and anticholinergic drugs affect transmission at synapses utilizing the transmitter acetylcholine. During normal transmission, acetylcholine is rapidly destroyed by the enzyme cholinesterase. Anticholinesterase drugs such as physostigmine and diisopropyl fluorophosphate (DFP) inactivate cholinesterase, and so indirectly prevent the destruction of acetylcholine. In submaximal dosage these drugs inactivate not all but only a part of the cholinesterase present and, hence, only slow down but not stop the destruction of acetylcholine. The overall effect at such submaximal levels of anticholinesterase is to increase by some constant the lifetime of any acetylcholine emitted into the synapse and to increase, thereby, the acetylcholine synaptic concentrations resulting from a given rate of emission. Up to a certain level, the greater this concentration the greater is the efficiency of transmission, that is, the conduction across the synapse. Above that level, which is set by the sensitivity of the postsynaptic membrane, any further increase in acetylcholine concentration produces a synaptic block (Goodman & Gilman, 1965; Feldberg & Vartiainen, 1934; Volle & Koelle, 1961). Thus the application of a given dosage of anticholinesterase will (by protecting acetylcholine from destruction) have different effects on the efficiency of synaptic conduction depending on the rate of acetylcholine emission during transmission and on the sensitivity of the postsynaptic membrane. At low levels of emission of acetylcholine or low sensitivity of the postsynaptic membrane, an application of anticholinesterase will render transmission more efficient. Such a property is used to good effect in the treatment of myasthenia gravis. In the treatment of this disorder, anticholinesterase is used to raise the effective concentration of acetylcholine at the neuromuscular junction and, so, to reduce apparent muscular weakness. On the other hand, the same dose of anticholinesterase that caused muscular contraction in the myasthenic patient produces paralysis in a man with normal levels of function at the neuromuscular junction.

If there are changes with time after learning in the level of acetylcholine emitted at the modified synapse, then such a synapse should show either facilitation or block depending on when in time after learning we inject the same dose of anticholinesterase. A similar argument with regard to the action of anticholinesterase can be applied if we assume that instead of a presynaptic increment in transmitter, it is the postsynaptic membrane which becomes more sensitive to transmitter as a function of time after learning. But the use of an anticholinesterase does not allow us to decide which of these alternative versions of the hypothesis of the increment of synaptic conductance actually holds for the learning situation. Later, however, I shall indicate how the use of other types of drugs, such as the cholinomimetics, allows us to surmise that postsynaptic sensitization is the more likely mechanism.

The first two experiments (Deutsch, Hamburg, & Dahl, 1966; Deutsch & Leibowitz, 1966) show that facilitation or block of a memory can be obtained with the same dose of anticholinesterase simply as a function of time of injection since original learning, as might be expected if synaptic change formed the substrate of memory.

II. EXPERIMENTAL INVESTIGATIONS

In the first experiment, rats were trained on a simple task.[2] Then an intracerebral injection of anticholinesterase was made at different times after

[2] The rats were Sprague Dawley males approximately 350 grams at the start of the experiment.

initial training, the time being varied from one group of subject to another. After injection, all rats, irrespective of the group to which they were assigned, were retested 24 hours after injection. Thus, what was varied was the time between training and injection. The time between injection and retest was kept constant. Any difference in remembering between groups was therefore due to the time between initial training and injection.

Rats were placed on an electrified grid in a Y-maze. The lit arm of the Y was not electrified and its position was changed randomly from trial to trial. The rats therefore learned to run into the lit arm. The criterion of learning was met when they had chosen the lit arm 10 trials in succession, whereupon training was concluded.

Then, at various times after training, the rats were injected intracerebrally with DFP dissolved in peanut oil.[3] This dose did not increase the number of trials to criterion in a naive group of rats, thus showing that learning capacity during training was not affected by the drug in the amounts used. At 24 hours after injection, the rats were retrained to the same criterion of 10 successive trials correct. The number of trials to criterion in this retraining session represented the measure of retention.

The first group was injected 30 minutes after training. Its retention was significantly worse than that of a control group injected only with peanut oil.[4] By contrast, a group injected with DFP 3 days after training showed the same amount of retention as did the control group. Thus, up to this point, it seems that memory is less susceptible to DFP the older it is. In fact, a subsidiary experiment (Deutsch & Stone, unpublished) has established that injections of DFP on habits 1 and 2 days old have no effect, showing that the initial stage of vulnerability lasts less than 1 day. Beyond 3 days, however, the situation seems to reverse itself: the memory is more susceptible to DFP the older it is because a DFP group injected 5 days after training showed only slight recollection at retest, and a further group injected 14 days after training showed complete amnesia. The score of the group trained 14 days before injection was the same as the score of the previously mentioned naive group which has not been trained before but had simply been injected with DFP 24 hours prior to testing. The amnesia of the DFP group trained 14 days before injection was not due to normal forgetting, since other controls showed almost perfect retention over a 15-day span. Similar results have been obtained by Hamburg (1967) with

---

[3] The Ss were placed in a stereotaxic instrument under nembutal anesthesia. They were intracerebrally injected in two symetrically placed bilateral loci. The placements were: anterior 3, lateral 3, vertical +2, and anterior 3, lateral 4.75, vertical −2, according to the atlas of DeGroot (1957). 0.01 ml of peanut oil containing 0.1 percent of diisopropyl fluorophosphate (DFP) was injected in each locus.

[4] Except as otherwise stated, the results quoted are significant beyond the 1 percent level. The tests used were the t-test, Mann-Whitney U test, and analysis of variance.

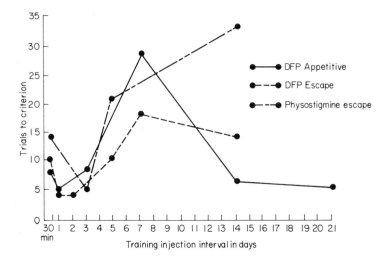

Fig. 3-1. The effect of anticholinesterase injection on memories of different age, shown in three separate experiments. Trials to criterion during retest are plotted against the time which elapsed between retest and original learning. A larger number of trials to criterion during retest signifies a greater amnesia. The time between injection and retest was constant. The differences past the 7-day point probably represent differing rates of forgetting in the three situations. The three experiments are Deutsch *et al.* (1966), Hamburg (1967), and Wiener and Deutsch (1968).

intraperitoneal injections of the anticholinesterase physostigmine, using the same escape habit. Biederman (1970) confirmed the shape of the amnesic function with physostigmine in an operant situation. He used a latency measure of forgetting and a bar press response.

To make sure that we were not observing some periodicity in fear or emotionality interacting with the drug, another experiment employing an appetitive rather than an escape task was conducted. The rats were taught to run a reward of sugar-water, the position of which always coincided with the lit arm of a Y-maze (Wiener & Deutsch, 1968). As seen in Fig. 3-1, the results when compared to the maze results from the preceding experiments show a very similar pattern of amnesia as a function of time of learning before injection. It is therefore most likely that we are, in fact, studying memory. The divergences in the curves after 7 days are probably due to differences in rates of forgetting among the three groups.

In this first set of experiments which dealt with the effects of the anticholinesterases DFP and physostigmine on habits which are normally well retained, the effects of these drugs were to decrease the retention of a habit, depending on its age. Thus, one of the predicted effects of an anticholinesterase was verified. However, the other predicted effect, facilitation, was not shown.

The reason for this is that the habit which was acquired was so well retained without treatment over 14 days that one could not, on methodological grounds, show any improvement of retention subsequent to injection of the drug. It may be the case that 1-, 2-, and 3-day-old habits were facilitated instead of merely being unaffected, but the design of the experiment would not allow us to detect this because there is an effective ceiling on performance. Therefore, an attempt was made to obtain facilitation where it was methodologically possible to detect it, namely, where retention of the habit by a control group was imperfect. For example, it was found that 29 days after learning, the escape habit described above was almost forgotten by a group of animals injected with peanut oil only 24 hours before. On the basis of this observation, a second kind of experiment was devised.

Rats were divided into four groups. The first two groups were trained 14 days before injection, the second two groups 28 days before injection. One of the 28-day and the 14-day groups were injected with the same dose of DFP, the remaining 28-day and 14-day groups were injected with the same volume of pure peanut oil instead. The experimental procedure and dosage were exactly the same as previously described.

On retest, poor retention was exhibited by the 14-day DFP group and 28-day peanut oil group. By contrast, the 28-day DFP group and the 14-day peanut oil group exhibited good retention. The results of anticholinesterase injection show a large and clear facilitation of an otherwise almost forgotten 28-day-old habit while they confirm the obliteration of an otherwise well-remembered 14-day-old habit already demonstrated in the previous experiments (Fig. 3-2A). The same facilitation of a forgotten habit was shown by Wiener and Deutsch (1968) using an appetitive habit and by Squire (1970) using physostigmine-injected mice. Biederman (in press) showed an improvement in memory in pigeons when physostigmine is injected 28 days after a line tilt discrimination was partly learned. A well-learned color discrimination acquired by the same subjects showed no such improvement under the same conditions. Thus, these results also lend strong support to the notion that forgetting is due to a reversal of the change in synaptic conductance which underlies learning (Fig. 3-2B). It must be emphasized, however, that both the block and facilitation of a memory are temporary, wearing off as the injected drug wears off.

So far it has been shown that the anticholinesterase drugs DFP and physostigmine have different effects on memories of different age. Though their actions on memory are consistent with, and plausibly interpreted by their anticholinesterase action, some other property besides their indirect action on acetylcholine could, in some unknown manner, produce the same results. It was, thus, desirable to conduct an independent check on the hypothesis that the effects observed are due to an effect on acetylcholine. This check can be provided by the use of an anticholinergic drug. An anticholinergic drug (like atropine or scopolamine) reduces the effective action of a given level of acetyl-

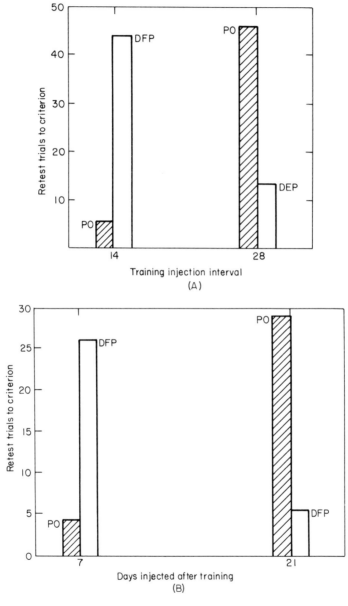

Fig. 3-2A,B. The effect of injection of the anticholinesterase DFP (diisopropyl fluorophosphate) and PO (peanut oil) the drug vehicle on well retained or almost forgotten habits. Trials to criterion are plotted against time between retest and original training. It can be seen that when controls remember well, DFP injected animals forget. When controls forget, DFP injected animals remember well. (From Deutsch & Leibowitz, 1966; Wiener & Deutsch, 1968.)

choline at the synapse without actually changing the level itself. It does this apparently by occupying some of the receptor sites on the postsynaptic membrane without producing depolarization. It thus prevents acetylcholine from reaching such receptor sites and so attenuates the effectiveness of this transmitter. We would therefore expect an anticholinergic to block conduction at a synapse where the postsynaptic membrane is relatively insensitive, while simply diminishing conduction at synapses where the postsynaptic membrane is highly sensitive. If the interpretation of the effects of DFP is correct, we would then expect the reverse effect with the administration of an anticholinergic drug. That is, we would expect the greatest amnesia with anticholinergics precisely where the effect of anticholinesterase was the least; and we would predict the least effect where the effect of anticholinesterase on memory was the largest. It will be recalled that the least effect of anticholinesterase was on habits 1 to 3 days of age.

In a third set of experiments (Wiener & Deutsch, 1968; Deutsch & Rocklin, 1967) the anticholinergic agent employed was scopolamine, and it was injected using exactly the same amount of oil and location as in the previous experiments using DFP.[5] The same experimental procedure was also used. A group injected 30 minutes after training showed little if any effect of scopolamine. However, a group injected 1 and 3 days after training showed a considerable degree of block. Groups injected 7 and 14 days after training showed little if any effect. The results from the appetitive and escape situations were very similar.

As far as the experimental methodology will allow us to discern, the effect, then, of an anticholinergic is the mirror-image of the anticholinesterase effect (Fig. 3-3). There is an increase of sensitivity between 30 minutes and 1 to 3 days, followed by a decrease of sensitivity. This further confirms the notion that there are two phases present in memory storage. Finally, it is of interest to not that amnesia can result in man from anticholinergic therapy (Cutting, 1964).

The experiments already outlined support the idea that at the time of learning some unknown event stimulates a particular group of synapses to alter their state and to increase their conductivity. At this point we may ask why such an increase in synaptic conductivity does not manifest itself with the passage of time when no drugs are injected. Why has it not been noted that habits are better remembered a week after initial learning than, say, three days after such learning? There are various possible answers. One is that the phenomena we have described are some artifact of drug injection. Another is that animal training has,

---

[5] Deutsch and Rocklin used an injection of scopolamine at the same loci as in footnote 4. Peanut oil (0.01 ml) containing 0.58 percent of scopolamine was injected in each placement. Wiener and Deutsch used only the first locus, but doubled the amount injected at that site (both of scopolamine and DFP).

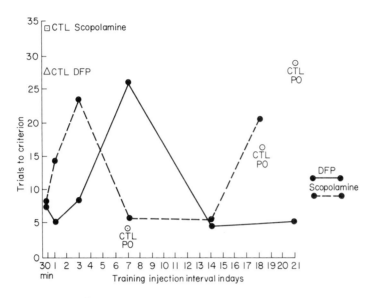

Fig. 3-3. The effects of the injection of the anticholinergic scopolamine compared with that of the anticholinesterase DFP and control injections of PO (peanut oil) on the retention of an appetitive task at various times after original learning. The time between injection and retest was constant. Also indicated are the number of trials to criterion when rats were injected with scopolamine (CTL scopolamine) or DFP (CTL DFP) before original learning to give an estimate of actual amount of amnesia produced. (From Wiener & Deutsch, 1968.)

in general, stretched over days in other studies, blurring in time the initiation of a memory. In addition, and partly as a consequence of the foregoing, it is difficult to find studies where the age of the habit, measured in days, has been used as an independent variable in studies of retention. However, should we not have seen such an improvement in recall in our control groups? This would have been unlikely for the methodological reasons that our animals were trained to the very high criterion of 10 out of 10 trials correct. Given a score which was initially almost perfect, it was thus well nigh impossible to observe any subsequent improvement in retention that might in fact actually exist. To rid ourselves of this methodological limitation, we devised a study in which rats were initially undertrained using escape from shock. The rats were given 15 trials. We then waited to see how many trials it would take these rats on some subsequent day to reach our strict criterion (Huppert & Deutsch, 1969). No drugs were used. We found that the rats took only about half the number of trials to reach criterion when they waited 7 or 10 days than when they waited 1 or 3 days (Fig. 3-4). Huppert (personal communication) has now shown an analogous improvement using an appetitive task. Finally, Dr. J. L. McGaugh has

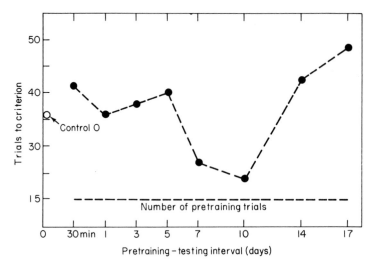

Fig. 3-4. The effects of delay between original partial training (15 trials) and subsequent training to criterion. Plotted are trials to criterion in subsequent training against time since original partial training. Control 0 indicates the number of trials to criterion taken by a group which received its training all in one session.

pointed out that there are old animal studies which purport to find similar effects (Anderson, 1940; Bunch & Magdsick, 1933; Bunch & Lang, 1939; Hubbert, 1915). This shows that our conclusions about the varying substrate of memory were not due to some pharmacological artifact.

We may now ask ourselves whether the inferred modification of a synapse represents an all-or-none, or a graded process. In other words, can a synapse be modified only once during learning, or does a repetition of the same learning task after some learning has already occurred further increase conductance at a single synapse. If we postulate an all-or-none process then how, according to such a model, can we explain empirical increases in "habit strength" with increased training? Possibly they are due to a progressive involvement of fresh synapses and a spread involving more parallel connections in the nervous system. In support of a graded process, we may hypothesize that successive learning trials modify the same synapses in a cumulative way by producing an increase either in the rate at which conductance increases or in the upper limit of such conductance, or both.

There are tests of these two alternatives. If, with increased training, a synapse becomes more conductive, then a habit should become increasingly more vulnerable to anticholinesterase with increased training. Furthermore, the memory of the same habit should be facilitated when its level of training is very low. In other words, we should be able to perform the same manipulations of

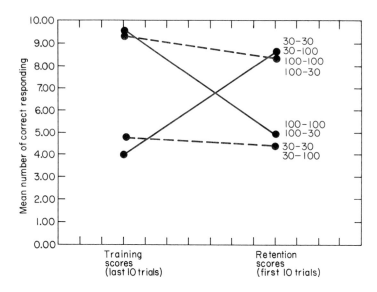

Fig. 3-5. The effects of anticholinesterase injection (DFP) on the retention of well-learned and poorly learned habits. The mean number of correct responses of the last 10 of 30 trials for two groups are shown on the left. One group had to learn to run to alley illuminated by bulb with 30v; the other had to learn the same task except that the bulb had 100v across it. As can be seen from the last 10 trials, the dim light of the 30v group posed a difficult task which produced little learning by the end of the 30 trials. The group learning the brighter cue (100v) displayed excellent acquisition. Because of the different rates of acquisition of the 100v and 30v habits, half of each group was shifted to retest on the other brightness and half was retrained on the same brightness (30-30, 100-100 retested on the same brightness, 30-100 trained on 30, retested on 100, 100-30 trained on 100, retested on 30). The scores of animals trained on the same brightness are combined. Half the animals were injected with DFP, the other half with peanut oil (PO). There is little change in the scores of the peanut oil animals. However, there is a complete crossover of the drug injected animals, showing block of the well-learned habit and facilitation of the poorly learned habit.

memory by varying the level of training as we were already able to perform when we varied time since training.

If, on the other hand, increases in training simply involve a larger number of synapses but no increase in the level of transmitter at any one synapse, then increases in training should not lead to an increased vulnerability of a habit to anticholinesterase. Rather, the opposite should be the case. As the number of synapses recruited is increased, some of the additional synapses will, by chance variation, be less sensitive to a given level of anticholinesterase. Thus, a larger number of synapses should be left functional after anticholinesterase injection when we test an overtrained habit. Three experiments (Deutsch & Leibowitz, 1966; Deutsch & Lutzky, 1967; Leibowitz, Deutsch, & Coons, in preparation) show a large and unequivocal effect. Poorly learned habits are enormously facilitated and well learned habits are blocked (Fig. 3-5). This supports the hypothesis that a set of synapses underlying a single habit remains restricted and each synapse within such a set simply increases in conductance as learning proceeds.

So far the results presented have been interpreted in terms of the action of drugs on synapses which alter their conductance as a function of time since training and amount of training. We can use the model we have developed to generate a somewhat different kind of prediction. An anticholinesterase in submaximal concentrations simply slows down the rate of destruction of acetylcholine. Since we have hypothesized that amnesia is due to a block resulting from an acetylcholine excess, we should predict no amnesia if we spaced our trials so that all or most of the acetylcholine emitted on the previous trial is destroyed by the time the next trial comes along. It has been shown by Bacq and Brown (1937) that (with an intermediate dose of anticholinesterase) block at a synapse occurred only when the intervals between successive stimuli were shortened. Accordingly, an experiment was performed where we varied the interval during retest between 25 and 50 seconds (Rocklin & Deutsch, unpublished). Using a counterbalanced design it was found that rats tested under physostigmine at 25-second intervals showed amnesia for the original habit. Those tested at a 50-second intertrial interval under physostigmine showed no amnesia.

In a second experiment the rats during retest had to learn an escape habit reverse of the one they had learned during training. Therefore, to escape shock during retest they had to learn not only to run to the dark alley but also to inhibit the original learning of running to the lit alley. Thus, provided that the original habit was remembered at the time the reversal was being learned, the time to learn the reversal should take longer than the time to learn the original habit. But if the original habit was not remembered, there should be no difference in trials to criterion between original learning and retest. The results showed that at 50 seconds between trials animals in both the physostigmine and the saline control groups took almost twice as long to reverse as it took them to learn the original habit, indicating in fact that they remembered the original habit (Fig. 3-6). At 25 seconds between trials, the physostigmine animals learned the reversal as quickly as the original habit, whereas the saline animals again took much longer. This second experiment shows that the amnesia of the 25-second physostigmine group in the first experiment is not due to disorientation or an incapacity to perform or learn, but to an amnesia. We might explain the high relearning scores of the same habit of the rats run at 25-second intervals under physostigmine by saying that the rats were somehow incapacitated by the physostigmine if they had to run at 25-second intervals. However, it is difficult to see how such incapacitation could produce abnormally low learning scores of the reversal habit. This dependence of the amnesia on the precise interval of

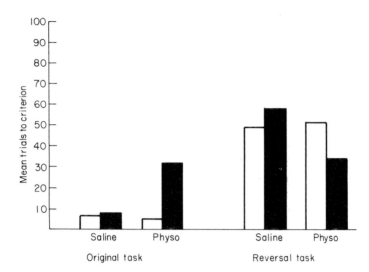

Fig. 3-6. The effect of massing and spacing trials during retest on anticholinesterase-induced amnesia. On the left, retest consisted of relearning the original habit (run to light, avoid dark). On the right, retest consisted of unlearning the original habit. On retest the animal had to learn to run to dark and avoid light (reversal). (ITI, intertrial interval; PHYSO, physostigmine.)

trials during retest should of course not be seen with anticholinergics or cholinomimetics, but only with anticholinesterases. This further prediction from the hypothesis should be tested.

So far, then, it seems that the drugs we are using to block or facilitate memory have their effect on synaptic conductance. However, what is it that changes when synaptic conductance alters? As mentioned previously, the two main hypotheses are (1) that the amount of transmitter emitted at the presynaptic ending increases or (2) that the postsynaptic ending increases in its sensitivity to transmitter. To test this idea, carbachol (carbamylcholine) was injected before retest. This drug is a cholinomimetic. It acts on the postsynaptic membrane much like acetylcholine. However, it is not susceptible to destruction by the enzyme acetylcholinesterase. Therefore, by injecting this drug, we can test the sensitivity of the postsynaptic membrane. It seems that 7-day-old habits are blocked by a dose of this cholinomimetic which leaves a 3-day-old habit unaffected (Table 3-1). This would indicate that it is probably the postsynaptic membrane that has increased its sensitivity and so increased synaptic conductance.

One of the questions that often arises is why it is that we do not block all cholinergic synaptic activity with the drugs we use. As was seen above, rats learn appetitive tasks at a normal rate under doses of drug which under some

TABLE 3-I

*The Effect of Carbachol Injection on Recall
of Habits that Were Three and Seven Days Old.
Criterion was Seven Correct Trials in Succession.*[a]

	Medium number of trials to criterion	
Treatment	3 days	7 days
Carbachol	6.0 (15)	20 (15)[b]
Saline	4.0 (8)	0 (7)

[a]Numbers in parentheses indicate number of rats tested.

[b]$P < .01$ compared with saline, Mann-Whitney U test.

circumstances produce complete amnesia. There is very little in the overt behavior of the rat to indicate that it has been drugged. The doses of drugs used produce no apparent malaise or incoordination. Clearly, the dose we use only seems to affect what one might call the "memory" synapses. It would therefore seem that these are therefore more sensitive to our drugs. Such an abnormal sensitivity may be more apparent than real. We know that there are some levels of training and times after training where a habit is unaffected by the dosage of drug we use, and this shows that "memory" synapses are not always affected. It therefore seems more plausible to think of the "memory" synapses as traveling through a much larger range of postsynaptic sensitivity, while normal synapses remain fixed somewhere in the middle of the range of sensitivity variation of the memory synapse. In other words, the "memory" synapse has to swing from extreme insensitivity to transmitter to extreme sensitivity in order to manifest those changes in conductance which we have demonstrated. It will therefore be much more susceptible to anticholinergic agents when conductance is low and to anticholinesterases and cholinomimetics when conductance is high. In the middle of the range, sensitivity to all agents will resemble that of a normal synapse and only grossly toxic doses will affect memory. This speculation, of course, will have to be further tested. The experiments so far reported implicate the cholinergic system in memory. It is, of course, possible that other systems such as the adrenergic will also turn out to have a similar function, and this, too, we hope to test.

When an animal is rewarded for performing a habit such a habit will be learned or acquired. However, when the habit is no longer rewarded, the animal will cease to perform the habit. Another kind of learning takes place, and this is called extinction. If initial learning consists of the formation of some synaptic (or other) connection, does extinction consist of the weakening or uncoupling of

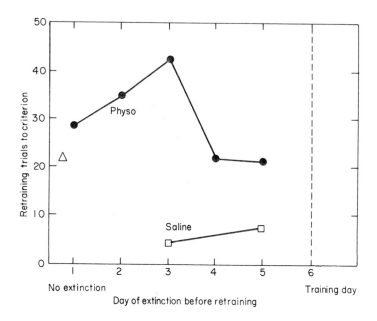

Fig. 3-7. The effect of physostigmine on retraining after extinction. The time between original learning and retraining is the same for all groups. When time of extinction is close to original learning, there is amnesia but no difference from the group receiving no extinction. At extinction 3 days before learning, the number of trials to relearn is almost double (SALINE, scores of controls injected with saline; PHYSO, scores of animals injected with physostigmine.)

this connection? Or is it the formation of some other connection which then works to oppose the effects of the first ("learning") connection? If extinction consists of weakening the connection set up in original learning, then an extinguished habit should be similar to a forgotten habit pharmacologically. We have already shown that an almost forgotten habit is facilitated by anticholinesterase. We would, then, on the "weakening" hypothesis of extinction, expect an injection of an anticholinesterase to produce less amnesia of an extinguished habit than of the same unextinguished habit. If, on the other hand, during extinction there is another habit acquired which inhibits the expression of the original habit, another pattern of results should be discernible after injection with an anticholinesterase. If original learning occurs 7 days before anticholinesterase injection and retest, there should be amnesia for the original habit. If extinction of the habit is given close in time to its acquisition, there should be amnesia for both the original learning and extinction. If, on the other hand, original learning is 7 days before injection and retest, the extinction is 3 days before injection and retest; the original habit should be lost but the extinction habit retained. (As we noted above, 3-day-old habits are unaffected by our dose of anticholinesterase.) When extinction was given to rats close in time to the original training, both the original training and extinction were blocked by physostigmine (Deutsch & Wiener, 1969). These rats took the same number of trials to relearn as control animals, which were trained, not extinguished and then drugged. However, when extinction was placed 3 days before injection and retest, it took the rats during retest after drug injection approximately twice as many trials to learn as control animals (unextinguished and drugged), showing that extinction has been retained while the original habit was blocked (Fig. 3-7). This supports the idea that extinction is the learning of a separate habit opposing the performance of the initially rewarded habit.

It has also been suggested (Carlton, 1969) that different systems such as excitatory or inhibitory systems are subserved by different transmitters. Habits acquired during extinction have been viewed as inhibitory. However, the last experiment we have outlined also shows that extinction placed close to original learning is equally as vulnerable to anticholinesterase as original learning. Habits can probably not be classified into synaptically inhibitory and excitatory on the basis of behavioral excitation or inhibition. However, as all habits compete for behavioral expression, there must be excitation and reciprocal inhibition connected with all habits.

III. CONCLUSIONS

A simple hypothesis can explain the results obtained to date if we disregard those results when we wait 30 minutes after original learning to inject. The hypothesis is that, as a result of learning, the postsynaptic endings at a specific set of synapses become more sensitive to the transmitter. This sensitivity increases with time after initial learning and then declines. The rate at which such sensitivity increases depends on the amount of initial learning. If the curve of transmission plotted against time is displaced upward with anticholinesterases, then the very low portions will show facilitation and the high portions will cause block (fig. 3-8). The middle portions will appear unaffected (unless special experimental tests are made). If the curve of transmission is displaced down with anticholinergics, then the middle portion will appear unaffected and only the very early or late components will show block.

Taken together, then, the results which have been obtained are evidence that synaptic conductance alters as a result of learning. So far it seems (1) that cholinergic synapses are modified as a result of learning and that it probably is the postsynaptic membrane which becomes increasingly more sensitive to acetylcholine with time after learning up to a certain point. (2) After this point, sensitivity declines, leading to the phenomena of forgetting. (3) There is also good evidence that there is an initial phase of declining sensitivity to cholin-

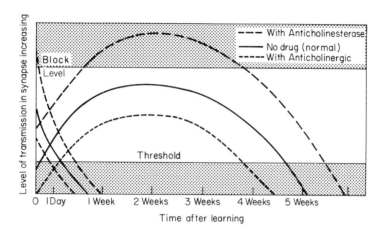

Fig. 3-8. The hypothesized changes in "memory" synapses with time after training and with pharmacological intervention.

esterase or increasing sensitivity to anticholinergics. This could reflect the existence of a parallel set of synapses with fast decay serving as a short-term store. (4) Increasing the amount of learning leads to an increase in conductance in each of a set of synapses without an increase in their number. (5) Both original learning and extinction are subserved by cholinergic synapses.

REFERENCES

Anderson, A. C. *Journal of Comparative Psychology*, Vol. 30, 1940, 399-412.

Bacq, Z. M., and Brown, G. C. *Journal of Physiology (London)*, 1937, Vol. 89, 45-60.

Biederman, G. B. *Quarterly Journal of Experimental Psychology*, 1970, Vol. 22, 384-388.

Biederman, G. B. *Psychonomic Science* (in press).

Bunch, M. E., and Lang, E. S. *Journal of Comparative Psychology*, 1939, Vol. 27, 449-459.

Bunch, M. E., and Magdsick, W. K. *Journal of Comparative Psychology*, 1933, Vol. 16, 385-409.

Carlton, P. L. In J. T. Tapp (Ed.), *Reinforcement and behavior*. New York: Academic Press, 1969.

Cutting, W. C. *Handbook of pharmacology . . . The actions and uses of drugs*. New York: Appleton-Century-Crofts, 1964.

DeGroot, J., Verhandel. Konink. Ned. Akad. Wettenschap. Afdel-Natuurk. Sect. II, 52 (1957).

Deutsch, J. A., Hamburg, M. D., and Dahl, H. *Science*, 1966, Vol. 151, 221-223.

Deutsch, J. A., and Leibowitz, S. F. *Science*, 1966, Vol. 153, 1017.

Deutsch, J. A. and Leibowitz, S. F. *Science*, 1966, Vol. 153, 1917.

Deutsch, J. A. and Lutzky, H. *Nature*, 1967, Vol. 213, 742.

Deutsch, J. A. and Rocklin, K. *Nature*, 1967, Vol. 216, 89-90.

Deutsch, J. A., and Stone, J., unpublished.

Deutsch, J. A., and Wiener, N. I. *Journal of Comparative & Physiological Psychology*, 1969, Vol. 69, 179-184.

Feldberg, W., and Vartiainen, A. Further observations on the physiology and pharmacology of a sympathetic ganglion. *Journal of Physiology*, 1934, Vol. 83, 103-128.

Goodman, L. S., and Gilman, A. *The pharmacological basis of therapeutics*. New York: Macmillan, 1965.

Hamburg, M. D. *Science*, 1967, Vol. 156, 973-974.

Hubbert, H. B. The effect of age on habit formation in the albino rat, *Behavior Monograph*, 1915, Vol. 2, no. 6.

Huppert, F. A., personal communication.

Huppert, F. A., and Deutsch, J. A. *Quarterly Journal of Experimental Psychology*, 1969, Vol. 21, 267-271.

Leibowitz, S. F., Deutsch, J. A., and Coons, E. E. (in preparation).

Rocklin, K., and Deutsch, J. A., unpublished.

Russell, W. R., and Nathan, P. W. *Brain*, 1946, Vol. 69, 280-300.

Sharpless, S. K, *Annual Review of Physiology*, 1964, Vol. 26, 357-388.

Squire, L. R. *Psychonomic Science*, 1970, Vol. 19 (1), 49-50.

Talland, G. A. *Deranged memory*. New York: Academic Press, 1965.

Tanzi, E. *Rivista sperimentale di Freniatria*, 1893, Vol. 19, 149.

Volle, R. L., and Koelle, G. B. The physiological role of acetylcholinesterase (AChE) in sympathetic ganglia. *Journal of Pharmacological Experimental Therapy*, 1961, Vol. 133, 223-240.

Wiener, N. I., and Deutsch, J. A. *Journal of Comparative & Physiological Psychology*, 1968, Vol. 66, 613-617.

CHAPTER

4

DRUG FACILITATION OF LEARNING AND MEMORY[1]

RONALD G. DAWSON[2]

and

JAMES L. McGAUGH

[1] This research was supported by Research Grant MH 12526 from the National Institute of Mental Health, United States Public Health Service, and Biomedical Sciences Support Grant FR-07008-05 from the National Institutes of Health, United States Public Health Service.

[2] Now at the University of Western Australia, Department of Psychology, Nedlands, W. A. 6009, Australia.

77

The ability of organisms to modify their behavior as a result of environmental encounters no doubt represents the most sophisticated advance in evolution. The development of the capacity to learn allows an organism not only to
escape harmful situations and approach desirable objects, but also to store some
representation of these events which can aid adaptation at a future time. If we
are to understand the nature of learning and memory, we must be able to
identify not only what is stored, that is, what neurobiological processes underly
memory, but, in addition, we must be able to explain how events are selected for
storage, and how they are recalled.

This chapter is concerned primarily with an analysis of studies of facilitation of learning and memory by the use of a variety of pharmacological agents.
We discuss the basis for the selection of these agents, the problems of interpretation of such experiments, and the implications of such research for theories of
learning and memory. In particular, we attempt to show how the findings of this
research may lead to an analysis of mechanisms which underly memory storage.
Much of the earlier research on this problem has been reviewed elsewhere (cf.
McGaugh & Petrinovich, 1965; McGaugh, 1968). Also see chapters in this
volume.

The impetus for much of the early research concerning drug influences on
behavior was gained from the successes achieved from drug applications in the
field of medicine. The emphasis was on drugs which might alleviate human
behavioral disorders (e.g., reviews by Herz, 1960; Ross & Cole, 1960; Cook &
Kelleher, 1963) as well as on an attempt to understand the behavioral effects of
common drugs such at alcohol, barbiturates, morphine, and caffeine (e.g., Macht
& Leach, 1929; Bernhardt, 1936a, b).

More recent research has had more of a theoretical focus. A major guiding
assumption has been that a knowledge of drug effects on behavior, coupled with
an understanding of the mechanism or mechanisms of action of a drug, may
provide insight into the physiological mechanisms which underlie the behavior
(cf. Russell, 1960, 1964).

I. METHODOLOGICAL DIFFICULTIES

With these considerations in mind, there has been considerable recent
interest in drugs which either improve or disrupt learning and memory in
animals. In addition, there has been a particular interest in drugs whose mecha

nisms of action are at least partially understood, and which for theoretical reasons might be expected to have an effect on learning and memory. One example of this approach is the investigation of the possible effects upon learning and memory of drugs which influence RNA and protein synthesis (see Agranoff, 1968; Barondes, 1968; Glassman, 1969; Booth, 1967).

Of course, knowledge of the mechanism of action of drug is of little use in analyzing the physiological bases of learning and memory if the drug cannot be shown to affect learning and memory in the behavioral situation. Good behavioral effects are essential. In addition, the finding that a drug whose mechanism of action is partially known affects learning and memory does not allow one to conclude that the behavioral effect is due to the known action of the drug. The behavioral effects could be due to unknown actions of the drug. These and other problems of interpretation may become more clear from the following example.

Let us suppose that rats are given injections of a drug each day 15 minutes prior to a series of training trials on a task such as shuttle box avoidance. Learning in this situation may be inferred from an increased tendency of the animal to cross from one side of the box to the other at the onset of a signal in order to avoid a punishing footshock. Let us assume that animals given the drug improve in avoidance from day to day more rapidly than animals injected with a control solution. Also assume that in previous biochemical experiments the drug was found to increase the rates of RNA synthesis in the brain. The "obvious" conclusion would seem to be that the drug facilitates learning by increasing the rates of RNA synthesis in the brain; what does this conclusion assume? On the behavioral side of things, it assumes that the improvement in performance is a true facilitation of learning. However, many factors contribute to the performance level of the animal, including nonassociative (general alertness, reactivity to stimuli, and motivation) factors. The drug may have affected these processes and thus influenced performance indirectly. For example, in studies using strychnine sulfate, Cholewiak, Hammond, Siegler, and Papsdorf (1968) and Benevento and Kandell (1967) suggest that their observations of facilitation of classical or Pavlovian conditioning may be due to an enhancement of sensitization, rather than, or in addition to, effects upon learning per se. In these experiments, enhanced responding was evidenced under the drug during both acquisition and extinction phases of conditioning. If the drug had improved learning, then both the learning of acquisition and extinction conditions should have been facilitated. Further, the enhancing effect of the drug on performance might well be specific to only one particular testing situation.

Unfortunately, our definitions of learning are not so precise that learning can be inferred from any single task because of the possible confounding from such nonassociative factors. However, there are a variety of criteria which help in delineating the associative from the nonassociative influences on performance. For example, there should be at least some generality in the effect: the drug should enhance learning in a variety of training tasks including both active and passive avoidance, as well as appetitive learning. Such evidence would eliminate the interpretation that the behavioral changes were due to a specific motivational or reactivity effect. Discrimination learning or some other more complex task and latent learning (where obvious reward effects are absent) should also be improved. Furthermore, the associative factors from one experiment should transfer to another situation (cf. Oliverio, 1968). For example, if a subject learned to make an avoidance response to a specific tone in the shuttle box, there should be some transfer to a different avoidance situation where the subject must make some other type of avoidance response to the tone. Unfortunately, learning cannot be assessed in a simple manner. Care must always be taken to show that improvement in performance is not due to nonspecific sensory and motivational processes. These points may become clearer in the later portion of this chapter after specific findings are reviewed in detail.

Assuming that proper behavioral experiments are conducted, other questions still remain to be answered before it can be concluded that drug effects on learning have a particular neurobiological basis. First it is possible that the drug may not affect the central nervous system because it is unable to pass the blood-brain barrier, or, possibly because of an inappropriate choice of route of administration, it may do so in limited amounts, or in an altered structural form. Metabolites of a drug may have different modes of action than the drug itself. These considerations would make it very unlikely that the behavioral effects seen were due to a central action of the drug, or that a central action was similar to the assumed action of the drug. When one considers the complexity of biochemical processes in the central nervous system, the occurrence of a single mode of action of a drug is extremely unlikely. A further problem is that all drugs have "side effects"; that is, effects other than the one under investigation which is, hopefully, the "main effect." Care must always be taken to rule out the possibility that the effect of a drug on learning is due indirectly to some "side effect." This is not an easy task, as we will show below.

To return to the experiment in question, one in which a drug that affects RNA synthesis is being examined for its effects on learning, let us now assume that, in a learning experiment, the drug in the doses used did not affect behavior. On the basis of such results it is inappropriate for several reasons to draw the conclusion that there is no relationship between rates of RNA synthesis and learning. Perhaps we were using too much or too little drug; dose is a critical variable in any drug experiment. The route of application of the drug may have been inappropriate. The time of injection may have been such that the drug did not have its peak effect at the time of training. The task may have been inappropriate; for example, suppose that the drug depressed motor performance, but did improve learning under some conditions. Active avoidance may have been hindered because the subject was sluggish, yet the subjects may have shown a large improvement had they been tested after the drug administration was discontinued.

II. PERFORMANCE EFFECTS

As we emphasized above, the primary consideration in such studies is that of characterizing a drug effect as being upon associative processes as opposed to a host of other nonassociative effects. However, the essential prerequisite is the identification of a performance effect. Following Lashley's (1917) initial experiments showing facilitation of maze learning with pretrial injections of the analeptic drug strychnine sulfate, a large number of studies have shown that it is possible to enhance performance with drugs. Many of these studies have been concerned primarily with the beneficial effects of drugs on the performance of learned responses. In such studies, the focus is usually on motivational or perceptual effects of the compounds, rather than on problems of learning and memory. For example, Hearst and Whalen (1963) found that rats' performance on a task which required them to press a lever upon presentation of a signal in order to avoid a shock was improved by injections of amphetamine (3 mg/kg). The improvement was only temporary, however. Performance returned to the preexperimental level on subsequent tests without the drug. Hearst and Whalen suggested that the improvement may have been due to an interference with "freezing" behavior typically displayed by rats on this task. Enhanced performance under amphetamine has also been reported in a variety of active avoidance situations (Bovet & Oliverio, 1967; Dews, 1953; Kriekhaus, Miller, & Zimmerman, 1965; Rech, 1966). However, in these experiments it has not been possible to dissociate effects of the drug on learning from effects such as decreased freezing behavior, increased general activity, or decreased fatigue. In another study, Gonzales and Ross (1961) found that chlorpromazine (1.0 – 40 mg/kg) improved discrimination-reversal learning in rats. They suggested that the drug may have alleviated the emotional consequences of lack of reward during the first few trials, when rats typically are still responding to the previously positive stimulus. If their suggested interpretation is correct, improvement in learning was an indirect result of the tranquilizing effect of chlorpromazine, rather than a direct effect on the drug on associative mechanisms.

Although these studies were primarily concerned with nonassociative explanations they do point to the problems inherent in the utilization of pretrial injection procedures. Thus, although there are a great number of studies which purport to show facilitation of learning with pretrial injections of central nervous system (CNS) stimulants (see McGaugh & Petrinovich, 1965), the studies do not provide clear evidence that the effects are due to influences on learning.

III. STATE DEPENDENCY

A second problem of interpretation which is encountered in studies in which subjects are either trained or tested while drugged is that of state dependent learning. Overton (1971) showed that the drug state in which an animal acquires a response is critical in determining animal's performance on a subsequent retest. Animals trained while drugged may subsequently show evidence of learning of the task only when tested under the drug. That this phenomenon is due to true dissociation and not to some simple performance effect is indicated by experiments in which animals were trained to perform two opposite response tendencies, one under the drug state and one under the nondrug state (Overton, 1964). Although some authors have attempted to explain this phenomenon in terms of drug produced stimulus changes (Bindra, 1959), this argument is not strongly supported. Overton (1971) has pointed out that in other experiments where the stimulus situation is changed drastically from one task to the next, it is very difficult to teach animals two clearly opposing response tendencies. A somewhat stronger argument against the stimulus change interpretation comes from studies showing lack of state dependency when peripherally acting drugs are used (see Kumar, Stolesman, & Steinberg, 1970). Drug states appear to involve marked reorganizations of neural activity or perhaps firing patterns. John (1967) has suggested that reconstitution of these firing patterns, by drug injection, is a necessary prerequisite for recall of the learned response.

These two phenomena, enhancement or disruption of performance and drug induced state dependency, may interact in the learning situation: a drug may either depress or improve performance, by an associative or other effect and may or may not have a state-dependent effect. In order to tease these two factors apart one must look at performance in both drugged and nondrugged states, and also examine transfer of performance across these two states. The use of such an analysis allows one to determine the relative contribution of these two variables. However, the question of the basis of a performance effect cannot be answered by this design.

IV. POSTTRAINING INJECTIONS

Another approach to the problem of distinguishing learning and performance effects in drug studies was developed from studies using electroconvulsive shock (ECS) to disrupt memory (Duncan, 1949). These experiments showed that if animals were given ECS shortly following a learning experience, performance on a subsequent test was poor. Extensive subsequent research (see Glickman, 1961; McGaugh, 1966) has supported the view that the disruption of performance was a result of amnesia for the previous learning experience. Further, the evidence from these studies indicates that the impairing effect is time dependent, that is, the closer the ECS is administered in time following the learning, the greater the result disruption. These findings have been interpreted as supporting the view (Hebb, 1949) that following learning, memory is first held in some labile state, which subsequently gradually consolidates into a more permanent form (cf. McGaugh & Dawson, 1970).

Following these findings, the assumption was made that if CNS stimulants do in part improve learning when injected before learning, they may also improve the conversion of memory from the labile into the permanent form when injected after training—during the critical period for memory consolidation. This was subsequently shown to be the case (McGaugh, 1959). The subsequent extension of these experiments however (see McGaugh & Petrinovich, 1965; McGaugh, 1968) has led to a shift in attention from the acquisition phase of learning to the postlearning phase. The major reason for this shift in emphasis is that the utilization of a posttrial injection procedure avoids many of the problems of interpretation inherent in the pretrial method, since the drug is not present in the animal either at the time of training or at the time of retesting. In addition, evidence that a given drug has posttrial facilitative effect adds some credence to the idea that a pretrial facilitation may in part have been due to an associative effect of the drug. The effects of posttrial facilitation of learning will be discussed further below. However, one major point should be made here. Posttrial facilitation has also been shown to be a time-dependent phenomenon (cf. ECS disruption), that is, the closer the drug injection is to the learning trial the greater the facilitative effect. These results thus add additional support for the notion that memory storage is time-dependent.

A. Considerations Governing the Choice of Drugs

The preceding sections raised several methodological questions and introduced the phenomenon of memory storage facilitation. At this point it is relevant to examine the considerations which governed the choice of drugs used in such research. As far as the CNS stimulants are concerned, the answer was behavioral: CNS stimulants were found to influence learning and memory in the behavioral situations. However, there have been other choices. When it was discovered that the neuron was an extremely active biochemical machine (see Schmidt, 1967), and when it was recognized that memory, if it is to be at least somewhat permanent, must have some biochemical base (Gerard, 1955), it was argued that memories (i.e., acquired information) may be coded in DNA and RNA somewhat analogous to the way that morphological characteristics (i.e., genetic information) are coded in these nucleic acids. Katz and Halstead (1950) actually preempted these arguments with their proposal that changes in brain nucleoproteins might underly memory storage. In very elegant experiments

Hydén and his collaborators (see Hydén, 1967a, b, for a review), provided evidence in favor of this idea. This evidence has been critically evaluated (Dingman & Sporn, 1964) and a number of alternatives to the direct molecular coding of memory have been advanced (Briggs & Kitto, 1962; Bogoch, 1968; John, 1967; Moore & Mahler, 1965). A detailed discussion of these experiments is beyond the scope of this chapter (see Chapters 1 and 2 in this volume and Glassman, 1969). However, these views led to the argument that drugs which affect RNA or protein synthesis might also affect memory storage.

Following the pioneering experiments of Curtis and Cole (1942) and Hodgkin and Huxley (1952a−c), great interest was generated concerning the contribution of ionic mechanisms to nervous conduction. Subsequently, the use of a variety of ionic solutions (particularly KCl) either applied to the cortex (Bures & Buresova, 1963; Albert 1966a) or into subcortical structures (Carlton, 1963) has had quite interesting mechanistic implications in the area of memory storage, although the mechanisms of action of these treatments are as yet unclear at a cellular level. Finally, the delineation of peripheral transmitter substances, their mode of action (cf. Eccles, 1957, 1964) and the drugs which affect them has led to an interest in attempting to manipulate experimentally levels of central neural transmitters and examining their effects upon learning and memory. Although this is not an exhaustive list it serves to illustrate the theoretical basis for the choice of a variety of drugs. These choices range from the mainly behavioral (e.g., CNS stimulants) to the mainly mechanistic (e.g., drugs affecting RNA synthesis). In the following sections the success of these choices in answering questions of mechanism will be explored in more detail.

B. CNS Stimulants

Following the initial demonstration that posttrial injections of strychnine sulfate facilitate learning (McGaugh, 1959), the question was one of establishing the nature and generality of such results. One important suggestion (Cooper & Krass, 1963) was that even though the drugs were injected following the trial they may have still been in the animal in appreciable amounts on the retest. In support of this contention, Cooper and Krass reported that the learning of female rats given strychnine sulfate either 72 or 24 hours prior to maze training was superior to that of noninjected controls. These findings are, however, inconsistent with previous research (e.g., Paré, 1961; McGaugh, Thomson, Westbrook, & Hudspeth, 1962), where delayed posttrial injections produced less facilitation than immediate posttrial injections, even though the delayed injections were closer to the subsequent (i.e., next day's) learning. Yet the question of dose was not solved by this argument and a more definitive study was needed. Greenough and McGaugh (1965) gave rats two training trials in a Lashley III maze, followed 1 week later by five retention trials. Strychnine injections were given either 2 days before training, immediately after training, or 2 days prior to the retention test. According to the interpretation advanced by Cooper and Krass, animals injected two days prior to training or retesting should perform significantly better than animals injected immediately following training. This prediction was not upheld. There were no significant differences across injection procedures. Rats injected immediately following training were superior to groups injected prior to training or testing. Posttrial facilitation, therefore, cannot be explained as due to the hangover of drug from 1 day's training to the next.

The use of posttrial injections also left open the possibility that subjects performed better because the injections were rewarding. However, Westbrook and McGaugh (1964), using the strychnine-like compound 1757 I.S. showed in a latent learning paradigm that this was unlikely. In this study, rats of the Tryon maze bright (S_1) and maze dull (S_3) strains were dosed with injections of either 1757 I.S. (1.0 mg/kg) or a control solution each day for 5 days, within 1 minute after each training trial on a 6-unit alley U-maze. All animals were both hungry and thirsty. Half of the animals were rewarded in the goal box and half were not. On the fifth trial and on 5 successive trials, all animals were rewarded in the goal box. No further drug injections were given; instead, all animals were given injections of the control solution after each trial. There was no difference in the performance of nonrewarded drug and control groups; neither improved. If 1757 I.S. injections had been rewarding one would have predicted that this group would perform better than the control group. The rewarded groups did improve as was expected, and the drug group made less errors than the controls. On trials 6–10, when reward was given to all groups, the previously nonrewarded drug group now performed at the same level as the drug group which had been rewarded all along, and both groups were significantly better than the control group treated the same way with respect to reward. This last group performed as well as the control group which had been rewarded all along. The important observation was that although both drug and control groups exhibited latent learning, the facilitation effect appeared upon introduction of reward, but not on prior trials in the group given no reward on the first trials. If the 1757 I.S. injections had been rewarding one would have expected that the drug group would have performed better than the control group prior to the introduction of reward. Thus, this effect seems to be due to facilitation of learning.

Following these initial studies a series of experiments investigated posttrial facilitative effects of CNS stimulants in a variety of tasks. Hudspeth (1964) reported that posttrial injections of strychnine sulfate (0.20 mg/kg) facilitated rats' learning of visual discrimination and oddity learning tasks (see also Shaeffer, 1968). Strychnine has also been shown to facilitate delayed alternation behavior in rats (Petrinovich, Bradford, & McGaugh, 1965). Visual discrimination has also been facilitated by posttrial caffeine injection (30 mg/kg; Paré, 1961) and posttrial strychnine injection (Krivanek & Hunt, 1967; McGaugh & Krivanek, 1970). Single posttrial strychnine injections have also been reported to facilitate inhibitory avoidance learning (Franchina & Moore, 1968; Franchina & Grandolfo, in press), active avoidance learning (Bovet, McGaugh, & Oliverio, 1966), and conditional stimulus transfer in a two way avoidance task in mice (Oliverio, 1968).

Thus, posttrial injections of a number of stimulants, including strychnine, 1757 I.S., picrotoxin, pentylenetetrazol, bemigride, caffeine, nicotine, and amphetamine appear to facilitate learning over a wide range of experimental conditions. There are, however, several reports which have failed to obtain strychnine facilitation (e.g., Louttit, 1965; Prien, Wayner, & Kahan, 1963; Shaeffer, 1968; Stein & Kimble, 1966). The reasons for these negative results are not altogether clear. They do at least suggest that there is a limit to the generality of the effect but whether this limit represents some subtle procedural difference, an animal strain difference, an inappropriate choice of drug dose, or the choice of a particular task is not obvious. Recently the implication of environmental factors in drug facilitation experiments raises an additional complication to the possible demonstration of drug facilitation.

In an interesting study, Shandro and Shaeffer (1969) studied the effects of prior rearing environment upon the effects of posttrial strychnine application. In general, facilitation of maze performance was seen in groups reared in an enriched environment, but not in groups reared in an impoverished environment. Similar results have been obtained by LeBoeuf and Peeke (1969) and Peeke, LeBoeuf and Herz, (1971). Thus, the environmental conditions during rearing appear to be an important factor influencing the susceptibility to drug facilitation. Further, Calhoun (1966) and subsequently Hunt (personal communication) have shown that the degree of stimulation provided in the posttraining environment is also crucial. Facilitative effects of posttrial strychnine injections upon discrimination learning were seen if rats were placed in a quiet environment, but not if they were subject to a great deal of sensory stimulation following learning. The unique characteristics of sensory responsiveness of strychnine animals (e.g., convulsions can be triggered by sensory stimuli at preconvulsive drug dosages) makes one question the generality of this effect.

A consideration of the above factors may help to explain previous negative results or to establish some boundaries for the phenomenon. However, the robust nature of the effect in a wide variety of situations and with a wide range of drugs is beyond question. More recently, McGaugh and Krivanek (cf. Krivanek & McGaugh, 1968, 1969; McGaugh and Krivanek, 1970) have explored the effects of several CNS stimulants on appetitive discrimination learning in mice. These experiments will be discussed in some detail since they reveal the importance of dosage of drug in relation to the behavioral effects observed.

The procedures are essentially identical for each of the series of experiments. Mice were injected each day immediately after the last three trials on a visual discrimination problem in which the subject had to choose between a black and a white alley to obtain food. Figure 4-1 shows the mean number of errors for saline control groups and groups injected with different concentrations of strychnine sulfate. The dose response curve is clearly biphasic. Greatest facilitation is found with the lower doses (0.25 − 0.100 mg/kg IP) and the higher doses (1.0 − 1.25 mg/kg IP). Smaller effects were found with intermediate doses (0.20 − 0.80 mg/kg IP). Figure 4-2 shows the results of a similar investigation of the posttrial dose response effects of pentylenetetrazol. In this case, with doses up to 10.0 mg/kg, errors decreased as a function of increasing drug dose. Drug doses from 10 mg/kg − 20 mg/kg had similar facilitative effects. A similar effect is found with posttrial injections of d-amphetamine (fig. 4-3) with the exception that the highest dose used, 2.5 mg/kg, was not as effective as lower doses.

In a subsequent series of experiments the effects of time of administration of a selected facilitative dose of each of these drugs were investigated in the same discrimination situation. In all three cases the closer the drug injection followed the learning trials, the greater the facilitative effect. However, there were indications of differential drug effectiveness. Strychnine (0.1 mg/kg and 1.0 mg/kg) produced significant facilitation if injected within 1 hour following each

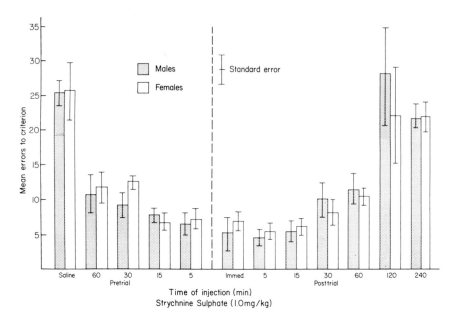

Fig. 4-1. The effect of posttraining administration of strychnine sulphate on visual discrimination learning in mice. Mean number of errors made by saline control groups and experimental groups (N per group = 12) receiving a range of drug doses. (From McGaugh, 1968.)

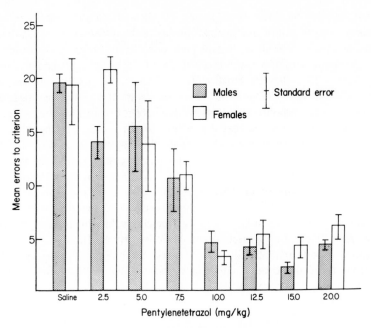

Fig. 4-2. The effect of posttraining administration of pentylenetetrazol on visual discrimination learning in mice. Mean number of errors made by saline control groups and experimental groups (*N* per group = 12) receiving a range of drug doses. (From Krivanek & McGaugh, 1968.)

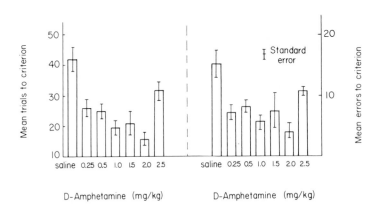

Fig. 4-3. The effect of posttraining administration of D-amphetamine on visual discrimination learning in mice. Mean number of errors made by saline control groups and experimental groups (*N* per group = 6) receiving a range of drug doses. (From Krivanek & McGaugh, 1970.)

block of training trials, whereas pentylenetetrazol (15 mg/kg) was only effective if administered within 15 minutes. *d*-Amphetamine showed an even steeper gradient, since it was effective if administered immediately following training, but not if administered after 15 minutes.

These studies clearly indicate the need for caution in selecting an appropriate drug dose, and, as well, they reveal the differential treatment effectiveness as indicated by the time of injection gradients. As was previously mentioned, it would be a significant contribution if one could infer the duration of neural processes underlying memory storage from such gradients. For instance, one might assume that the labile phase of memory is essentially complete at that point at which a facilitative drug is no longer effective; however, these studies suggest three different times depending upon the choice of drug. A similar argument holds for studies which have attempted to assay time-dependent processes in memory storage by the use of techniques which disrupt memory storage. With these techniques estimates have ranged from minutes to hours (Dorfman & Jarvik, 1968; Quartermain, Paolino, & Miller, 1965; Miller, 1968; Weissman, 1963). The point is that treatment effectiveness, whether of a facilitative or of a disruptive nature is always reflected in the observed temporal gradients, in addition to the underlying processes which are being influenced by the treatment. At the present time estimates of the duration of memorial processes are not possible, yet the overwhelming evidence suggests that memory is stored in a time dependent fashion and is not an all-or-none event (For further discussion, see Cherkin, 1969; McGaugh, 1966; McGaugh & Dawson, 1970).

In contrast to the strict time dependent gradient of treatment effectiveness, Hunt and Bauer (1969) have recently shown, with posttrial injections of pentylenetetrazol, that the extent of facilitation observed was a joint function of the amount of drug and the time of injection. Animals were injected either immediately or 15 minutes following discrimination training. Groups given 7.5 mg/kg of drug performed better if injected immediately, than if injected after 15 minutes. However, groups given 10 mg/kg performed better if the injection was delayed. A similar effect was also obtained on a position discrimination task. Here pentylenetetrazol (10 mg/kg) was given either immediately, 5 minutes or 10 minutes following training, and the greatest facilitation was obtained with the 10-minute injection. These results raise problems for a strict time dependent relationship at all facilitative drug doses, and require further explanation.

C. Drugs which Affect RNA and Protein Synthesis

As we have previously mentioned, the major impetus for the study of the effects on memory drugs which influence RNA and protein synthesis has foundation in the experiments of Hydén (1967). Although this research is discussed at some length in other chapters, several points are of interest in this section. The great advantages, in terms of interpretation, are that the mechanisms of action of these drugs are known, at least to some extent. For example, tricyanoaminopropene (TCAP), which has been shown to stimulate nucleoprotein production in rabbit brain (Hydén & Hartelius, 1948), and increase ribosomal RNA synthesis in neurons in the lateral vestibular (Deiters) nucleus in this animal (Hydén & Egyházi, 1962), has also been shown to facilitate maze learning in rats (Schmidt & Davenport, 1967). However, the generality of the facilitating effects of TCAP has not been extended to other learning situations (Brush, Davenport, & Polidora, 1966; Otis & Pryor, 1968). A second drug, Mg pemoline, which has also been reported to increase RNA synthesis, has also been shown to facilitate learning with both pre- and posttrial injections (Plotnikoff, 1966a, b, 1967). However, the specificity of the behavioral effects is in question (Beach & Kimble, 1967; Bowman, 1966; Stein, Brink, & Patterson, 1968), as are the chemical effects (Stein & Yellin, 1967). Most importantly, the effects of such drugs which may affect RNA synthesis must be rationalized alongside the finding that RNA synthesis may be severely curtailed (up to 95 percent) in both goldfish (Agranoff, 1968) and mice (Barondes & Cohen, 1967a, b) without the appearance of an effect upon memory. These findings make significant the suggestion that Mg-pemoline and possibly other agents which affect RNA synthesis may improve performance via a general stimulation effect rather than via a specific increasing of RNA synthesis (Bowman, 1966; Talland, 1966).

Following a similar rationale, levels of RNA have also been artificially increased by injection of an alkaline hydrolyzate of yeast RNA. In rats chronic oral administration of the extract has been shown to speed up acquisition of a pole climbing task and prolong its retention (Cook & Davidson, 1968). However, the generality of this effect did not extend to Sidman avoidance learning even with a 3-month pretreatment with the drug (Cook & Davidson, 1968). Moreover, the chronic treatment procedures leave open the possibility that these effects were due to influences upon performance. The likelihood of this alternative is given credence by the findings of yeast RNA-induced increased activity and responsiveness to shock in operant conditioning experiments in well-trained animals (Brown, 1966a, b). Moreover, the problem of mechanisms is extremely difficult to attack when very large quantities of drug are needed to obtain the effect. Under these circumstances it is unlikely that a posttrial treatment procedure could be used to examine the effect of the drug.

Suffice it to say the attempts to facilitate learning by increasing brain RNA and protein synthesis have produced equivocal results. Attempts to interfere with these processes have been far more rewarding. Initial experimentation reported that the learning of various kinds of tasks was impaired by drugs impairing RNA synthesis (e.g., Dingman & Sporn, 1961; Chamberlain, Rothschild, & Gerard, 1963; Corning & John, 1961). These studies did not, however, give good reason to assume that the drugs acted by influencing time dependent processes involved in memory consolidation; that is, injections were not systematically manipulated over time following learning. In fact, the findings of these early studies did not provide particularly convincing evidence that the drugs acted by selectively impairing the neurochemical processes involved in learning (McGaugh & Petrinovich, 1965). The danger of such specific interpretations is evident from an experiment of the effects of puromycin upon learning. Bitemporal injections of puromycin have been shown to produce retrograde amnesia (Flexner, Flexner, & Stellar, 1963). However, such injections have also been reported to produce abnormal brain activity (Cohen *et al.*, 1966). Thus, in this particular instance, one is left with the likelihood that amnesia resulted from the abnormal electrical activity rather than from inhibition of protein synthesis.

As mentioned previously, other studies have shown that learning is unimpaired with doses of actinomycin D, which produced up to 95 percent inhibition of RNA synthesis (Barondes & Jarvik, 1964; Cohen & Barondes, 1966). However, these results are worthy of further consideration since the drug does appear to prevent the retention of information for more than a day or so (Appel, 1964; Agranoff, Davis, Casola, & Lim, 1967), although acquisition is unaffected. A similar absence of an effect of inhibition of cerebral protein synthesis by cycloheximide and acetoxycycloheximide (AXM) upon acquisition of T-maze learning has been reported by Barondes (Barondes, 1968; Barondes and Cohen, 1967b, 1968). In this situation the memory for the task decays gradually over the next 6 hours. Similar findings have also been obtained following puromycin and AXM injections in goldfish (Agranoff, 1968).

These results add to the growing mechanistic picture of memory storage. They suggest that although short term storage of information may not require RNA or protein synthesis, longer term storage may be dependent upon these processes. Avoiding the specific interpretation of these results, they do suggest that memory may be held in more than one form in the course of its consolidation.

D. Transmitter Substances

Perhaps the greatest breakthrough in contemporary neurophysiology was the finding that neurons communicate with each other at specialized junctions (synapses) through the release of chemical transmitter substances which diffuse across the synaptic cleft to influence the postsynaptic element of the next neuron. The initial impetus for this discovery came from the observations (Loewi, 1921) that the perfusate obtained after vagal stimulation of frog heart could be used to stimulate an isolated heart preparation. The chemical was later identified as acetylcholine. Subsequently, this research was extended to the peripheral autonomic nervous system and skeletal musculature (e.g., Cannon and Uridil, 1921). Norepinephrine has been isolated as the transmitter for all autonomic preganglionic junctures and, with one exception (sweat glands), for all postganglionic sympathetic junctures. Acetylcholine has been shown to fulfill this role at the postganglionic parasympathetic junctures as well as the neuro-muscular junction (Fatt, 1954; Fatt and Katz, 1951, 1952; Nachmanson, 1955). In its progress this research led to the development of several criteria which prospective transmitter substances must fulfill (see Thompson, 1967). Although few of these criteria have been met in isolating prospective central transmitter substances (see Mandell and Spooner, 1968), there is sufficient evidence for the two previously mentioned substances to indicate their importance in neural functioning. Moreover, the attempts to provide adequate tests for prospective candidates has led to the isolation of a variety of substances which have, in one preparation or another, been shown to mimic the excitatory or inhibitory effects typically seen when neural impulses cause postsynaptic cell firing.

Typically, the methods used to attempt to change synaptic events by drugs have followed one or more of the following rationales: the effective transmitter availability at synapses might be increased either by injections of drugs which mimic the transmitter substance (e.g., carbachol mimics acetylcholine in periph-eral synapses), or by preventing transmitter breakdown with anticholinesterase drugs (DFP and physostigmine antagonize acetylcholinesterase which breaks down acetylcholine). The effective transmitter may be decreased by anticho-linergic drugs either by blocking the postsynaptic membrane and preventing depolarization by the transmitter (atropine and scopolamine block cholinergic synapses), or by preventing release, or antagonizing the transmitter when re-leased (tetanus toxin prevents the release or availability of transmitter, pre-sumably glycine, in the spinal cord; Curtis and De Groot, 1968).

Two systems have attracted the most attention, the cholinergic system, whose central transmitter is assumed to be acetylcholine, and the adrenergic system, whose central transmitter is assumed to be norepinephrine. It is not by coincidence that these two substances were the ones initially isolated at periph-eral synapses. Incidentally, these "systems" may not be as distinct as was originally thought. Even at the synaptic level the dichotomy between them may be semantic rather than one that might lead to any clear central distinction. Specifically, the two "systems" may not be amenable to separate manipulation. Suffice it to say in the examples which follow, the assumption has been that the two systems could be manipulated separately.

Whitehouse (1964) has shown that atropine, an anticholinergic drug, impairs discrimination learning in rats. Moreover, the impairment persisted even after subjects were taken off the drug. Therefore it appears that performance was not simply depressed because subjects were drugged. Buresova, Bures, Bohdanecky, and Weiss (1964) also found impairment of a passive avoidance task with atropine. Bohdanecky and Jarvik found a similar effect with sco-polamine (1967). However, since in these experiments subjects were drugged prior to the learning experience, it is possible that the drug influenced behavior by affecting attentional or motivational factors. Herz (1959) made the interesting observation that the anticholinergics, atropine (10 mg/kg) and scopolamine (1 mg/kg), depressed rats' performance of avoidance responses only during the earlier stages of training. No effects were found on performance if the avoidance response was well established. These results may also be explained as a consequence of effects of the drugs on attentional factors, which may be assumed to be more at play during the early stages of learning.

Under some circumstances, anticholinesterases (i.e., drugs which prevent the breakdown of acetylcholine) have been shown to facilitate learning, when administered shortly before (Bures, Bohdanecky, & Weiss, 1962) or shortly after (Stratton & Petrinovich, 1963) learning. In line with these findings there is some evidence that anticholinergics may cause memory disruption. Carlton and Vogel (1965) reported that when rats were exposed to a stimulus which was subsequently used as a conditioning stimulus, its effects were attenuated as a result of the prior exposure. Subjects which were exposed while drugged with scopolamine did not show the attenuation. These authors suggested that prior exposure to the stimulus resulted in habituation and scopolamine prevented this. Further, they suggested that the cholinergic system may in part mediate behavioral inhibition. This notion might also explain why anticholinergics are effective in disrupting performance of passive avoidance learning (Buresova, 1964) and early stages of learning (Herz, 1959) when presumably irrelevant responding is in the process of being eliminated. However, Warburton and Groves (1969) have recently shown that scopolamine does not completely prevent habituation, but, rather, simply retards it. They suggest that the results of Carlton and Vogel may be explained by assuming that the animals suffered amnesia for the prior exposure to the CS rather than that they failed to habituate to it. This notion is supported by their observation that there was no carry over of habituation in scopolamine treated subjects from day to day, while control subjects showed significantly faster habituation on the second day.

This brief reference to anticholinergic drug effects is in no sense complete (see other chapters in this volume); it should serve to illustrate the complexities of interpretation even when somewhat "specific" manipulations are attempted. However, from these studies it does appear that anticholinergic drugs may affect performance both by affecting substrates underlying behavioral inhibition and also by preventing memory storage. Unfortunately, there is at present little evidence of posttrial effects of these drugs which might solidify the latter assumption.

E. Ions

Since the discovery of the ionic basis of nervous condition (see Thompson, 1967, for a review), several experimenters have attempted to influence neural activity through the use of a variety of ionic solutions. The procedures typically used in behavioral research have been either direct injection into the brain or ventricles, or topical cortical application of the solutions.

In one study, Sachs (1962) investigated the effects of intraventricular injections of calcium (22.5 μ CaCl$_2$, 0.25 percent) and potassium (25 μ KCl, 0.375 percent) on avoidance learning in cats. The cats were trained on successive days, 10 minutes following injection to a strict avoidance criterion (18 of 20 correct responses) in a shuttlebox. The rate of learning of the KCl group was superior to controls injected with saline, while the CaCl$_2$ group was inferior to the control groups. Although the KCl groups showed clear behavioral signs of increased alertness and arousal, this was not associated with an increased occurrence of spontaneous shuttling behavior. This measure typically indicates that the expected response may be occurring by chance with greater frequency as a result of increased activation. An interesting finding was that KCl groups made many fewer errors than controls following the first successful avoidance response. Prior to the first avoidance KCl and control groups made as many errors. This observation also suggests that KCl did not make the avoidance response more probable, but rather accentuated the consequences of the first avoidance response.

In apparent contrast with these findings are the results of topical application of KCl solutions on the cortex in rats. The technique (Leao, 1947) typically results in the production of a negative wave of depression which spreads over the cortex. However, the spread does not extend across sulci. Therefore, in the rat it is possible to selectively depress one hemisphere independently of the other. This technique has also been shown to disrupt memory storage with posttrial application in a time-dependent fashion (Bures & Buresova, 1963; Albert, 1966a).

By way of summarizing, Fig.4-4 illustrates the several times at which drugs have typically been introduced into animals in behavioral tasks. The problems in interpretation of treatments administered prior to learning (A) have been discussed. These problems are particularly relevant when one attempts to interpret the research concerned with manipulation of the cholinergic system, injections of ionic solutions, or pretrial manipulations of RNA and protein synthesis which have been discussed above. The interpretation of posttrial injection procedures (B, C & D) avoids the confounding of attentional, motivational, and other performance variables with the associative components. The results of this research come particularly from investigations of the effects of CNS stimulants on memory storage. The general interpretation of these findings is that memory storage proceeds in a time-dependent fashion, illustrated by the rising curve in that section of the figure. Also depicted in the figure is the possibility of injection of drugs both prior to training (A) and prior to retesting (E). This relates to the question of state dependent learning (Overton, 1967) mentioned

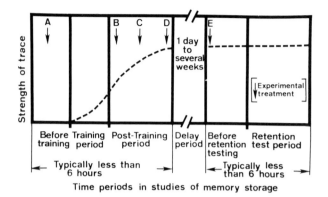

Fig. 4-4. Times of experimental treatment in studies of memory storage. Treatments administered at points A and E may be used to assess the proactive effects of the treatment upon training and retest performance respectively. Treatments administered at points B, C, and D may be used to assess the temporal gradient of effectiveness of the treatment, without the confounding of performance effects, since subjects are neither trained nor tested under the influence of the treatment. (From McGaugh, 1968.)

previously. However, such state dependent considerations need not apply to posttrial drug procedures since subjects are neither trained nor tested while drugged. As a consequence of the relative ease of interpretation of the results of experiments of learning and memory facilitation with CNS stimulants, the question of their mechanism of action would appear to be a much simpler one to tackle. For this reason in the following sections we will deal almost exclusively with these drugs.

V. THE QUESTION OF MECHANISM

This question has been approached in two distinct ways. The first has been an attempt to extend and combine the research from both memory facilitation and disruption research in the hope of answering several conceptual questions. For example, might the disruptive effects of ECS be prevented by affecting more efficient storage with stimulant drugs administered following the trial but prior to the ECS treatment? These types of experiments have been performed in a behavioral context. The second approach has been to attack, at the systems level, the question of how these drugs might act in the CNS. One method has been to stimulate specific brain centers following learning in the hope of localizing critical areas involved in memory storage. A second method has been to investigate the neurophysiological changes either in the whole animal or in specific isolated preparations following drug manipulation.

VI. BEHAVIORALLY ORIENTED RESEARCH

Recent research has shown that it is possible appreciably to attenuate the disruptive effects of a variety of treatments or appreciably shorten the time during which disruption can be produced with a variety of CNS stimulants. This capability has been demonstrated with strychnine prior to ECS (Bivens & Ray, 1966; McGaugh & Hart, in preparation), magnesium pemoline prior to ECS (Stein & Brink, 1960), TCAP prior to ECS (Essman, 1966), and anodal polarization prior to cathodal polarization (Albert, 1966b). Although it is possible that these treatments act merely by reducing the effectiveness of the disrupting treatment, several authors prefer the argument that these treatments act by maintaining a sufficiently high level of neural activity for consolidation of memory to proceed (McGaugh & Hart, in preparation; Stein and Brink, 1969). John (1967) has put forward an interesting theoretical argument for assuming that this might be the case.

One interesting, though unexpected outcome of the study by McGaugh and Hart (in preparation) was that even if strychnine was administered following ECS, memory was shown to persist. Normally, ECS would have produced amnesia in that situation. These results cannot be interpreted as an effect upon the ECS treatment since the effect was still evident when the drug was injected 3 hours following ECS. A similar result has been obtained when anodal polarization was applied following disrupting cathodal polarization (Albert, 1966b) and with amphetamine or footshock (FS) after inhibition of cerebral protein synthesis (Barondes and Cohen, 1968). In all of these studies, stimulation applied within a few hours following treatment with an amnesic agent appeared to restart or accelerate consolidation. One interesting experimental finding which bears upon this hypothesis is that following ECS (Geller and Jarvik, 1968; McGaugh and Landfield, 1970) and protein synthesis inhibition (Barondes and Cohen, 1968), recall is possible shortly after the treatment but decays gradually over the following several hours. It may be that the stimulants arrest or reverse this memory decay.

The results of the above studies are extremely interesting and await further confirmation. They point, however, to important conceptual notions about memory storage, and suggest that the labile state of memory might not only serve a retrieval function for a short period of time following learning, but also a template function for long term storage. Disruption might conceivably occur through the removal of the substrates upon which the template acts.

Notice that these speculations are conceptual and have little direct relevance to the understanding of memory storage at the neurophysiological systems level. An attempt at such an understanding has been made by stimulating localized regions of brain. Denti and her colleagues (Denti, 1965; Bloch, Denti & Schmaltz, 1966; Denti, McGaugh, Landfield, & Shinkman, 1970), for example, found significant facilitation of learning with immediate posttrial stimulation of the mesencephalic reticular formation. Significant facilitation has also been achieved by implantation of strychnine (Alpern, 1968) or posttrial injections of pentylenetetrazol (Grossman, 1969) into discrete brain regions. In all these studies, where comparisons can be made with operated and unoperated controls, the stimulated groups performed at a level intermediate to the controls. Therefore it is arbitrary whether the effect is termed facilitation or compensation for a lesion effect.

These experiments bring up an extremely important theoretical point, however, since the discrete manipulations have been made in regions which have been implicated in the control of arousal (see Routtenberg, 1968). In addition, time dependent disruption of memory has been reported following stimulation (Wyers, Peeke, Williston, & Herz, 1968) and lesions of arousal systems (Hudspeth & Wilsoncroft, 1969; Dorfman et al., 1969). Does the finding that a wide variety of drugs have been shown to facilitate memory storage in many tasks indicate that there are many mechanisms involved in storage, or is there some common relationship between these results? The findings from discrete CNS manipulations would appear to suggest that the state of arousal of the animal is critical for efficient storage.

Some insight into this question has been given by the electrophysiological data of Luttges (1968). This investigator drew from the behavioral literature on the dose response effects of CNS stimulants in rats and selected two drugs, megimide and strychnine, which had been shown to exert both disruptive and facilitative effects upon memory storage, depending upon the dosage of drug used. Most importantly, the drugs have quite different central mechanisms of action. Luttges argued that effects common to both drugs, injected in facilitatory doses, might be used to assess a common facilitatory mechanism. Effects common to both drugs injected in disruptive doses might likewise be used to assess a common disruptive mechanisms. Effects common to both facilitative and disruptive doses might be assumed to be incidental to the main effects.

Subsequently, Luttges examined the effects of intraperitoneal injections of these drugs on spontaneous and evoked electrical activity in a number of cortical and subcortical areas in chronically prepared unanesthetized rats. Summarized briefly, the results reveal a minimal effect of either drug in lower sensory relays. Strychnine effects appear greatest as changes in the evoked and spontaneous activity in the reticular formation, with some changes in the posterior hypothalamus. Megimide injections appear to cause changes in the posterior hypothalamus mainly and the cortex to a lesser extent. Despite the apparent differences between the systems which change following strychnine as opposed to metrazol injections, there is some communality between facilitatory and disruptive effects of both drugs. With facilitative doses of both drugs, the reticular formation appeared to be activated along with the posterior hypothalamus.

On the basis of these results, Luttges suggested that facilitative doses of these drugs may produce high states of internal activation in the absence of high amounts of external stimulation, thus decreasing the possibility for retroactive interference. Disruptive doses also produced high levels of activation, but in the absence of control over external stimuli. In this instance it appears that two conceivable mechanisms for more efficient storage, namely enhanced internal processing and decreased external interference, are inextricably related.

Dawson (unpublished observations) has recently extended these findings to the behavioral situation using the same facilitative and disruptive doses of strychnine. Rats were injected with the drug, or a control solution. Subsequently, their startle responses to a series of discrete white noise bursts were measured. The results indicate that while the initial response to the drug was directly related to the dose of drug administered, subjects given facilitative doses habituated rapidly over trials while subjects given the disruptive dose did not. This suggests that although the initial effect of the drug increases responsivity, facilitative doses are conducive to the appearance of a high degree of behavioral inhibition (reducing external interference?) while the disruptive dose is not.

In summary, although these results require further confirmation and extension, they point to the necessity of distinguishing between general and specific effects of CNS manipulations. If it can be shown that an optimum state of arousal is critical for the storage of information, then lesions, or stimulation of discrete brain regions might influence storage by changing the state of arousal of the organism in some general manner, rather than by being critically involved in the storage of specific information. Since the isolation of specific structural involvement in storage is implicit in the utilization of discrete central structural manipulations, it is crucial to distinguish between these two possibilities.

VII. LEARNING SITUATIONS INDIRECTLY
RELATED TO LEARNING AND MEMORY

Some insight into the mechanisms of action of drugs implicated in memory oriented research has been gained from the study of a variety of phenomena whose relationship to learning and memory is at present obscure. For example, Chamberlain et al. (1963) showed that following unilateral cerebellar lesions, a postural asymmetry developed in the hind limbs. Spinal transection was effective in preventing a permanent asymmetry if performed within 45 minutes of the cerebellar lesion. Subsequently, it was shown that TCAP injections shortened the time in which the spinal transection was effective and injections of 8-azaguanine, an RNA synthesis inhibitor, lengthened the fixation time to 70 minutes. The suggestion is that these drugs act by increasing or decreasing RNA synthesis. These findings have recently been extended by Giurgea, Daliers, and Moruvieff (1969). These investigators confirmed the effects of TCAP and 8-azaguanine on fixation time and also showed that strychnine and nicotine shorten fixation time. However, a great number of psychotropic drugs (chlorpromazine, amphetamine, caffeine, picrotoxin, scopolamine) had no effect. These results make it exceedingly difficult to predict an effect from a given class of drugs.

A related phenomenon has been reported by Morrell (1964). When a localized area of cortex is subjected to cooling, a primary epileptogenic focus is produced. Over a period of weeks, a secondary focus starts up in the contralateral hemisphere at a point homotypic with the primary focus, presumably as a result of collosally transmitted activity. After a period of time, the secondary focus becomes independent of continued excitation from the primary focus and can be shown to retain its heightened excitability after collosal transections, even following long periods of inactivity of the secondary focus. Obviously, some change has taken place in this secondary region which persists even during periods of inactivity. Morrell noticed an increase in the RNA content of cells within the secondary focus and has interpreted this finding in a very cautious way. Yet it is attractive to speculate that the RNA increases reflect biochemical changes which might subserve some type of "memorial" function.

The results of these experiments generally "fit" the notion of RNA synthesis involvement in the long term consequences of storage: however, it is hard to conceive of many circumstances where RNA synthesis rates might not change following sustained neural bombardment. In any event, the specification of the conditions under which sustained changes occur in isolated systems would surely provide some clues as to the possible extent of such effects in the central nervous system. For example, it would be unlikely that sustained optic nerve firing would produce drastic changes in the levels of RNA in the nerve itself since this fibre pathway operates normally at a high frequency. Systems which do not normally support high firing rates or have relatively long recovery cycles would appear to be much more susceptible to changes in rates of synthesis or availability of substrates. One further point is that there is very little overlap of drugs used in such isolated preparations with drugs used to facilitate learning and memory, and for this reason it is difficult to extend the analogy too far.

In contrast to this state of affairs, a striking parallel is apparent between the effects of drugs on learning and memory, and the effects of such drugs upon recovery of behavioral functioning following brain lesions. In certain instances, particularly when lesions are inflicted early in the life of animals, a loss of a particular function, for example, tactile discrimination (Benjamin and Thompson, 1959), is apparent shortly following the lesion, but the animal subsequently recovers the capacity to perform at a later time. In several instances, it has been shown that pharmacological manipulations following the lesion or between successive lesions can speed up or retard recovery.

In one study, Cole, Sullins, and Isaac (1967) showed that chronic *d*-amphetamine injections administered between successive unilateral visual cortical ablations speeded up the recovery of avoidance responding to visual stimuli in rats. A similar effect has been obtained by injecting animals chronically with strychnine sulfate between successive visual cortical lesions (Petrinovich, 1963). Furthermore, Watson and Kennard (1945) have provided evidence that sedatives delay recovery of function. Although the mechanisms underlying these effects are obscure, the findings are consistent with the notion that CNS stimulants enhance functioning while CNS depressants retard it. It would be interesting to investigate the extent of the parallel between memorial and recovery phenomena, however. On the basis of memory research one would predict that disruptive doses of stimulant drugs should retard functional recovery if the processes involved in the phenomena in question are to any degree parallel.

At the cellular level an attempt has been made to explain the mechanism of action of a variety of CNS stimulants. It is generally assumed for example that strychnine acts by blocking postsynaptic inhibition and picrotoxin acts by blocking presynaptic inhibition (Eccles, Schmidt, & Willis, 1963). The release from inhibition is therefore assumed to be the basis of the stimulant effects of these two drugs. However, these findings have as yet been of little use in elucidating either the communalities or differences in action of these drugs in the behaving animal. Apart from the obvious jump in complexity, there are several other reasons for this situation. The pharmacological dichotomy of effects of these two drugs is not universally supported. For example, Kellerth and Szumski (1966) have demonstrated instances of postsynaptic inhibition in the spinal cord which are resistant to strychnine but which are blocked by picrotoxin. Curtis and DeGroot (1968) also report that blocking of postsynaptic inhibition by strychnine may be specific to the type of transmitter substance released by the presynaptic inhibitory nerve terminals. This finding might explain strychnine resistant postsynaptic inhibition (Kellerth and Szumski, 1966a). In addition, the criteria for identifying presynaptic inhibition are still in question (Granit, 1968; Kellerth and Szumski, 1966b.)

Therefore, the possibility that presynaptic inhibition may have specific neuroanatomical and neurophysiological characteristics which might be blocked specifically by picrotoxin seems remote. A similar set of circumstances appears to hold for postsynaptic inhibition and strychnine. As a result, it seems unlikely that one will be able to build on such synaptic and anatomical foundations in order to predict strychnine or picrotoxin behavioral effects. The analysis of the neurophysiological relationships between structures in the whole animal would appear to be a more rewarding approach where, in addition, behaviorally appropriate drug doses may be studied.

VIII. SUMMARY

In the preceeding sections we have discussed both the general and specific problems of drug research and the rationale for the experimental value of drugs as tools to study learning and memory. At this point an evaluation seems to be in order.

The rationale behind drug research was that the discovery of mechanisms of drug action might be combined with analysis of relevant learning phenomena in order to understand the mechanisms underlying learning and memory. Experiments in which pretrial injection procedures have been used have proven difficult to interpret, in that a clear associative effect of the drug is always obscured by other performance factors. The use of posttrial injection procedures, however, has been extremely productive. The results of such research indicate that appropriate doses of a wide variety of CNS stimulants facilitate learning when administered following learning in a wide variety of tasks. Since the drugs in these experiments are not present in the animals either at the time of training or retesting, these effects cannot be due to changes in activity, alertness, or attention, or to changes in motivation. Nor can these experiments be confounded by "state dependency" notions. Although it is conceivable that these drugs act solely by somehow reducing external interference following learning, this does not appear to be the case. In fact there is some evidence to suggest that facilitative drugs produce a state of increased internal excitability while also reducing external excitability.

One source of confusion in the isolation of possible mechanisms of memory has been that such a wide variety of drugs have been shown to facilitate memory storage. Does this result indicate that memory storage may be facilitated by a variety of mechanisms, or is there some communality of drug effects at one level or another? Several of the facilitative drugs have been investigated intensively and distinct modes of action have been ascribed to them; for example, picrotoxin has been shown to block presynaptic inhibition while strychnine blocks postsynaptic inhibition. However, the university of these results have been disproved. Therefore it does not seem likely that the simple analysis of areas in which pre- and postsynaptic inhibition predominant in the CNS will lead to a better understanding of facilitative mechanisms.

One suggestion is that both disruptive and facilitative drugs may exert their effects by a direct effect upon arousal level—which in turn affects memory storage. Unfortunately, the evidence directly bearing upon this hypothesis is sparse. All of the drugs which affect memory storage can be shown to influence arousal but careful dose-response correlations are not available at present. The question must be asked, do the same doses which facilitate memory storage increase arousal level to some functional optimum and do disruptive doses cause a displacement from optimum conditions of arousal?

Obviously, at some level the concept of optimum arousal can be considered equivalent to that of efficient processing or storage; however, the distinction has some implications for procedures which attempt to localize structures intimately involved in memory storage. Structures which to date have been implicated in storage, in that their removal or stimulation results in time dependent facilitation or disruption of memory, are also intimately involved in arousal systems of the forebrain and brain stem. In order to dissociate between areas which store information and areas which are secondarily involved we must be able to distinguish between arousal systems which actively participate in ongoing storage processes and ones which are peripheral to storage.

Perhaps the most important finding which has arisen from this area of research is that memory storage processes have been shown to be time dependent; that is, the closer the treatment follows the learning trial, the greater the effect. This is true for both disruptive and facilitative treatments. This finding is extremely important for studies in which discrete brain regions are manipulated since it suggests that in order to implicate any structure in memory storage, experimental manipulation of the region should produce a time dependent effect. Structures that affect memory but do not produce time dependent effects may be the sites of storage, but they may be also simply necessary for input or output processing.

A second critical finding is that memory appears to involve more than one process. The strongest information for this notion comes from studies in which restarting of consolidation has been achieved by injection of stimulant drugs after disruption of memory. These results suggest that some form of template, which can subserve retrieval survives after disruption, decays over approximately a 6-hour period, but it can be reactivated if the CNS is stimulated during this decay period. Another line of evidence in favor of at least two memory processes comes from the finding that while protein synthesis inhibition does not appear to impair acquisition of short-term holding of information, it does appear to be necessary for the long term storage of information.

One of the major problems in attempting to equate short-term memory with some notion of circulation of neural impulses and longer term storage with the laying down of a biochemical substrate is that it is exceedingly difficult to distinguish between biochemical processes necessary for the general well-being and repair of cells, and those processes which might subserve a memorial function. In addition, it is difficult to conceive of a mechanism whereby short-term memory could be preserved following ECS—even for a short time, if we assume that seizure activity induced by ECS essentially disrupts ongoing neural circulation patterns. This latter observation makes it very likely that there are biochemical factors involved in even short-term events, which can to some degree reconstitute specific patterns of information.

If one were to accept the notions put forward by John (1967) to attempt to understand memory mechanisms, then the picture would be somewhat like the following: let us suppose that at the biochemical level, memory in neurons is represented by some deviation from a homeostatic equilibrium. This may result in either the availability of more transmitter substances, for greater firing potential, or less availability of transmitter for lesser firing potential. Let us also suppose that there are several different mechanisms which may be displaced from a homeostatic equilibrium either in the same or in different neurons. These different mechanisms may have different rates of homeostatic imbalance and recovery from that imbalance, depending, for example, upon the availability of a variety of neural substrates.

Suppose that during and shortly following a learning experience, more and more cells are recruited into the storage process. As they are recruited they are displaced from a homeostatic equilibrium. This displacement reflects first systems which change quickly, then, as consolidation continues, it reflects systems which change more slowly. CNS stimulants may, in part, act to increase the numbers of cells participating in storage and, in part, to accelerate the involvement of systems which normally take a long time to become displaced from their homeostatic equilibrium. Perhaps they subserve the second function by increasing the available substrate concentrations necessary for these changes. ECS may block, in a random fashion, much of the storage specific firing and also deplete relevant neural substrates. However, the homeostatic imbalances in short-term storage cells may be sufficient to reinstitute firing or to preserve firing above the random noise created by ECS. However, these imbalances are presumably only short-term ones and would therefore be expected to revert back to equilibrium in a short time. This would be seen in the animal as short-term memory initially following ECS followed by short-term decay. Long-term memory presumably may not be formed either because ECS has removed relevant substrates or because cells which exhibit long-term effects do not have the biochemical potential to reinstitute firing after ECS. The former case appears conducive to explanation of the post-ECS reinstitution of memory if CNS stimulants replace neural substrates.

Needless to say, this is only one of a variety of speculative models. Its advantages are: it attempts to incorporate most of the available behavioral data and it considers the neuron as a biochemical machine which obeys the fundamental biochemical characteristic of homeostasis. The general model does have some suggestions for future research. First, it directs attention to attempts to correlate the duration of availability of memory with specific time courses of neural events. For example, Richard Thompson (personal communication) has pointed out the interesting correlation between measures of retention of short-term material and the characteristics of recovery cycles of cells in cat cortex. Decay of short-term memory after a brief visual presentation (Averbach & Sperling, 1960) has a remarkably similar time course to the recovery of primary sensory evoked potentials (approximately 200 msec). Similarly, short-term memory (Peterson, 1966) for word association has a similar time course to the recovery cycle for novelty cells in cat association cortex (approximately 8 sec). Second, it points to the characterization of the time course of biochemical events in individual neurons as an important consideration; for example, do individual neurons have one or several mechanisms of different durations by which transmitter availability is changed? The utilization of model systems would appear to provide an excellent means of asking this question (cf. Eisenstein, 1967; Kandel, 1967; Thompson and Spencer, 1966). Third, it brings the question of substrates for neural activity to focus with regard to treatments which facilitate or disrupt memory; for example, might the amnesic effects of ECS be alleviated by artificially increasing the availability of CNS transmitter substances or their precursors?

Obviously, the assumption that changes in transmitter availability are the necessary and sufficient conditions for retrieval of memory is simplistic; however, the notion has considerable empirical support (Deutsch, 1969). Nevertheless, the argument of homeostatic changes and memory might be extended to cover a wide variety of other possible biochemical changes.

In summary, memory and learning are all-pervasive phenomena, yet do not exist in isolation from the methods used to assess them or from the ongoing processes of day to day neural functioning. Through the use of drugs, in particular the CNS stimulants, some rather molar questions have been answered. The questions of further localization may demand a more serious consideration of the brain as an ongoing biological machine. We have attempted to outline some of these considerations and also suggest how, through the use of drugs, these more specific questions may be approached.

REFERENCES

Agranoff, B. W. Biological effects of antimetabolites used in behavioral studies. In: D. H. Efron *et al.* (Eds.), *Psychopharmacology: A review of progress*, PHS Publ. No. 1836. Washington, D.C. U.S. Government Printing Office, 1968. Pp. 909-917.

Agranoff, B. W., Davis, R. E., Casola, L., & Lim, R. Actinomycin D blocks formation of memory of shock avoidance in the goldfish. *Science*, 1967, Vol. 158, 1600-1601.

Albert, D. J. The effect of spreading depression on the consolidation of learning. *Neuropsychologia*, 1966, Vol. 4, 49-64. (a)

Albert, D. J. The effects of polarizing currents on the consolidation of learning. *Neuropsychologia*, 1966, Vol. 4, 65-77. (b)

Alpern, H. P. Facilitation of learning by implantation of strychnine sulphate in the central nervous system. Unpublished doctoral dissertation, University of California, Irvine, 1968.

Appel, S. A critical appraisal of the role of RNA information storage in the nervous system. In: J. Gaito (Ed.), *Symposium of the Role of Macromolecules in Complex Behavior*. Manhattan, Kansas: Kansas State University, 1964.

Averbach, E., & Sperling, G. Short term storage of information in vision. In E. O. Cherry (Ed.), *Fourth London symposium on information theory*. London and Washington, D.C.: Butterworth, 1960.

Barondes, S. H. Effect of inhibitors of cerebral protein synthesis on "long-term" memory in mice. In D. H. Efron *et al.* (Eds.), *Psychopharmacology: A review of progress*. PHS Publ. No. 1836. Washington, D.C.: U.S. Government Printing Office, 1968. Pp. 905-908.

Barondes, S. H., & Cohen, H. D. Comparative effects of cycloheximide and puromycin on cerebral protein synthesis and consolidation of memory in mice. *Brain Research,* 1967, Vol. 4, 44-51. (a)

Barondes, S. H., & Cohen, H. D. Delayed and sustained effect of acetoxycycloheximide on memory in mice. *Proceedings of the National Academy of Sciences,* 1967, Vol. 58, 157-164. (b)

Barondes, S. H., & Cohen, H. D. Arousal and the conversion of "short-term" to "long-term" memory. *Proceedings of the National Academy of Sciences,* 1968, Vol. 61, 923-929.

Barondes, S. H., & Jarvik, M. E. The influence of actinomycin-D on brain RNA synthesis and on memory. *Journal of Neurochemistry,* 1964, Vol. 11, 187-195.

Beach, G., & Kimble, D. P. Activity and responsivity in rats after magnesium pemoline injections. *Science,* 1967, Vol. 155, 698-701.

Benevento, L. A., & Kandel, G. L. Influence of strychnine on classically conditioned defensive reflexes in the cat. *Journal of Comparative & Physiological Psychology,* 1967, Vol. 63, 117-120.

Benjamin, R. M., & Thompson, R. F. Differential effects of cortical lesions in infant and adult cats on roughness discrimination. *Experimental Neurology,* 1959, Vol. 1, 305-321.

Bernhardt, K. S. Phosphorous and iron deficiencies and learning in the rat. *Journal of Comparative Psychology,* 1936, Vol. 22, 273-276. (a)

Bernhardt, K. S. Vitamin A deficiency and learning in the rat. *Journal of Comparative Psychology,* 1936, Vol. 22, 277-278. (b)

Bindra, D. Stimulus change, reactions to novelty and response decrement. *Psychological Review,* 1959, Vol. 66, 96-103.

Bivens, L. W., & Ray, O. S. Effects of electroconvulsive shock and strychnine sulphate on memory consolidation. *Proceedings of the Fifth International Congress of the Collegium Internationale Neuropsychopharmacologicum,* 1966, 1030-1034.

Bloch, U., Denti, A., & Schmaltz, G. Effets de la stimulation reticulaire sur la phase de consolidation de la trace amnesique. *Journal de Physiologie,* 1966, Vol. 58, 469-470.

Bogoch, S. *The biochemistry of memory.* Oxford University Press, London and New York, 1968.

Bohdanecky, Z., & Jarvik, M. E. Impairment of one-trial passive avoidance learning in mice by scopolamine, scopolamine methylbromide, and physostigmine. *International Journal of Neuropharmacology,* 1962, Vol. 6, 217-222.

Booth, D. A. Vertebrate brain ribonucleic acids and memory retention. *Psychological Bulletin,* 1967, Vol. 68, 149-177.

Bovet, D., McGaugh, J. L., & Oliverio, A. (1966) Effects of post trial administration of drugs on avoidance learning of mice. *Life Sciences,* Vol. 5, 1309-1315.

Bovet, D., & Oliverio, A. Decrement of avoidance conditioning performance in inbred mice subjected to prolonged session: Performance recovery after rest and amphetamine. *Journal of Psychology,* 1967, Vol. 65, 45-55.

Bowman, R. Magnesium pemoline and behavior. *Science,* 1966, Vol. 153, 902.

Briggs, M. H., & Kitto, C. B. The molecular basis of memory and learning. *Psychological Review,* 1962, Vol. 69, 537-541.

Brown, H. Effect of ribonucleic acid (RNA) on the rate of lever pressing in rats. *Psychological Record,* 1966, Vol. 16, 173-176. (a)

Brown, H. Effect of ribonucleic acid (RNA) on reversal of a probability matching problem in pigeons. *Psychological Record,* 1966, Vol. 16, 441-448. (b)

Brush, F. R., Davenport, J. W., & Polidora, V. J. TCAP negative results in avoidance and water maze learning and retention. *Psychonomic Science,* 1966, Vol. 4, 183-184.

Bures, J., Bohdanecky, Z., & Weiss, T. Physostigmine induced hippocampal theta activity and learning in rats. *Psychopharmacologia,* 1962, Vol. 3, 254-263.

Bures, J., & Buresova, O. Cortical spreading depression as a memory disturbing factor. *Journal of Comparative & Physiological Psychology*, 1963, Vol. 56, 268-272.

Buresova, O., Bures, J., Bohdanecky, Z., & Weiss, T. Effect of atropine on learning, extinction, retention, and retrieval in rats. *Psychopharmacologia,* 1964, Vol. 5, 255-263.

Calhoun, W. H. Effect of level of external stimulation on rate of learning and interaction of this effect with strychnine treatment in mice. *Psychological Report*, 1966, Vol. 18, 715-722.

Cannon, W. B., & Uridil, J. E., Some effects on the denervated heart of stimulating the nerves of the liver. *American Journal of Physiology*, 1921, Vol. 58, 353-364.

Carlton, P. L. Cholinergic mechanisms in the control of behavior by the brain. *Psychological Review*, 1963, Vol. 70, 19-39.

Carlton, P. L., & Vogel, J. R. Studies of the amnesic properties of scopolamine. *Psychonomic Science*, 1965, Vol. 3, 261-262.

Chamberlain, T. J., Rothschild, G. H., & Gerard, R. W. Drugs affecting RNA and learning. *Proceedings of the National Academy of Science*, 1963, Vol. 49, 918-925.

Cherkin, A. Kinetics of memory consolidation: Role of amnesic treatment parameters. *Proceedings of the National Academy of Science*, 1969, Vol. 63, 1094-1101.

Cholewiak, R. W., Hammond, R., Siegler, I. C., & Papsdorf, J. D. The effects of strychnine sulphate on the classically conditioned nictating membrane response of the rabbit. *Journal of Comparative & Physiological Psychology,* 1968, Vol. 66, 77-81.

Cohen, H. D., & Barondes, S. H. Further studies of learning and memory after intracerebral actinomycin-D. *Journal of Neurochemistry,* 1966, Vol. 13, 207-211.

Cohen, H. D., Ervin, F., & Barondes, S. H. Puromycin and cycloheximide: Different effects on hippocampal electrical activity. *Science*, 1966, Vol. 154, 1557-1558.

Cole, D. D., Sullins, W. R., Jr., & Isaac, W. Pharmacological modification of the effects of spaced occipital ablations. *Psychopharmacologia* (Berl.), 1967, Vol. 11, 311-316.

Cook, L., & Davidson, A. B. Effects of yeast RNA and other pharmacological agents on acquisition, retention and performance in animals. In D. H. Efron *et al.* (Eds.), *Psychopharmacology: A review of progress 1957-1967.* PHS Publ. No. 1836. Washington, D.C.: U.S. Government Printing Office, 1968. Pp. 931-946.

Cook, L., & Kelleher, R. T. Effects of drugs on behavior. *Annual Review of Pharmacology*, 1963, Vol. 3, 205-222.

Cooper, R. M., & Krass, M. Strychnine: Duration of the effects on maze learning. *Psychopharmacologia*, 1963, Vol. 4, 472-475.

Corning, W. C., and John, E. R. Effect of ribonuclease on retention of a conditioned response in regenerated planarians. *Science*, 1961, Vol. 134, 1363-1364.

Curtis, H. J., & Cole, K. S. Membrane resting and action potentials from the squid giant axon. *Journal of Cellular & Comparative Physiology,* 1942, Vol. 19, 135-144.

Curtis, D. R., & DeGroot, N. C. Tetanus toxin and spinal inhibition. *Brain Research*, 1968, Vol. 10, 208-212.

Dawson, R. G. Unpublished observations.

Denti, A. Facilitation of conditioning by reticular stimulation in the fixation phase of memory. Unpublished dissertation, University of Paris, France, 1965.

Denti, A., McGaugh, J. L., Landfield, P. W., & Shinkman, P. Facilitation of learning with posttrial stimulation of the reticular formation. *Physiological Behavior,* 1970, Vol. 5 659-662.

Deutsch, J. A. The physiological basis of memory. *Annual Review of Psychology*, 1969, Vol. 20, 85-104.

Dews, P. B. Measurement of the influence of drugs on voluntary activity in mice. *British Journal of Pharmacology*, 1953, Vol. 8, 46-48.

Dingman, W., & Sporn, M. B. The incorporation of 8-azaguinine into rat brain RNA and its effect on maze-learning by the rat; an inquiry into the biochemical bases of memory. *Journal of Psychiatry Research*, 1961, Vol. 1, 1-11.

Dingman, E., & Sporn, M. B. Molecular theories of memory. *Science*, 1964, Vol. 144, 26-29.

Dorfman, L. J., Bohdanecka, M., Bohdanecky, Z., and Jarvik, M. E. Retrograde amnesia produced by small cortical stab wounds in the mouse. *Journal of Comparative & Physiological Psychology*, 1969, Vol. 69, 324-328.

Dorfman, L. F., & Jarvik, M. E. A parametric study of electro-shock induced retrograde amnesia in mice. *Neuropsychologia*, 1968, Vol. 6, 373-380.

Duncan, C. P. The retroactive effect of electroshock on learning. *Journal of Comparative & Physiological Psychology*, 1949, Vol. 42, 32-44.

Eccles, J. C. *The physiology of nerve cells*. Baltimore, Maryland: Johns Hopkins Press, 1957.

Eccles, J. C. *The physiology of synapses*, Berlin: Springer, 1964.

Eccles, J. C., Schmidt, R., & Willis, W. D. Pharmacological studies on presynaptic inhibition. *Journal of Physiology*, 1963, Vol. 168, 500-530.

Eisenstein, E. M. The use of invertebrate systems for studies on the bases of learning and memory. In G. C. Quarton, T. Melnechuk, and F. O. Schmitt, (Eds.). *The neurosciences*. Rockefeller: New York, 1967.

Essman, W. B. Effect of Trycyanoaminopropene on the amnesic effect of ECS. *Psychopharmacologia*, 1966, Vol. 9, 426-433.

Fatt, P. Biophysics of functional transmission. *Physiological Review*, 1954, Vol. 34, 674-710.

Fatt, P., & Katz, B An analysis of the end-plate potential recorded with an intra-cellular electrode. *Journal of Physiology*, 1951, Vol. 115, 320-370.

Fatt, P., & Katz, B. Spontaneous threshold activity at motor nerve endings. *Journal of Physiology*, 1952, Vol. 117, 109-128.

Flexner, J. B., Flexner, L. B., & Stellar, E. Memory in mice as affected by intracerebral puromycin. *Science*, 1963, Vol. 141, 57-59.

Franchina, J. J., & Grandolfo, P. Effects of strychnine and stimulus change on response withholding. Submitted for publication.

Franchina, J. J., & Moore, M. H. Strychnine and the inhibition of previous performance. *Science*, 1968, Vol. 160, 903-904.

Geller, A., & Jarvik, M. E. The time relations of ECS-induced amnesia. *Psychonomic Science*, 1968, Vol. 12, 169-170.

Gerard, R. W. Biological roots of psychiatry. *Science*, 1955, Vol. 122, 225-230.

Giurgea, C., Daliers, J., & Moruvieff, F. Pharmacological studies on an elementary model of learning: The fixation of an experience at spinal level. Paper presented at Fourth International Congress of Pharmacology, Basel, Switzerland, 1969.

Glassman, E. The biochemistry of learning: An evaluation of the role of RNA and protein. *Annual Review of Biochemistry*, 1969, Vol. 38, 605-646.

Glickman, S. E. Perseverative neural processes and consolidation of the memory trace. *Psychological Bulletin*, 1961, Vol. 58, 218-233.

Gonzales, R. C., & Ross, S. The effects of chlorpromazine on the course of discrimination-reversal learning in the rat. *Journal of Comparative & Physiological Psychology*, 1961, Vol. 54, 645-648.

Granit, R. The case for presynaptic inhibition by synapses on the terminals of motor neurons. In C. Von Euler, S. Skoglund, & U. Soderberg, (Eds.). *Structure and function of inhibitory neuronal mechanisms*. Pergamon: London, 1968.

Greenough, W. T., & McGaugh, J. L. The effect of strychnine sulphate on learning as a function of time of administration. *Psychopharmacologia*, 1965, Vol. 8, 290-294.

Grossman, S. P. Facilitation of learning following intracranial injections of pentylenetet-razol. *Physiological Behavior,* 1969, Vol. 4, 625-628.

Hearst, E., & Whalen, R. E. Facilitating effects of d-amphetamine on discriminated avoid-ance performance. *Journal of Comparative & Physiological Psychology,* 1963, Vol. 56, 124-128.

Hebb, D. O. *The organization of behavior.* New York: Wiley, 1949.

Herz, A. Uber die wirkung von scopolamin, benactyzin and atropin auf das reaktive verholten der ratte. *Archives of Experimental Pathology,* 1959, Vol. 236, 110-112.

Herz, A. Drugs and conditioned avoidance responses. *International Review of Neurobiology,* 1960, Vol. 2, 229-277.

Hodgkin, A. L., & Huxley, A. F. Currents carried by sodium and potassium ions through the membrane of the giant axon of *holigo. Journal of physiology,* 1952, Vol. 116, 449-472. (a)

Hodgkin, A. L., & Huxley, A. F. The components of membrane conductance in the giant axon of *holigo. Journal of Physiology,* 1952, Vol. 116, 473-496. (b)

Hodgkin, A. L., & Huxley, A. F. A quantitative description of membrane current and its application to conduction and excitation in nerve. *Journal of Physiology,* 1952, Vol. 117, 500-544. (c)

Hudspeth, W. J. Strychnine: Its facilitating effect on the solution of a simple oddity problem by the rat. *Science,* 1964, Vol. 145, 1331-1333.

Hudspeth, W. J., & Wilsoncroft, W. E. Retrograde amnesia: Time dependent effects of rhinencephalic lesions. *Journal of Neurobiology,* 1969, Vol. 2, 221-232.

Hunt, E. B., & Bauer, R. H. Facilitation of learning by delayed injections of pentylenetet-razol. *Psychopharmacologia,* 1969, Vol. 16, 139-146.

Hunt, E. B. Personal communication.

Hydén, H. RNA in brain cells. In G. C. Quarton, T. Melnechuk, & F. O. Schmitt, (Eds.), *The Neurosciences.* Rockefeller: New York, 1967. (a)

Hydén, H. Biochemical changes accompanying learning. In G. C. Quarton, T. Melnechuk, and F. O. Schmitt, (Eds.). *The Neurosciences.* Rockefeller: New York, 1967. (b)

Hydén, H., & Egyházi, E. Nuclear RNA changes of nerve cells during a learning experi-ment with rats. *Proceedings of the National Academy of Science,* 1962, Vol. 48, 1366-1373.

Hydén, H., & Hartelius, H. Stimulation of nucleoprotein production in nerve cells by malonitrile and its effect on psychic function in mental disorders. *Acta Psychiatrica Neurologica Scandinavian,* 1948, Vol. 48, 1-117.

John, E. R. *Mechanisms of memory.* New York: Academic Press, 1967.

Kandel, E. R. Cellular studies of learning. In E. C. Quarton, T. Melnechuk, & F. O. Schmitt (Eds.), *The Neurosciences.* Rockefeller: New York, 1967.

Katz, J. J., & Halstead, W. C. Protein organization and mental function. *Comparative Psychological Monographs,* 1950, Vol. 20, 1-39.

Kellerth, J. -O., & Szumski, A. J. Aspects on the relative significance of pre- and post-synaptic inhibition in the spinal cord. In C. Von Euler, S. Skoglund, and V. Doderberg (Eds.), *Structure and function of inhibitiory neuronal mechanisms.* London: Pergamon, 1968.

Kellerth, J. -O., and Szumski, A. J. Two types of stretch-activated postsynaptic inhibitions in spinal motoneurons as differentiated by strychnine. *Acta Physiological Scandinavian,* 1966, Vol. 66, 133-145.

Kellerth, J.-O., & Szumski, A. J. Effects of picrotoxin on stretch-activated post-synaptic inhibitions in spinal motoneurones. *Acta Physiologica Scandinavica,* 1966b, Vol. 66, 146-156.

Kriekhaus, E. E., Miller, N. E., & Zimmerman, P. Reduction of freezing behavior and improvement of shock avoidance by d-amphetamine. *Journal of Comparative & Physiological Psychology*, 1965, Vol. 60, 36-40.

Krivanek, J., & Hunt, E. B. The effects of posttrial injections of pentylenetetrazol, strychnine, and mephenesin on discrimination learning. *Psychopharmacologia*, 1967, Vol. 10, 189-195.

Krivanek, J., & McGaugh, J. L. Effects of pentylenetetrazol on memory storage in mice. *Psychopharmacologia*, 1968, Vol. 12, 303-321.

Krivanek, J., & McGaugh, J. L. Facilitating effects of pre- and posttrial amphetamine administration on discrimination learning in mice. *Agents and Actions*, 1969, Vol. 1, 36-42.

Kumer, R., Stolesman, I. P., & Steinberg, H. Psychopharmacology. *Annual Review of Psychology*, 1970, Vol. 21, 595-628.

Lashley, K. S. The effects of strychnine and caffeine upon the rate of learning. *Psychobiology*, 1917, Vol. 1, 141-170.

Leao, A. A. P. Further observations on the spreading depression of activity in the cerebral cortex. *Journal of Neurophysiology*, 1947, Vol. 10, 409-414.

LeBoeuf, B. J., & Peeke, H. V. S. The effect of strychnine administration during development on adult maze learning in the rat. *Psychopharmacologia*, 1969, Vol. 16, 49-53.

Loewi, O. Uber humorale Ubertragbarkeit der Herznerven-Wirkung. *Pflugers Archiv fuer Gesamte die Physiologie*, 1921, Vol. 189, 239-242.

Louttit, R. T. Central nervous system stimulants and maze learning in rats. *Psychological Record*, 1965, Vol. 15, 97-101.

Luttges, M. Electrophysiological dose-response effects of megamide and strychnine. Unpublished doctoral dissertation, University of California, Irvine, 1968.

Macht, D. I., & Leach, M. C. Effect of Methyl and ethyl alcohol mixtures on behavior of rats in a maze. *Proceedings of the Society of Experimental Biological Medicine,* 1929, Vol. 26, 330-331.

Mandell, A. J., & Spooner, C. E. Psychochemical research studies in man. *Science*, 1968, Vol. 162, 1442-1453.

McGaugh, J. L. Some neurochemical factors in learning. Unpublished doctoral dissertation, University of California, Berkeley, 1959.

McGaugh, J. L. Time-dependent processes in memory storage. *Science*, 1966, Vol. 153, 1351-1358.

McGaugh, J. L. Drug facilitation of memory and learning. In D. H. Efron *et al.* (Eds.), *Psychopharmacology: A review of progress*. Washington, D.C.: Public Health Service Publ. No. 1836. Pp. 891-904.

McGaugh, J. L., & Dawson, R. G. Modification of memory storage processes. In W. K. Honig & P. H. R. James (Eds.), *Animal Memory*. Academic Press: New York, 1971. Pp. 215-242.

McGaugh, J. L., & Hart, J. D. Strychnine attenuation of retrograde amnesia induced by electroconvulsive shock. In preparation.

McGaugh, J. L., & Krivanek, J. Strychnine effects on discrimination learning in mice: Effects of dose and time of administration. *Physiology and Behavior*, 1970, Vol. 5, 1437-1442.

McGaugh, J. L., & Landfield, P. W. Delayed development of amnesia following electroconvulsive shock. *Physiology and Behavior*, 1970, Vol. 5, 1109-1113.

McGaugh, J. L., & Petrinovich, L. F. Effects of drugs on learning and memory. *International Review of Neurobiology*, 1965, Vol. 8, 139-196.

McGaugh, J. L., Thomson, C. W., Westbrook W. H., & Hudspeth, W. J. A further study of learning facilitation with strychnine sulphate. *Psychopharmacologia*, 1962, Vol. 3, 352-360.

Miller, A. J. Variations in retrograde amnesia with parameters of electroconvulsive shock and time of testing. *Journal of Comparative & Physiological, Psychology*, 1968, Vol. 66, 40-47.

Moore, W. J., & Mahler, H. R. Introduction to molecular psychology. *Journal of Chemistry Education*, 1965, Vol. 42, 49-60.

Morrell, F. Modification of RNA as a result of neural activity. In M. A. B. Brazier, (Ed.), *Brain Function* II. *RNA and Brain function, Memory and learning*. Los Angeles: University of California, 1964. Pp. 183-202.

Nachmanson, D. In J. F. Fulton (Ed.), *Textbook of physiology*. Chapter 10. Philadelphia, Pennsylvania: Saunders, 1955.

Oliverio, A. Effects of nicotine and strychnine on transfer of avoidance learning in the mouse. *Life Sciences*, 1968, Vol. 7, 1163-1167.

Otis, L. S., & Pryor, G. T. Lack of effect on TCAP on conditioned avoidance learning in rats. *Psychonomic Science* 1968, Vol. 11, 95-96.

Overton, D. A. State-dependent or "dissociated" learning produced with pentobarbital. *Journal of Comparative & Pysiological Psychology*, 1964, Vol. 57, 3-12. (a)

Overton, D. A. Differential responding in a three-choice maze controlled by three drug states. *Psychopharmacologia*, 1964, Vol. 11, 376-387. (b)

Overton, D. A. Discrimination Control of Behavior by Drug States. In G. Thompson and R. Dickens (Eds.), *Stimulus Properties of Drugs*. Appleton-Century-Crofts, Inc.: New York, 1971. Pp. 87-110.

Paré, W. The effect of caffeine and seconal on a visual discrimination task. *Journal of Comparative & Physiological Psychology*, 1961, Vol. 54, 506-609.

Peeke, H. V. S., LeBoeuf, B. & Herz, M. J. The effect of strychnine administration during development on adult maze learning in the rat. II. Drug administration from day 51 to 70. *Psychopharmacologia,* 1971, Vol. 19, 262-265.

Peterson, L. R. Short-term verbal memory and learning. *Psychological Review*, 1966, Vol. 73, 193-207.

Petrinovich, L. F. Reorganization of memory traces following cortical destruction. Paper presented to American Psychological Association, 1963.

Petrinovich, L. F., Bradford, D., & McGaugh, J. L. Drug facilitation of memory in rats. *Psychonomic Science*, 1965, Vol. 2, 191-192.

Plotnikoff, N. Magnesium pemoline: Enhancement of memory after electroconvulsive shock in rats. *Life Sciences*, 1966, Vol. 5, 1495-1498. (a)

Plotnikoff, N. Magnesium pemoline: Enhancement of learning and memory of a conditioned avoidance response. *Science*, 1966, Vol. 151, 703-704. (b)

Plotnikoff, N. Pemoline and magnesium hydroxide: Memory consolidation following acquisition trials. *Psychonomic Science*, 1967, Vol. 9, 141-142.

Prien, R. F., Wayner, M. J., Jr., & Kahan, S. Lack of facilitation in maze learning by picrotoxin and strychnine sulphate. *American Journal of Physiology*, 1963, Vol. 204, 488-492.

Quartermain, D., Paolino, R. M., & Miller, N. E. A brief temporal gradient of retrograde amnesia independent of situational change. *Science*, 1965, Vol. 149, 1116-1118.

Rech, R. H. Amphetamine effects on poor performance of rats in a shuttle box. *Psychopharmacologia*, 1966, Vol. 9, 110-117.

Routtenberg, A. The two-arousal hypothesis: Reticular formation and limbic system. *Psychological Review*, 1968, Vol. 75, 51-80.

Ross, S., & Cole, J. O. Psychopharmacology. *Annual Review of Psychology*, 1960, Vol. 11, 415-438.

Russell, R. W. In: L. Uhl & J. G. Miller (Eds.), *Drugs and behavior*, New York: Wiley, 1960.

Russell, R. W. Psychopharmacology. *American Review of Psychology*, 1964, Vol. 15, 87-114.

Sachs, E. The role of brain electrolytes in learning and retention. Unpublished doctoral dissertation. University of Rochester, New York, 1962.

Schmitt, F. O. Molecular neurobiology in the context of the neurosciences. In G. C. Quarton, T. Melnechuk, & F. O. Schmitt, (Eds.), *The Neurosciences*, Rockefeller: New York, 1967.

Schmidt, M. J., & Davenport, J. W. TCAP: Facilitation of learning in hypothyroid rats. *Psychonomic Science*, 1967, Vol. 7, 185-186.

Shandro, N. E., & Schaeffer, B. H. Environment and strychnine: Effects on maze behavior. Paper presented at Western Psychological Association Meeting, Vancouver, B.C., 1969.

Shaeffer, B. H. Strychnine and maze behavior: Limited effects of varied concentrations and injection times. *Journal of Comparative Physiological Psychology*, 1968, Vol. 66, 188-192.

Stein, D. G., & Brink, J. J. Prevention of retrograde amnesia by injection of magnesium pemoline in dimethylsulfoxide. *Psychopharmacologia*, 1969, Vol. 14, 240-247.

Stein, D. G., & Kimble, D. P. Effects of hippocampal lesions and posttrial strychnine administration on maze behavior in the rat. *Journal of Comparative & Physiological Psychology*, 1966, Vol. 62, 243-249.

Stein, D. G., Brink, J. J., & Patterson, A. H. Magnesium pemoline: Facilitation of maze learning when administered in pure dimethylsulfoxide. *Life Sciences*, 1968, Vol. 7, 147-153.

Stein, H. H., & Yellin, T. O. Pemoline and magnesium hydroxide: Lack of effect on RNA and protein synthesis. *Science*, 1967, Vol. 157, 96-97.

Stratton, L. O., & Petrinovich, L. F. Post-trial injection of an anticholinesterase drug and maze learning in two strains of mice. *Psychopharmacologia*, 1963, Vol. 5, 47-54.

Talland, G. A. Improvement of sustained attention with Cylert. *Psychonomic Science*, 1966, Vol. 6, 493-494.

Thompson, R. F. *Foundations of Physiological Psychology*. Harper and Row: New York, 1967.

Thompson, R. F. Personal communication.

Thompson, R. F., & Spencer, W. A. Habituation: A model phenomenon for the study of neural substrates of behavior. *Psychological Review*, 1966, Vol. 173, 16-43.

Warburton, D. M., & Groves, P. M. The effects of scopolamine on habituation of acoustic startle in rats. *Communications in Behavioral Biology,* 1969, Vol. 3, 289-293.

Watson, C. W., & Kennard, M. A. The effect of anticonvulsant drugs on recovery of function following cerebral cortical lesions. *Journal of Neurophysiology*, 1945, Vol. 8, 221-231.

Weissman, A. Effect of electroconvulsive shock intensity and seizure pattern on retrograde amnesia in rats. *Journal of Comparative & Physiological Psychology*, Vol. 56, 806-810.

Westbrook, W. H., & McGaugh, J. L. Drug facilitation of latent learning. *Psychopharmacologia*, 1964, Vol. 5, 440-446.

Whitehouse, J. M. The effects of atropine on discrimination learning in the rat. *Journal of Comparative & Physiological Psychology*, 1964, Vol. 57, 13-15.

Wyers, E. J., Peeke, H. V. S., Williston, J. S., & Herz, M. J. Retroactive impairment of passive avoidance learning by stimulation of the caudate nucleus. *Experimental Neurology*, 1968, Vol. 22, 350-366.

CHAPTER

5

ELECTROCONVULSIVE SHOCK AND MEMORY

J. ANTHONY DEUTSCH

The original impetus behind the many investigations employing electro-convulsive shock (ECS) as a tool has been the hope that "consolidation" of the memory trace could be studied. Muller and Pilzecker (1900) and Hebb (1949) had suggested that a temporary perseveration of neural activity occurred after the reception of a sensory message and that during this perseveration a change or consolidation into permanent memory gradually took place. It was suggested that the memory trace shortly after being laid down was liable and susceptible to destruction, but that it soon changed state and became impervious to disruption. If this suggestion is correct, it should be possible to impair or even improve the process of learning by various types of treatment which might influence the temporary perseveration of neural activity after a learning trial. Such effects have indeed been found. It has been shown that learning can be impaired by the administration of electroconvulsive shock after a learning trial (Duncan, 1949; Thompson & Dean, 1955; Thomson, McGaugh, Smith, Hudspeth, & Westbrook, 1961). In this procedure a brief current is passed between the ears of the rat so that a convulsive seizure followed by unconsciousness occurs. By showing that the loss of memory also occurred when the current was applied to an animal under ether anesthesia and no seizure followed, McGaugh (1966) demonstrated that the loss of memory obtained was not due to the seizure caused by the electroconvulsive shock (ECS). Effects similar to that of ECS have been shown, for instance, in the case of hypoxia (oxygen lack) (Thompson & Pryer, 1956) and when depressant drugs were administered (Leukel, 1957; Pearlman, Sharpless, & Jarvik, 1961). Cerf and Otis (1957) found that narcosis, produced by heating goldfish at various intervals after a learning trial, produced decrements in learning that were larger the closer the narcosis had been to the preceding trial. Such a temporal relation has also been demonstrated in the case of ECS. The closer the ECS to the end of a preceding learning trial, the more severe the learning loss. To measure the supposed rapid increase in consolidation after a learning trial, the use of ECS was greatly favored by most investigators because its application could be precisely pinpointed in time. In contrast, the application of drugs or heating produces a gradual onset of the effects of the agent on the central nervous system, which is somewhat indeterminate in time. (This argument, of course, assumes unjustifiably that it is the actual passage of electric current rather than its biochemical sequelae, which produces amnesia.) The use of ECS in the study of memory was also brought into vogue by observations on human patients. Here the disturbances produced by the therapeutic use ofECS produced apparent memory disruption (Williams, 1950, 1969; Cronholm, 1969).

If the time that it took the memory trace to consolidate could be measured, some clue to its physical identity might be found. However, no constant time over which ECS disrupts memory after training has been found. For instance, Quartermain, Paolino, and Miller (1965), and Chorover and Schiller (1965) have found an interval in the order of seconds. On the other hand, Kopp, Bohdanecky, and Jarvik (1967) have found effects 6 hours after training, and McGaugh (1966) reported effects on memory 3 hours after training. Some of these discrepancies are due to amount of current passed through the animal.

It has been shown in many studies that increased current intensity and increased duration of ECS produces increasing amnesia (McGaugh, 1966; Jarvik & Kopp, 1967; Dorfman & Jarvik, 1968; Pagano, Bush, Martin, & Hunt, 1968; Alpern & McGaugh, 1968; Zornetzer & McGaugh, 1970). There is another factor which might alter the gradient of retrograde amnesia in ECS. Misanin, Miller, and Lewis (1968) have reported that if animals are familiar with the environment in which they are subsequently shocked, memory of the shock is not eliminated by ECS, or ECS is only effective in producing amnesia when ECS is administered very close to the shock. However, this effect of environmental familiarity is not always found for reasons which are not well understood, as, for instance, in two experiments by Dawson and McGaugh (1969). Thomson *et al.* (1961) have demonstrated different effects of ECS on learning in rats that were descendants of the Tryon maze-bright strain and of the Tryon maze-dull strain. In the maze-dull strain, ECS produced a learning decrement after a much longer interval than that observed in the maze-bright strain. This evidence indicated to Thomson *et al.* that the process of consolidation takes a longer time in the Tryon maze-dull strain. Such results are of particular interest because it has been shown in McGaugh's laboratory (1961) that the maze-dull strain is only inferior to the maze-bright strain in learning mazes if the trials are massed. If the trials are spaced, the difference in learning rate between the two strains disappears. It is, of course, possible that such results are only coincidental. It could be argued that the maze-dull strain is in some way more sensitive to a given level of electric shock. Against this argument there is the finding of Woolley *et al.* (1960) that the maze-bright animals have lower thresholds in terms of current for seizures than the maze-dull rats, but such a finding is not conclusive because the threshold being measured is for seizure and not for effects on memory processes.

Whether ECS effects are seen at all may be influenced by competing responses. Gerbrandt, Buresova, and Bures (1968) report failure to find an effect of ECS on memory of a discrimination training using hooded rats. In a subsequent experiment, Bures and co-workers (1964) found such an effect only in albino rats. They did find an adverse effect of ECS on the memory of a reversal habit when overtraining was given on the original habit. This effect was observed both in hooded and albino rats.

The picture of two qualitatively different processes—one susceptible to ECS and the other an invulnerable consolidated memory trace—seems no longer so plausible. That some change is occurring during the footshock-ECS interval has been made clear. However, ECS seems to be capable of interfering with memory up to an ill-defined point on a merely quantitatively changing continuum. The notion of a quantitatively changing continuum is supported by the amnesic effects of other agents. For instance, fluorothyl (hexafluorodiethyl ether) when compared in efficacy to ECS by Bohdanecky, Kopp, and Jarvik (1968), showed an effect longer after training than did ECS. The curves of amnesic effect of these two agents presented by Bohdanecky *et al.* (1968) run parallel and, except for the degree of amnesic effect, seem qualitatively similar.

I. OTHER EXPLANATIONS OF ECS EFFECTS

On the basis of their experimental findings, Coons and Miller (1960) put forward an ingenious argument about the effects of ECS on the retention of a habit. They point out that the work demonstrating "loss of memory" for a given habit after ECS is vitiated by the fact that if the shock were felt, it would produce avoidance of a response which could be mistaken for amnesia. Accordingly, these workers used a somewhat complex design in which ECS, if felt, would facilitate learning. The results of their study support their contention. However, more recent results (McGaugh, 1961, using ECS; and Pearlman *et al.*, 1961, using anesthetic drugs to produce amnesia) do not support Coons and Miller's contention. Abt *et al.* (1961) and McGaugh (1961) created a simpler situation by placing a rat on a small restrictive platform raised slightly above a much larger platform. Very shortly the rat stepped off the small platform and onto the larger platform where it obtained an electric shock. When these same animals were placed on the small platform a second time they stayed there when no amnesic agent had been applied. If an amnesic agent was applied immediately after the animal stepped off the small platform and the animal was then placed on the platform a second time, he would step off again. As in the studies already quoted, the effect of the amnesic agent diminished when application was postponed in relation to the crucial response. In this situation, the effects of ECS and shock to the feet should summate if the animal is avoiding the electroshock. The same argument could be applied to the more complex situation devised by Pearlman *et al.* (1961) when an animal "forgot" that it had been punished after pressing a lever. In each of these cases the amnesic agent, instead of increasing fear or avoidance, produced what is most plausibly interpreted as an amnesia. This conclusion is strengthened by the result of an experiment conducted by McGaugh and Madsen (1964). These investigators showed that rats did eventually learn to avoid a place when they were given ECS on successive occasions. However, such learning was slow compared with the learning of rats when the shock administered was of a lower intensity but was not strong enough to produce a convulsion. They further showed that when this shock in amounts insufficient to produce a convulsion was followed 5 seconds later by ECS, the ECS slowed down acquisition of avoidance learning of the place where such insufficient shocks were given. Supporting evidence has been reported by Quartermain *et al.* (1965).

It has also been shown that the loss of memory effect cannot be attributed to possible punishing effects of electroconvulsive shock because the same shock applied across the hindlegs of rats under the same conditions produces no such decrement of learning (Duncan, 1949) except at the shortest interval used (20 seconds).

Perhaps the most damaging criticism of ECS as a tool is that it does not produce a retrograde memory deficit at all. Routtenberg and Kay (1965) and Kopp *et al.* (1967) have provided evidence that ECS causes decreased latencies and thus could produce an appearance of amnesia in tests where an increase in latency is taken as evidence of retention. However, such findings by themselves could not explain why somewhat small differences in time of ECS after learning (the retrograde effect) should produce differences in amount of amnesia. However, Schneider and Sherman (1968) have now shown why this explanation in terms of reduced latency could fit the retrograde effect. Schneider and Sherman found that the critical variable to produce an appearance of amnesia was the interval between footshock and ECS. When rats were shocked upon stepping off a platform, ECS 0.5 seconds later produced amnesia 24 hours later. ECS administered 30 seconds or 6 hours later produced no amnesia. However, if a second footshock was given 0.5 seconds before the ECS (given either 30 seconds or 6 hours later), "amnesia" was produced.

Schneider (personal communication) states that the combination of foot-shock and ECS can be given outside the test situation, either before or after the step-off task, and apparent amnesia for the step-off task will still result. It seems that some interaction between footshock and ECS is responsible for the quasi-retrograde amnesia normally observed. It is difficult to see how this explanation could be extended to situations where there is an apparent amnesic effect of ECS even where shock is not used before ECS, such as in the study of Peeke and Herz (1967). However, the "amnesia" in their experiment may have been a simple performance decrement due to ECS as no retrograde action of the ECS was demonstrated. There does seem to be an interaction between ECS and footshock. Coons and Miller (1960) showed that ECS side effects were greater if ECS was administered sooner after footshock.

Another experiment casting doubt on the retrograde amnesic nature of ECS was performed by Misanin *et al.* (1968) who propose a hypothesis which would cover ECS results found in appetitive situations. They trained rats to lick when thirsty. The rats were then exposed to a burst of intense white noise. The offset of this noise coincided with footshock. A control group showed that 24 hours later such noise depressed the rate of licking. The rate of licking was equally unaffected in the group given ECS immediately after the noise-footshock training and in the group where ECS was administered 24 hours later, immediately after a second exposure to the noise. When the white noise was omitted just prior to ECS treatment 24 hours later, memory was not significantly affected, as judged by depression in the rate of licking. The authors explain the result by assuming that ECS has an effect on memory when the memory trace is activated and "that the memory system must be in a state of change at the time of ECS." However, Dawson and McGaugh (1969) repeated the Misanin *et al.* (1968) experiment and were not able to find the same effect. Reactivation of the memory trace before ECS did not produce amnesia. Dawson and McGaugh state, "We have been unable to discover any procedural details that could explain our failure to replicate the findings of Misanin *et al.* (1968)."

II. THE PERMANENCE OF ECS EFFECTS

Turning back again to the original hypothesis which appeared to motivate research with ECS, it was hoped to show that there was a phase during which memory was labile and so subject to destruction by ECS. If this were the case, the application of ECS at some interval after learning should lead to a permanent amnesia for the habit learned (Duncan, 1949). Chevalier (1965) found no diminution of ECS amnesia after a month. Zinkin and Miller (1967) found an apparent recovery of memory after ECS under conditions of repeated testing of a single group. Luttges and McGaugh (1967) found no such effect if separate groups were tested at different time intervals, so that each mouse was retested only once. No apparent recovery of memory occurred after 1 month, even though control animals had not forgotten the task. Kohlenberg and Trabasso (1968) on the other hand, found that mice given ECS performed at the same level as controls 48 hours after treatment, but were markedly inferior after only 24 hours. It is to be noted here that there was a considerable degree of forgetting in the controls after 48 hours. Such a trend can also be seen in the data of McGaugh and Alpern [quoted by McGaugh (1966)]. There are, therefore, discrepancies both in the time course of memory after ECS and without ECS.

Some of the differences with respect to recovery of memory after ECS are resolved by Peeke and Herz (1967) who showed an apparent recovery in mice 72 hours after learning, when such mice had been tested 24 and 48 hours after learning, but no such recovery when mice were tested only 72 hours later. Schneider and Sherman (1968) present data which suggest that recovery of memory after ECS occurs when there is stronger initial learning, as produced by increasing the number of footshocks, but not when such learning is weaker. Another possible reason for this discrepancy in the ECS data has been given by Pagano *et al.* (1969). They have shown that whether memory returns after ECS treatment depends upon the intensity of ECS. Relatively low ECS intensity permitted a return of memory of a step-down task within 24 to 48 hours. There was amnesia at one hour after ECS, in contrast with the results of Geller and Jarvik (1968). Such amnesia was only observed when ECS was administered 0.5 second after footshock. No amnesia was observed when the footshock-ECS interval was 30 seconds. On the other hand, high ECS intensity led to an amnesia which lasted for 48 hours, the longest time after ECS that the rats were tested.

III. IS ECS AMNESIA IMMEDIATE?

An interesting sidelight on the initial hypothesis of consolidation which motivated work with ECS is cast by a study of Geller and Jarvik (1968). These workers found that memory remains for a few hours after ECS but disappears by 24 hours, the interval after which animals treated with ECS have been traditionally tested.

The persistence of a memory a short while after ECS and its disappearance only later, has been confirmed by McGaugh and Landfield (1970).

These results create somewhat of a paradox for the simple consolidation model. It is difficult to see how memory could persist after the labile stage of memory has been destroyed by ECS. There are alternate possibilities to explain Geller and Jarvik's result. The first would be to suppose that there were two processes involved, both beginning with the learning experience. The first would be transient and immune to ECS. The second process would normally be long-lasting but ECS could prevent its initiation. This type of explanation has been suggested in connection with the protein synthesis data. A second possible explanation would be to assume that there was a single process and that ECS accelerates forgetting. The data do not compel us to accept a two-stage model.

IV. EFFECTS OF ECS ON OLDER HABITS

Effects of ECS given after a longer time span have been reported by Hunt and Brady (1951) and a whole series of investigations designed to elucidate these effects has been reported by Hunt (1965). When a sound is used to signal impending unavoidable shock, the sound will suppress ongoing operant behavior, such as pressing a lever for water. This suppression of behavior caused by the sound can be eliminated by giving a rat a whole series of ECS treatments. Such treatments were applied four days after the end of training a rat to press a lever for a reward of water. The suppression of responding caused by the sound disappears for one or two weeks after the ECS treatments. The rat can be trained again during this period to reacquire the behavior. However, the loss of suppression of lever-pressing when the sound occurs is only temporary, and suppression reappears again spontaneously. Though this effect of the electroconvulsive shock looks like an amnesia in some respects, only the warning function of the sound seems forgotten. There is no amnesia for the lever-pressing habit for obtaining water. Other possible interpretations are discussed by Hunt (1965).

Another interesting phenomenon connected with ECS and older habits has recently been reported by Robbins and Meyer (1970) and Howard and Meyer (1971). The phenomenon could be related to that reported by Schneider and Sherman (1968). Rats were taught three two-choice visual discrimination problems one after another. Two different motivations were used. Some discriminations were motivated by shock avoidance and others by food approach. As soon as the rat had completed learning the third discrimination problem, ECS was administered. Twenty four hours later the rats were retested to establish their retention of the first or second discrimination. Either the first or second discrimination would have been motivated in the same way (shock or food) as the third discrimination immediately after the acquisition of which the rat was convulsed. Whether the first or second discrimination was similarly motivated to the third depended on the group assignation of the particular rat. It was found that the retention of a problem was impaired only if the problem had been learned under the same motivation as the problem that had been followed by ECS. Whether the problem had been learned first or second in the series made no difference to retention.

V. CHOLINERGIC SYSTEMS AND ECS

How does ECS operate to produce its effects on memory? While ECS undoubtedly has many behavioral effects many of which can be mistaken for effects on memory, on balance it seems reasonable that ECS does have some effect on memory. Recent research strongly suggests that ECS has its amnesic effect via a change in the cholinergic system. The release of bound acetylcholine as a result of ECS increases the activity of cholinergic neurons (Richter & Crossland, 1969). As a result of the release of such acetylcholine there may be induction of the enzyme acetylcholinesterase (Adams, Hobbit, & Sutker, 1969). Adams *et al.* found elevations in acetylcholinesterase levels after a series of four ECS treatments. In a behavioral assay for memory, they trained rats to avoid footshock when a light appeared. After training, three ECS treatments were administered. The rats were retested four hours later. Half an hour before retest the rats were injected with either physostigmine or scopolamine or saline. (Physostigmine increases acetylcholine levels, while scopolamine reduces the effect of a given level of acetylcholine on the postsynaptic ending). While ECS amnesia was not affected by saline, physostigmine enhanced and scopolamine reduced such amnesia. Physostigmine alone without ECS also produced some retention loss. These results suggest that ECS raises acetylcholine concentrations which then lead to synaptic block and consequent amnesia (see section on cholinergic synapse and memory). That ECS has effect on memory analogous to cholinergic drugs has been shown in a very interesting experiment by Wiener (1970). Wiener trained animals in a single session in a Y maze to escape shock by running to the lit alley to ten consecutive correct trials. Then at various times after training (5 minutes to 31 days) rats were given ECS and retested 24 hours later. The results of the retest were very similar to those obtained with anticholinesterases. There was an initial amnesic effect (5 minutes to 1 day) followed by no effect at 1 to 3 days. At 7 to 14 days there was again amnesia. At 31 days where controls show considerable forgetting, the ECS treated animals actually show facilitation much as they do as when they are treated with anticholinesterase. Wiener also found that scopolamine acted as a complete antidote against the amnesic effects of ECS while physostigmine augmented the effect of ECS.

Davis, Thomas, and Adams (1971) also studied the effects of cholinergic agents on ECS induced amnesia, but on a one trial passive avoidance habit. Physostigmine administered before the learning trial and ECS protected memory four hours later from disruption. Scopolamine injected prior to the retention trial served as an antidote to the memory disruption produced by ECS alone in the control group.

VI. ECS AMNESIA AS ACCELERATED FORGETTING

Because ECS experiments had been designed to show that a memory was initially in a labile state and that it needed some time to become fixed, it seemed quite adequate only to test animals 24 hours later. If animals could not remember at that time it was assumed that the short term labile memory had been knocked out before it had become fixed. If animals could remember 24 hours after ECS, it was assumed that fixation had taken place. However, these assumptions have now shown to be false. Geller and Jarvik's (1968) experiment showed that ECS did not knock the memory out immediately. Hughes, Barrett, and Ray (1970a,b) showed that while lower intensities of ECS or longer intervals between learning and ECS had no significant amnesic effect at 24 hours, they did produce premature forgetting at a later test time. It seems that there is a time just after the experience during which ECS simply accelerates forgetting. These results lead to a radically different model of memory consolidation. It looks as if there is a gradual change in the memory trace with time. Agents such as ECS, protein synthesis inhibitors, KCl, etc., alter the rate at which consolidation takes place; that is, they alter the slope of growth by some constant factor. The alteration may be so large that the slope of growth may actually become negative if the agent applied is strong enough. From this it follows that if an agent of a given strength is applied early during the process of growth, and then, if the slope of growth becomes negative, the memory trace will shrink to zero (Hughes et al., 1970b). If two agents of unequal strength are applied at the same point in the process of consolidation, then it will take longer for the memory trace to shrink to zero after the weaker agent (Hughes et al., 1970). While such a model is simpler than the two-stage consolidation hypothesis and can account for most of the experimental data somewhat more convincingly, both hypotheses have difficulty in explaining why, at least in some cases, memory returns after it has apparently been lost due to ECS. If ECS blocks retrieval temporarily instead of causing decay of storage, then we must begin to think in other terms. We may have to abandon the assumption, already made tenuous by Wiener's (1970) work, that the agent which produces its effect on memory is the electric current. It seems more likely that the electric current sets in train a gradually increasing biochemical imbalance. This imbalance interacts with the increasing strength of the underlying mnemonic trace in influencing retrievability of such a trace. Eventually biochemical balance may recover, leading to a gradual retrievability of the mnemonic trace.

REFERENCES

Abt, J. P., Essman, W. B., & Jarvik, M. E. Ether-induced retrograde amnesia for one-trial conditioning in mice. *Science*, 1961, Vol. 133, 1477-1478.

Adams, H. E., Hobbit, P. R., & Sutker, P. B. Electroconvulsive shock, brain acetylcholinesterase activity and memory. *Physiological Behavior*, 1969, Vol. 4, 113-116.

Alpern, H. P., & McGaugh, J. L. Retrograde Amnesia as a function of duration of electroshock stimulation. *Journal of Comparative Physiology*, 1968, Vol. 65, 265-269.

Bohdanecky, Z., Kopp, R., & Jarvik, M. E. Comparison of ECS and Flurothyl-induced retrograde amnesia in mice. *Psychopharmacologia (Berlin)*, 1968, Vol. 12, 91, 95.

Bures, J., Buresova, O., & Fifkova, E. Interhemispheric transfer of a passive avoidance reaction. *Journal of Comparative & Physiological Psychology*, 1964, Vol. 57, 326-30.

Cerf, J. A., & Otis, L. S. Heat narcosis and its effect on retention of a learned behavior in the goldfish. *Federation Proceedings*, 1957, Vol. 16, 20-21.

Chevalier, J. A. Permanence of amnesia after a single posttrial electroconvulsive seizure. *Journal of Comparative & Physiological Psychology*, 1965, Vol. 59, 125-27.

Chorover, S. L., & Schiller, P. H. Short-term retrograde amnesia in rats. *Journal of Comparative & Physiological Psychology*, 1965, Vol. 59, 73-78.

Coons, E. E., & Miller, N. E. Conflict versus consolidation of memory traces to explain "retrograde amnesia" produced by ECS. *Journal of Comparative & Physiological Psychology*, 1960, Vol. 53, 524-31.

Cronholm, B. Post-ECT amnesias in the pathology of memory. In A. Talland and N. Waugh (Eds.), *The pathology of memory*. New York: Academic Press, 1969. Pp. 81-89.

Davis, J. W., Thomas, R. K. Jr., & Adams, H. E. Interactions of scopolamine and physostigmine with ECS and one trial learning. *Physiology & Behavior*, 1971, Vol. 6, 219-222.

Dawson, R. G., & McGaugh, J. L. Electroconvulsive shock produced retrograde amnesia: analysis of the vamiliarization effect. *Communications in Behavioral Biology*, 1969, Vol. 4, 91-95.

Dorfman, L. J., & Jarvik, M. E. A parametric study of electroshock-induced retrograde amnesia in mice. *Neuropsychologia*, 1968, Vol. 6, 373-380.

Duncan, C. P. The retroactive effects of shock on learning. *Journal of Comparative & Physiological Psychology*, 1949, Vol. 42, 32-34.

Geller, A., & Jarvik, M. E. The time relations of ECS induced amnesia. *Psychonomic Science*, 1968, Vol. 12, 169-70.

Gerbrandt, L. K., Buresova, O., & Bures, J. Discrimination and reversal learning followed by a single electroconvulsive shock. *Physiology & Behavior*, 1968, Vol. 3, 149-53.

Hebb, D. O. *The organization of behavior*. New York: Wiley, 1949.

Howard, R. L., & Meyer, D. R. Motivational control of retrograde amnesia in rats. *Journal of Comparative & Physiological Psychology*, 1971, Vol. 74, 37-40.

Hughes, R. A., Barrett, R. J., & Ray, O. S. Retrograde amnesia in rats increases as a function of ECS-test interval and ECS intensity. *Physiology & Behavior*, 1970, Vol. 5, 27-30.

Hughes, R. A., Barrett, R. J., & Ray, O. S. Training to test interval as a determinant of a temporarily graded ECS-produced response decrement in rats. JCPP, 1970, Vol. 71, 318-324.

Hunt, H. F. Electro-convulsive shock and learning. *Transactions of the New York Academy of Sciences*, 1965, Vol. 27, 923-45.

Hunt, H. F., & Brady, J. V. Some effects of electro-convulsive shock on a conditioned emotional response ("anxiety"). *Journal of Comparative & Physiological Psychology*, 1951, Vol. 44, 88-98.

Jarvik, M. E., & Kopp, R. An improved one-trial passive avoidance learning situation. *Psychological Report*, 1967, Vol. 21, 221-224.

Kohlenberg, R., & Trabasso, T. Recovery of a conditioned emotional response after one or two electroconvulsive shocks. *Journal of Comparative & Physiological Psychology*, 1968, Vol. 65, 270-273.

Kopp, R., Bohdanecky, Z., & Jarvik, M. E. Proactive effect of a single ECS on step-through performance on naive and punished mice. *Journal of Comparative & Physiological Psychology*, 1967, Vol. 64, 22-25.

Leukel, F. A. A comparison of the effects of ECS and anesthesia on acquisition of the maze habit. *Journal of Comparative & Physiological Psychology*, 1957, Vol. 50, 300-306.

Luttges, M. E., & McGaugh, J. L. Permanence of retrograde amnesia produced by electroconvulsive shock. *Science*, 1967, Vol. 156, 408-10.

McGaugh, J. L. Facilitative and disruptive effects of strychnine sulphate on maze learning. *Psychological Report*, 1961, Vol. 8, 99-104.

McGaugh, J. L. Time-dependent processes in memory storage. *Science*, 1966, Vol. 153, 1351-58.

McGaugh, J. L. Time dependent processes in memory storage. *Science*, 1966, Vol. 153, 1351-1358.

McGaugh, J. L. & Alpern, H. P. Effects of electroshock on memory: amnesia without convulsions. *Science*, 1966, Vol. 152, 665-666.

McGaugh, J. L., & Landfield, P. W. Delayed development of amnesia following electroconvulsive shock. *Physiology & Behaviour*, 1970, Vol. 5, 1109-1113.

McGaugh, J. L., & Madsen, M. C. Amnesic and punishing effects of electroconvulsive shock. *Science*, 1964, Vol. 144, 182-183.

Misanin, J. R., Miller, R. R., & Lewis, D. J. Retrograde amnesia produced by electroconvulsive shock after reactivation of a consolidated memory trace. *Science*, 1968, Vol. 160, 554-555.

Misanin, J. R., Miller, R. R., & Lewis, D. J. Retrograde amnesia produced by electroconvulsive shock.

Muller, G. E., & Pilzecker, A. Experimentelle Beitrage zur Lehre vom Gedaechtmiss. *Zeitschrift für Psychologie Physiologie Sinnesorg*, 1900, Vol. I, 1-300.

Pagano, R. R., Bush, D. R., Martin, G., & Hunt, E. B. Duration of retrograde amnesia as a function of electroconvulsive shock intensity. *Physiological Behaviour*, 1969, Vol. 4, 19-21.

Pearlman, C. A., Sharpless, S. K., & Jarvik, M. E. Retrograde amnesia produced by anesthetic and convulsant agents. *Journal of Comparative & Physiological Psychology*, 1961, Vol. 54, 109-12.

Peeke, H. V. S. & Herz, M. J. Permanence of electroconvulsive shock produced retrograde amnesia. *Proceedings 75th Annual Convention of the American Psychological Association*, 1967, Vol. 2, 85-86.

Quartermain, D., Paolino, R. M., & Miller, N. E. A brief temporal gradient of retrograde amnesia independent of situational change. *Science*, 1965, Vol. 149, 1116-1118.

Richter, D., & Crossland, J. Variation in acetylcholine content of the brain with physiological state. *American Journal of Physiology*, 1969, Vol. 159, 247-255.

Routtenberg, A. & Kay, K. E. Effect of one electroconvulsive seizure on rat behavior. *Journal of Comparative & Physiological Psychology*, 1965, Vol. 59, 285-288.

Schneider, A. M. & Sherman, W. Amnesia: A function of the temporal relation of footshock to electroconvulsive shock. *Science*, 1968, Vol. 59, 219-221.

Thompson, R., & Dean, W. A. A further study on the retroactive effects of ECS. *Journal of Comparative & Physiological Psychology*, 1955, Vol. 48, 488-91.

Thompson, R., & Pryer, R. S. The effect of anoxia on the retention of a discrimination habit. *Journal of Comparative & Physiological Psychology*, 1964, Vol. 57, 321-25.

Thomson, C. W., McGaugh, J. L., Smith, C. E., Hudspeth, W. J., & Westbrook, W. H. Strain differences in the retroactive effects of electroconvulsive shock on maze learning. *Canadian Journal of Psychology*, 1961, Vol. 15, 69-74.

Wiener, N. I. Electroconvulsive shock induced impairment and enhancement of a learned escape response. *Physiology & Behaviour*, 1970, Vol. 5, 971-974.

Williams, M. Traumatic retrograde amnesia and normal forgetting. In G. A. Tallard and N. C. Waugh (Eds.), *The pathology of memory*. New York: Academic Press, 1969. Pp. 75-80.

Williams, M. Memory studies in ECT. *Journal of Neurology, Neurosurgery, & Psychiatry*, 1950, Vol. 13, 30-35, 314-319.

Woolley, D. W., Rosenzweig, M. R., Krech, D., Bennett, E. L., & Thomas, P. S. Strain and sex differences in threshold and pattern of electroshock convulsions in rats. *Physiologist*, 1960, Vol. 3, 182.

Zinkin, S., & Miller, A. J. Recovery of memory after amnesia induced by electroconvulsive shock. *Science*, 1967, Vol. 155, 102-104.

Zornetzer, S., & McGaugh, J. L. Effects of frontal brain electroshock stimulation on EEG activity and memory in rats: relationship to ECS-produced retrograde amnesia. *Journal of Neurobiology*, 1970, Vol. 1, 379-394.

CHAPTER

6

ELECTROPHYSIOLOGICAL ANALYSES OF LEARNING AND MEMORY

ARNOLD L. LEIMAN

and

CLIFFORD N. CHRISTIAN

I. INTRODUCTION

Nerve cells receive, generate, and conduct excitation. These properties form the basic vocabulary, and neural connections determine the complexity of the nervous system's language. Throughout the animal kingdom, from the most eloquent to the most reticent of nervous systems, from the brains of primates to the nerve nets of coelenterates, one can observe not only statements of the present but messages from the past. A facile but compelling explanation is near at hand: parameters of neural systems are subject to transitory or enduring modifications. The past, speaking the language of the nervous system, informs the present.

The way in which nervous systems accomplish the feat of memory is not understood. Although considerable advance has been made in the understanding of basic features of nervous conduction, synaptic transmission, and the computations of neural networks, our comprehension of storage mechanisms is composed of tantalizing hunches which occasionally verge on plausible models. Writing 40 years ago, Lashley said of the hypotheses proposed for memory: "This list of theories includes almost every conceivable change which could occur in a system made up of nerve cells . . . . No one more than another serves to unify and make more intelligible the diverse phenomena of learning [Lashley, 1934]." Such a list compiled today (Table 6-1) shows an increase in the range of conceivable change but no decrease in the wisdom of Lashley's judgment. Clearly, choices and exclusions are warranted. In writing this report we wish to convey in broad outlines the best guesses, strategies, and data which comprise current electrophysiological inquiries about memory. To this end, we present representative findings and approaches rather than provide the exhaustive rendering of other reviews (e.g., John, 1961, 1967; Morrell, 1961; Kandel & Spencer, 1968; Horn & Hinde, 1970).

A. The Scale of Inquiry: A Quest for Simplicity

The experimental approach to the neurology of the acquisition and retention of experience once seemed rather straightforward. After all, memory was somewhere in brains, and with scalpels, recording probes, and persistence, the textbook illustrations of the conditioned reflex would be reified in the form of relations among sets of neurons in an anatomically defined storage system. Frustrating years spent attempting to extirpate engrams, however, made some conclude that experiential traces were elusive and perhaps even diffusely distri-

TABLE 6-1

Samples of Proposed Memory Mechanisms

Structure modifications	Reference	Process modifications	Reference
Birth of neurons	Altman, 1966	Facilitation of synapses with successful use	Hebb, 1949
Directed growth of nerve processes and creation of synapses	Ariens Kappers, 1917	Frequency tuned nerve membranes	Landauer, 1964
Axon terminals swell during activity	Eccles, 1953	Long-term posttetanic potentiation	Eccles, 1953
Spine apparatus storage	Hamlyn, 1962	Perineuronal pattern recognition	Adey, 1969
Glial storage	Galambos, 1961	Facilitation of synapses with disuse	Sharpless, 1964
Destruction of synapses	Ranck, 1964	Turning off synapses	Young, 1966
Death of neurons	Dawkins, 1971	Coherence of population activity	John, 1967
		Heterosynaptic activity	Burke, 1966
		Tuning motor system to sensory frequencies	Loeb, 1902
		Neural holograms	Pribram, 1966
		Residual excitation in neurons	Ebbecke, 1919

buted (Lashley, 1950). Representations of learning and memory as a change in the properties of discrete circuits or connections were first regarded with scepticism and then dismissed with deprecation as "switchboard" theories.

Following a period of experimental quiescence, sophisticated electro-physiological monitoring systems were developed. Measures of performance in conditioning or discrimination learning were related to gross potentials recorded from chronically implanted electrodes. At this level of analysis there is a wealth of data concerning both changes in the characteristics of endogenous spontaneous activity, and modifications of the amplitude and waveform of evoked activity. These measures are not signals of information transaction but samples from an enormous aggregate of neurons. They are statistical representations of the spatial and temporal distribution of synaptic potentials and action potentials in very complex networks. And, although there is strength (that is, reliability) in numbers, there is ambiguity as well. Rather than specifying transactions at cellular connections, models of learning or memory formulated at this level of analysis emphasize such dimensions as the probabilities of discharge in populations of neurons (e.g., John, 1967).

The mammalian brain contains ten to twenty billion neurons, each with a myriad array of synapses. The depiction of this system, even in the most impressionistic terms, produces a portrait of bewildering complexity for the researcher seeking clues to the biology of memory. The quest for simplicity in neurophysiological approaches to this problem is taking several forms. Some experimenters emphasize the use of nervous systems organized more simply than mammalian brains. The successful use of bacteria in elucidating the molecular mechanisms of species inheritance has provided inspiration for the pursuit of learning or analogous processes in "miniaturized" nervous systems. Candidates for such small neuron assemblies include (1) invertebrate nervous systems, particularly components of such systems that include morphologically and functionally identifiable inputs and outputs, (2) surgically isolated portions of mammalian nervous systems, for example, isolated spinal cords, and (3) mammalian nervous tissue cultures. Other examples of structurally or functionally simple systems, perhaps with the ability to learn, include immature nervous systems and drug modified nervous systems. In these systems we may possibly discern the intimate details of neural transactions in circuits which, it is believed, can be described in detail. Learning mechanisms found at this level of analysis may provide a model of the elementary memory processes of more complex nervous systems. This aspiration is clearly buoyed by the evidence of basically similar signalling mechanisms in the nervous systems of all animals.

Some doubts about the feasibility of this approach can be answered with data already collected. It has been objected that any simple system is mneumonically nugatory; learning and memory are only to be found in tortuous webs of neural networks. This ignores the rapidly accumulating evidence, however, that

almost all nervous systems, and many neural subsystems, at least display habituation. Another difficulty is to bridge the gap between neurophysiology and
psychology. This entails the depiction of the relevant circuitry for behaviors
conforming to the psychologist's criteria of learning. A description of the
dynamics of a single synapse obviously falls far short of an explanation of the
elaboration and retention of complex learned responses. The resolution of this
difficulty awaits a demonstration of the strength of similarity between simple
and complex systems. A generalization from the one to the other must be
tempered by verification.

B. Electrical Signals in Nervous Systems

An electrode within a single nerve cell can register two principal forms of
activity: (1) action potentials (nerve impulses) and (2) graded or synaptic
potentials. The action potential is the characteristic form of the output of
axonal zones. It is a regenerative state which, once initiated, travels without
decrement to the terminal portions of the axon. Most neurons display this form
of response, although there is growing sentiment that amacrine cells in the retina
and certain neurons in the mammalian central nervous system are without
axonal processes and probably do not display action potentials. Graded potentials result from changes in membrane conductance at synaptic or receptive
zones. They are either excitatory (membrane depolarization) or inhibitory
(membrane hyperpolarization). They arise from local changes in ion permeability produced at most synapses by the release of transmitter from a presynaptic terminal. Nerve impulses in the terminal region of an axon produce the
release of a transmitter substance. The sequence of steps coupling the arrival
of an impulse with the liberation of transmitter is not understood, but
is known to require calcium ions. The transmitter substance is generally believed
to be contained in synaptic vesicles-inclusions found in the presynaptic axon.
The contents of these vesicles are probably released as a packet and diffuse
across the synaptic cleft. The sign of the result—depolarization or hyperpolarization—is not inherent in the type of transmitter, but apparently depends on some
feature of the postsynaptic membrane. Wachtel and Kandel (1971) have shown
that the same transmitter produces excitation and inhibition in some cells. The
magnitude of the postsynaptic graded potential is directly related to the amount
of released transmitter.

Many neurons function as neural accountants: they tally up their instan-
taneous inputs and respond if the total exceeds a fixed amount. A multipolar
cell in the mammalian nervous system is studded with many synapses. This
somatodendritic surface may be thought of as a receptive pole. Local depolarizations or hyperpolarizations are algebraically summed at the axon hillock and
at a critical depolarization level a nerve impulse is initiated. The complexities of

dendritic synaptic mechanisms have been examined by Purpura (1967) and Rall (1970).

The synapse we have considered is simply the functional connection of two neurons. When three neurons are considered, more elaborate functions are possible. A number of findings indicate that axons end on the presynaptic terminals of other axons, producing presynaptic facilitation or presynaptic inhibition. These processes vary the amount of transmitter released from the second axon ending, and, hence, modulate its effect on its postsynaptic neuron. Unusually long periods of inhibition can be produced in this way.

II. HABITUATION

The progressive waning of a response to a regularly repeated stimulus is one of the most elementary and ubiquitous forms of behavior modifiability exhibited in the animal kingdom. The types of behavior that attenuate are as extensive as the variety of animals displaying them and include species-characteristic escape or defensive responses, orientation to exteroceptive stimuli, exploratory behavior, startle responses, and polysynaptic reflexes. Habituation is the term most commonly used in discussions of this phenomenon, near cognates being "negative learning," negative adaptation, acclimatization, accommodation, stimulatory inactivation, inhibition, and fatigue (Harris, 1943). In many cases, habituation indicates that an animal is learning to distinguish between novel and familiar stimuli in its environment.

Habituation should be differentiated from other decremental processes. A waning in responsiveness may arise from the diminished sensitivity of a sensory receptor, as in light adaptation of photoreceptors. Response strength may decline because muscles fatigue, various behaviors are diminished in motivational states such as satiety, and hormones may attenuate some behaviors while potentiating others. Although these processes are types of biological memory and mediate adaptive changes in behavior, they are not habituation.

The defining characteristics of habituation have been described by Harris (1943) and Thompson and Spencer (1966). They include (1) decreased response magnitude with repeated stimulation; (2) response recovery in the absence of stimulation; (3) greater response decrement with a weaker stimulus; (4) generalization of habituation to stimuli similar to the repeated stimulus; and (5) dishabituation, the recovery of an habituated response after one presentation of a different stimulus. It should be noted that habituation is produced by nonreinforced stimuli; it is the decrement in the response to stimuli without consequence to the organism. Clearly, stimulus repetition per se may have a variety of outcomes other than habituation. The apparent simplicity of the usual habituation experiment, often involving stereotyped species-typical behaviors, has encouraged neurophysiologists to search for correlates of this memory process at the cellular level.

A. Habituation in Unicellular Animals

A surprisingly large variety of behaviors can be found in the class Protozoa. Single-celled animals, such as the *Amoeba* or *Paramecium*, can exhibit elaborate locomotor patterns associated with feeding, graded movements of approach or withdrawal elicited by mechanical, chemical, light or electrical stimuli, and some rudimentary experiential changes in behavior. Some investigators consider protozoan response modification as a possible model for plasticity in higher organisms. After observing the response of the unicellular *Stentor roeselii* to repetitive stimuli, Jennings (1906) commented,

> . . . after responding once or a few times to very weak stimulation, the organism becomes changed, so that it no longer reacts as before, and that this change is not due to fatigue either of the contractile apparatus or of the perceptive power. The behavior may then be of the same regulatory character as is the similar behavior in higher animals.

In the intervening years, numerous studies have described decremental processes in protozoans analogous to habituation in higher organisms. Most recently, Wood (1970a) investigated the response of *Stentor coeruleus* to repetitive mechanical stimulation. Animals are placed in a beaker attached to a solenoid that moves quickly downward, producing a general body contraction. Stimuli delivered once a minute result in a progressive decrease in the probability of response. This response decline endures for a period of 3 hours. The contraction threshold for electrical stimulation is not changed by repetitive mechanical stimulation, indicating some stimulus specificity in this decremental process.

Although the cellular organization of these animals includes elaborate cytoplasmic differentiation at an organelle level, there is little evidence for a specialized nervous system similar to that of multicellular animals. Rather, the protozoan has some of the properties of a single neuron. Microelectrode studies of protozoan cell membranes have found both resting potentials and action potentials associated with effector activation. Wood (1970b, c) examined the relation between intracellular potential changes in *Stentor* and the decreased response to repetitive stimulation. A mechanical stimulus elicited two principal electrical potential states: (1) a prepotential attributed to a receptor process, and (2) a spike potential correlated with cell contraction. The decreased probability of body contraction is accompanied by a decline in the prepotential amplitude and an increase in its latency. These changes are interpreted as a modification in receptor operations producing a decline in body contraction.

Being unicellular and integrating some features of their experience over long time periods, protozoans apparently make attractive model systems for the detailed physiological analysis of behavioral plasticity. On the other hand, the physiological operations of these animals are a quite different solution to the demands of successful adaptation than that which characterizes multicellular organisms with structurally differentiated nervous mechanisms.

B. Single Synapse Habituation

Major contributions to the understanding of basic neurophysiological mechanisms have partially depended on various "natural bonuses," notably the existence in certain animals of large structural elements which remain viable during *in vitro* isolation. Hodgkin and Huxley, in their incisive work on the action potential process, were greatly indebted to the squid giant axon. Similarly, studies of the mechanisms of synaptic transmission have involved preparations in which single synapses could be effectively isolated, such as nerve-muscle junctions and the giant synapse of the squid stellate ganglion. Decremental processes have been noted in these model synapses, although such changes have seldom been described in the context of habituation. Recently, however, Horn and Wright (1970) have examined the giant synapse of the squid stellate ganglion using conventional habituation stimulus paradigms. In this preparation, a single electrical shock delivered to the presynaptic element elicits, after some minimum delay, an excitatory postsynaptic potential and an action potential. Repetitive trials, consisting of 20 successive electrical pulses delivered within one-half second, are delivered to the presynaptic element. During the initial trial, each pulse elicits a spike of slightly increasing latency. If trials are presented every 10 seconds, spike latencies during each trial increase more rapidly, and later pulses gradually fail to elicit spikes. This decremental process lasts for seconds. As synaptic transmission diminishes, the time of initiation of the graded EPSP remains constant, but its slope decreases. Over one trial the magnitude of the graded response decreases until it is insufficient to initiate an impulse. Horn and Wright (1970) argue that this response decline is due to a presynaptic mechanism rather than a postsynaptic membrane alteration or postsynaptic inhibitory potential. They suggest that this simple form of transmission failure arises from a modification of the link between the action potential and the release of transmitter.

In the crayfish neuromuscular synapse a more prolonged monosynaptic depression has been similarly related to a presynaptic transmitter mechanism. Bruner and Kennedy (1970) have suggested that this process is a simple analog of habituation at a behavioral level, although its actual contribution to the behavior of these animals is as yet unspecified. The crayfish fast abdominal flexor is innervated, among others, by a motor giant neuron which can be uniquely excited. The decremental features of this neuromuscular synapse are more complex than those of the stellate ganglion in that attenuation or facilitation may be produced by changing stimulus frequency. A marked decrement in end plate potentials accompanies low frequencies of stimulation; three stimuli at one minute intervals result in a decline of responsiveness requiring five minutes to recover. A facilitatory or potentiation process becomes evident at higher stimulus frequencies, being maximal at two per second. Because the end plate potential declines when only one neuromuscular synapse is active, and no change in the postsynaptic membrane is observed, decrements are probably due to the presynaptic mechanism of a single synapse. Interestingly, the rate of attenuation is unaffected by changes in Mg^{++} or Ca^{++} concentrations sufficient to decrease the amount of transmitter released per end plate potential. Hence, the decremental process does not result from the simple depletion of presynaptic transmitter stores.

Although attenuation in these single identifiable synapses is in some respects isomorphic to behavioral habituation, there are several behavioral responses known to be mediated by monosynaptic neuronal circuits (involving, however, many parallel synapses) which do not display such decremental effects.

C. Invertebrate Giant Fiber System Habituation

The velocity of conduction of the nerve impulse in any fiber is directly related to its diameter. The large diameter nerve fibers of some invertebrates exhibit conduction velocities of from 5 to 30 meters per second. Presumably, the prime selectional advantage of these fibers is their capacity for rapid conduction, and with this possibility in mind, many investigators have frequently suggested and demonstrated the relation between the activation of invertebrate giant fibers and aspects of such species typical protective behaviors as escape, evasion, and defense. These behaviors in invertebrates are often mediated by the short latency, synchronous contraction of muscles. Giant fiber systems related to evasion behavior have been described in annelids, insects, crustacea, and molluscs. In all these animals, the giant fibers constitute a small percentage of the total fiber or connective system. However, the accessibility for recording purposes and the apparent simplicity of the elicited behavior make giant fiber systems good candidates for the examination of habituation mechanisms. Under some circumstances, the escape behaviors mediated by giant fiber systems wane with repetitive elicitation and in some animals this diminution of responsiveness can last for hours. Unfortunately, it is difficult to reconcile the ease of habituation with the presumed survival value of short latency responses. If they are important in protecting the animal it is not clear why fast escape responses should drop out so quickly. Perhaps laboratory habituation paradigms utilizing these behavior systems obscure the highly successful adaptive capabilities of evasive behaviors mediated by giant fibers.

1. Annelid Escape Behavior Habituation

Many polychaetes and most oligochaetes have giant fibers, which usually run the length of the ventral cord. Only species having these fibers emit the rapid withdrawal reflex, a fast contraction of longitudinal muscles elicited by sudden changes in stimuli. For tubiculous and burrowing annelids, the reflex serves to retract the anterior body into a tube or burrow. Although a slow, long latency evasive response persists after many repetitions of mild stimuli, the rapid withdrawal quickly habituates.

The rapid withdrawal of the earthworm *Lumbricus terrestris* decreases in strength and ceases after approximately 10 proddings of its anterior end (Roberts, 1962b). The response is associated with a burst of action potentials in the medial giant fiber (Roberts, 1962a). Electrical stimulation of the medial giant fiber causes muscle contraction, which quickly habituates. However, stimulation of the longitudinal muscle or the motor neurons innervating the muscle yields a contraction which habituates very slowly. Thus the attenuation does not involve neuromuscular fatigue but a decrement with repetition in the transmission from the giant fiber to the motor neuron. If the sensory nerves distal to the cord are stimulated, the number of action potentials elicited in the medial giant fiber also quickly decreases, indicating a decrement in transmission between the sensory and giant fibers.

By similar experiments, it can be shown that facilitation of the withdrawal response during the first few stimulus presentations is mediated by an increased transmission between the giant and motor neurons (Roberts, 1966). Thus, a short-term facilitation and a longer habituation of the withdrawal reflex involve plastic connections in the central nerve cord rather than in peripheral structures. Unfortunately, a precise location of these connections awaits an anatomical description of the synaptic junctions of the medial giant fiber.

A decrement in the sensory to giant connection mediates withdrawal response habituation in other annelids (Horridge, 1959; Gwilliam, 1969). Its adaptive significance is apparently the prevention of any one reflex dominating the response repertoire of the animal. Placing the plastic connection in the central nervous system permits a change in response while the sensory receptors maintain maximal sensitivity. The reason for the habituation of the giant to motor connection is less clear, but may involve the protection of the longitudinal muscles from fatigue.

2. Insects

Various insects also have a small number (4 to 8) of giant fibers. They course a considerable distance from the last abdominal ganglion to thoracic ganglia and perhaps to the brain (Hughes, 1965). Conduction velocity in this system may not be uniform along their length, since at least some of the giant fibers taper at the thoracic ganglia level (Spira, Parnas, and Bergmann, 1969). In cockroaches, locusts, and other insects these giant fibers form part of a circuit mediating evasive or escape behavior. In cockroaches, the giant fibers are second-order neurons activated by afferents on the tip of the abdomen (the anal cerci) and connected to thoracic motor cells controlling the leg muscles. Mechanical stimuli (e.g., puff of air or touch) delivered to the cerci elicit a startle movement. The latency of this response ranges between 28-90 msec (Roeder, 1963), with 10 percent of the reaction time taken by the giant fiber conduction time. Stimuli delivered at frequent intervals result in habituation of the startle response. Huber (1965) has shown that stimulus intervals of 1 minute do not elicit decrementing responses; at intervals of 30 seconds or 15 seconds habituation is evident. This decremental process can also be shown in an isolated abdomen preparation in which the measured response process is the giant fiber action potential. The cercal nerve response can unfailingly follow stimulus frequencies of at least one per second, hence the decrementing process seemingly does not involve the receptor interface. The initial labile element in this behavior thus appears to be the synapses between the cercal afferents and the giant fibers. In addition to habituation, this system displays a diurnal variation in responsiveness, suggesting a hormonal modulation.

3. Crustacea

The crayfish can quickly flex its abdomen to produce a rapid backward "darting" movement generally described as escape behavior. Presumably, this response is related to predator encounters, although there are no complete naturalistic descriptions of its characteristics in nonlaboratory settings. Under experimental conditions it can be elicited by visual, tactual, and proprioceptive stimuli, and is reported to be quite variable. This escape response rapidly habituates to light stimuli delivered to the eye and cannot be elicited by the less sensitive photoreceptor present in the sixth abdominal ganglion (Chow & Leiman, 1971). Krasne (1969) has described the characteristics of escape response decrement under conditions in which abdominal flexion is produced by lateral compression of the abdomen. In these studies, the animal was restrained by rigidly holding its thorax. A thread attached to the tail fin was connected to a transducer for recording the abdominal flexion. Failure of the response to an abdominal segment pinch was evident within ten trials separated by 5-minute intervals. Recovery from the habituated state is barely evident following an hour rest period and remains somewhat below baseline 6 hours later. Further studies by Krasne (1969) have analyzed a synaptic system which is probably a component of the mediating circuit. He studied an afferent portion of this circuit: synaptic potentials elicited in the lateral giant fiber by root stimulation. The elicited synaptic potential complex is composed of an initial stabile portion and later labile components. With frequencies of stimulation greater than 2 per second, the later components attenuate. The pathway involved in this later response is reasonably assumed to be polysynaptic.

D. Habituation in Identifiable Cells: The Case of Aplysia

The marine Gastropid *Aplysia* has come to play a particularly valued role in the plans and products of contemporary neurophysiology. It has an honored status because a number of nerve cells in its ganglia are extraordinarily large. The size of these neurons permits visual identification and prolonged intracellular recording. Thus, the same cell can be examined in all members of the species. Detailed circuitry relations have been established for a number of these identifiable cells (e.g., Frazier, Kandel, Kuppferman, Waziri, & Coggeshall, 1967).

Decrements in the synaptic transmission to identifiable cells have been described by several investigators. Bruner and Tauc (1966) used a simplified preparation consisting of an isolated *Aplysia* head with attached tentacles, connectives, and ganglia. A drop of water delivered to the head results in a tentacle contraction which wanes with successive stimulations. A period of rest or a scratching of the skin reinstrates the contraction. An electrophysiological correlate of this response is a complex excitatory postsynaptic potential in a giant cell of the left pleural ganglion. The amplitude of this synaptic potential declines with repetitive stimulation and declines more rapidly if previous habituation has occurred. The preparation may be further simplified by isolating the ganglia and electrically stimulating afferents of the cell. This produces a simpler synaptic potential which attentuates during repetitive stimulation, and is dishabituated by shocks delivered to the left pleural ganglion. After dishabituation, synaptic potentials are often greater in amplitude than before habituation, supporting the view that dishabituation is not a simple reversal of habituation but, rather, is a superimposed potentiation.

A prime advantage of miniaturized nervous systems is the possibility of exhaustively depicting a neuronal network that mediates a behavioral response exhibiting plasticity. To date, the sole example of this is an elegant series of studies which successively link a defensive behavior to a defined network (Pinsker, Kupferman, Castellucci, & Kandel, 1970; Castellucci, Pinsker, Kupferman, & Kandel, 1970). In *Aplysia*, gill withdrawal occurs spontaneously and can also be elicited by tactile stimulation. This later response habituates within five to ten trials, and may remain depressed from 10 minutes to 2 hours. Dishabituation can be produced by changing the locus of tactile stimuli. Because habituation does not change the magnitude of spontaneous gill contractions, it is not produced by generalized fatigue. The neural circuit for this behavior consists of four motor neurons within the abdominal ganglion that receive sensory input over both monosynaptic and polysnaptic pathways. Repetitive stimulation decreases both the spike discharges and the excitatory postsynaptic potentials elicited in these cells. During the decline in the input to these neurons, their ability to drive the response does not change, since stimulation by intracellular depolarization still elicits gill contractions. The plastic link is thus afferent to the motor neurons. This connection can be studied in an isolated abdominal ganglion connected by a nerve to a small piece of skin. Electrical stimulation of the skin evokes an electrical postsynaptic potential described by the investigators as "elementary" in form and probably monosynaptic. Evidence indicates that the tactile stimulus is conveyed to the motor neuron by a single sensory neuron. This monosynaptic pathway displays habituation, and dishabituation (the facilitation of the postsynaptic potential) is produced by a parallel polysynaptic pathway. Because the motor neuron membrane resistance does not change during habituation, this decremental process is attributed to an attenuation in the presynaptic terminals of the sensory neuron.

E. Spinal Cord Habituation in Mammals

The mammalian spinal cord consists of a well-defined peripheral input system of cutaneous and muscular afferents, tracts to and from the brain, an assembly of motoneurons, and an extensive interneuron pool. If the spinal cord is simplified by severing its connections to the brain, it can still mediate two classes of relatively stereotyped responses. First, monosynaptic reflexes including the stretch and tendon reflexes: stretch of a muscle activates muscle receptors whose central terminals synapse directly on the motoneuron of the same muscle, producing contraction. In polysynaptic reflexes, there is at least one interneuron between afferent and efferent neurons. In the flexion reflex, a limb is withdrawn when noxiously stimulated. The scratch reflex refers to scratching movements of the hind limb when an animal's flank surface is stimulated. The afferents for polysynaptic reflexes are a diverse group of cutaneous and muscle receptors, that conduct at much slower rates than those mediating monosynaptic reflexes.

Thus, an isolated spinal cord retains a circuitry capacity for a number of fundamental movement patterns. Although students of behavior have regarded this capability as a property of "hard-wired" systems listening obligingly and faithfully to the instructions of either the periphery or the brain, experiments from time to time have indicated a capacity for plasticity (Sherrington, 1906; Prosser & Hunter, 1936). Moreover, the accumulated knowledge about spinal mechanisms at the cellular level (e.g., Eccles, 1964) provide a basis for detailed electrophysiological inquiries about possible spinal memory processes.

The simplest spinal mechanism that could exhibit plasticity is the monosynaptic stretch reflex, and this mechanism does display a memory process that has been intensively examined for over twenty-five years—posttetanic potentiation. In its simplest form, this process refers to an enhancement in the amplitude of synaptic transmission following a period of high-frequency stimulation (e.g., 500 per second) of a synapse. This kind of memory process can last for hours. It has been noted that twenty minutes of tetanic stimulation delivered to the tibial nerve produces a potentiated ventral root response recorded at the seventh lumbar ventral root that lasts for two hours (Spencer and April, 1970). However, monosynaptic reflexes do not display habituation, although an initial depression may be noted with prolonged tetanic stimulation. Posttetanic potentiation of inhibitory interneurons may consistitute part of an habituation mechanism as has been argued by Wickelgren (1967b) and Wall (1970).

The habituation of polysynaptic reflexes is quite common and was initially described by Sherrington (1906) during the course of his studies of the flexion and scratch reflexes. Although he referred to this state as "fatigue," the properties he described closely resemble attributes of habituation. He noted, for example, that, "The reflex when tired out to stimuli at that spot is easily obtainable by stimulation two or more cm. away [Sherrington, 1906]." As a mediating mechanism he postulated a modification at the level of the synapse. To Sherrington, the biological advantage of "fatigue" mechanisms was to preclude the control of motor outputs by maintained excitation of a limited receptor area; "It favors the receptors taking turn about [Sherrington, 1906]."

Many years later, armed with microelectrodes, several investigators reexamined this spinal decremental process (Spencer, Thompson, & Neilson, 1966a-c; Wickelgren, 1967a, b; Groves & Thompson, 1970). They confirm the presence of attenuation at the spinal level and attest to the usefulness of this preparation for analytic studies of habituation mechanisms. By present understanding, the possible sites and mechanisms for a spinal decremental process are: (1) presynaptic terminal failure at one or many links; (2) postsynaptic membrane desensitization; and (3) the progressive increase in inhibition at any point in the neuronal chain. The principal objective of contemporary electrophysiological studies of spinal habituation is to find the locus of modification. Spencer *et al.* (1966a-c) studied the modifiability of a flexion reflex elicited by skin or peripheral nerve electrical stimulation. Reflex decrements were measured either as changes in the activity of flexor muscles (myograms) or the outputs of motor horn cells (intracellular measurements or ventral root mass response). The stimulus schedule in these experiments consisted of an initial series of ten control stimuli delivered at 1–4 minute intervals. Then, at ten second intervals, half second trains of stimuli at a rate of 50 per second were presented. The measure of habituation was the difference in the activity elicited by the initial control series and a repetition of this same series. Measured in this fashion, the duration of habituation was variable, ranging between 30 seconds and 20–30 minutes. Habituation effects are most prominent with weaker stimuli. Generalization of habituation was noted with skin stimuli although the receptive field for this effect was much narrower than the field for dishabituation. The experimenters argue that the dishabituation of response with an "extraneous stumulus" reflects a superimposed potentiation process rather than the reversal of the habituation process.

The synaptic nodal points possibly mediating this modification are: (1) skin receptors, (2) the terminals of primary afferent fibers, (3) interneuron linkages, (4) connections to the motor horn cells, and (5) the neuroeffector junction. Changes in skin receptor sensitivity are not related to flexion reflex decrements, since similar effects are obtained with direct electrical stimulation of the peripheral nerve. Some of the properties of afferent terminals and interneuron changes can be assessed by recording of the cord dorsum potential, a gross potential at the dorsal surface of the spinal cord, consisting of several distinct deflections (upon afferent stimulation) attributable to different pre- or postsynaptic processes. Decrements are noted in both interneuron activity and the response systems mediating presynaptic inhibition. However, strychnine and picrtoxin, which are believed to block postsynaptic and presynaptic inhibition, fail to modify this decremental process. This evidence supports the view that habituation need not involve the progressive buildup of an inhibitory synaptic process. Unfortunately, the pharmacological action of these drugs may not be the same in all regions of the nervous system. Moreover, the cord dorsum potential being the summation of an undefinable assembly of elements cannot provide us with a detailed cellular portrait.

Intracellular recordings of motorneurons during habituation reveal a decrement in both depolarizing and hyperpolarizing synaptic potentials. A transmission failure in the interneuron population interpolated between the afferent input and motor cells probably produces this effect. A single cell analysis of interneuron firing patterns during habituation discloses three types of afferent elicited activity (Groves & Thompson, 1970). One type shows no change and two types display plastic properties. Some plastic units, characteristically emitting short latency, high frequency discharges, show a progressive attenuation. The third class of neurons displays an initial sensitization (the increase in firing during early trials) and subsequent habituation. Interestingly, the flexion reflex itself displays sensitization followed by or superimposed on habituation.

The acknowledged parameters of signal processing in nervous systems indicate that there are at least two classes of spinal mechanisms potentially relevant to spinal habituation. The views described above emphasize a transmission failure attributable to a presynaptic mechanism. An alternative viewpoint promoted by Wickelgren (1967a, b) and Wall (1970) emphasizes a presumed process consisting of a progressive increment in an interneuron postsynaptic inhibitory process. The experiments of Wickelgren (1967a, b) are rather similar in approach to those of Spencer et al. (1966 a–c). An initial test series is followed by a series of twenty habituation trials followed by the repetition of the initial test series. Measurements are made of both ventral root evoked activity and single unit dorsal horn interneuron responses elicited by either skin or nerve stimulation. Decrements in motor unit responses are noted only in flexor motor units and cannot be attributed to primary afferent changes. Dorsal horn interneurons which show habituation have certain "static" characteristics which are quite dissimilar from those which fail to display decrements with successive stimulation. They respond with more spikes per stimulus, exhibit longer latencies, and can be driven by a wider range of stimuli delivered to the appropriate receptive field although receptive field size fails to distinguish these two classes. Units that habituate also exhibit a higher level of spontaneous activity. Wall (1970) argues that several parametric and anatomical features of the interneuron population in these experiments suggest a mediating mechanism consisting of the posttetanic potentiation of an "inhibitory side chain."

In addition to these short-term memory processes, several habituation experiments point to the existence of more enduring modifications at this level (e.g., Kozak & Westerman, 1961; Griffin, 1970). The mechanisms mediating these effects have yet to be explored in either biochemical or neurophysiological experiments.

F. Single Unit Habituation in the Brain

Novel stimuli often elicit a general autonomic activation and investigative behavior, known collectively as the orienting response. The habituation of this response represents one of the less complex forms of plasticity at the organismic level. It is one form of learning impressed on animals in laboratory settings which can also be observed in animals in their natural habitat. Moreover, it has been proposed that the habituation of the orienting response is the behavioral manifestation of the successful registration of a stimulus (Sokolov, 1960). As a novel stimulus is registered in memory, it becomes more familiar and fails to elicit orienting. Thus, the activity of single units in habituation paradigms has been monitored both to explain orienting behavior and to elucidate processes of sensory gating and memory encoding.

Single units which show response attenuation to repetitive stimuli can be found in many areas of the brains of both vertebrates and invertebrates. As a general rule, areas having greater stimulus specificity have fewer units habituating to repetitive stimuli. The primary sensory projection and receiving areas show little habituation, thus allowing fine grade sensory analysis before a signal is ignored as familiar. Although many sensory receptors show adaptation, neurons farther from the periphery are more likely to exhibit habituation, and to recover from habituation more slowly.

In the superior colliculus and brainstem reticular formation, units respond and rapidly habituate to both stressful stimuli and to such natural stimuli as taps to the skin and puffs of air (Bell, Sierra, Buendia, & Segundo, 1964; Horn & Hill, 1966b; Scheibel & Scheibel, 1965). Units in these structures have characteristically large receptive fields, and many are multimodal. About 75 percent of the units excited by stimuli show attenuation, and often cease to respond after five or six stimulus presentations. Single units with sensitive, restrictive fields show less habituation. Moreover, stimulation of certain small areas in large receptive fields often elicits responses which do not habituate. This raises the possibility that all units may have undiscovered stimulus configurations to which they do not attenuate. The significance of this fact to the experimenter may be that he has failed to find the optimal stimulus. Its significance to the animal remains to be discovered.

The neuroanatomy of the reticular formation explains the large receptive fields and multimodality of single units, but gives no clue to their plastic properties. Golgi stains show the typical large reticular neuron to have many long dendrites extending out in the transverse plain of the brain stem (Scheibel & Scheibel, 1967). Such a structure is well suited to sample the many diverse input channels which course through the reticular formation.

Recovery of an habituated response usually occurs after a few minutes. Many units show stimulus specificity, in that the attenuation to one stimulus does not decrease the response to a different stimulus. Although some investigators have failed, others have succeeded in showing unit dishabituation, perhaps as a result of using unanesthetized animals (Bell et al., 1964).

Most of the single cells in the hippocampus, both excitatory and inhibitory, show attenuation, which is often complete within 10 to 20 trials (Vinogradova, 1965). These units act like novelty detectors, for any change in the modality, intensity, or frequency of the habituated stimulus elicits a strong response. About one third of the single units in the caudate nucleus habituate, with a somewhat slower rate than in the hippocampus. Interestingly, hippocampal units give similar diffuse unspecific responses to all types of stimuli, whereas caudate units respond to different stimuli with different patterned phasic responses (Vinogradova, 1968).

Habituating units in the protocerebrum and optic lobes of the locust have wide visual fields, and are often also driven by auditory and somatic stimuli (Horridge, Scholes, Shaw & Turnstall, 1965). Similar units in the locust tritocerebrum have receptive fields including the entire contralateral visual field (Horn & Rowell, 1968). Habituating units in all these areas behave as novel movement detectors. They are maximally excited by moving objects but show rapid habituation if the object moves only within a small locus. Novel movement at another spatial location elicits a strong response. Attenuation can occur even with intertrial intervals of several minutes, and recovery may take many hours. No natural stimuli have been found which produce dishabituation, but the responsiveness, as well as the spontaneous activity, of tritocerebral units may be increased by the electrical stimulation of the contralateral neck connective (Rowell & Horn, 1967).

Although the neuronal circuitry involved in the attenuation of unit activity is unknown, plasticity need not involve inhibition by higher brain centers, for habituating units can be found in the mesencephalon of a decorticate animal (Horn & Hill, 1966a) or in a sectioned spinal cord (Spencer et al., 1966a-c). Nor is habituation due to the random failure of inefficient connections because the first stimulus is always maximally effective and, after attenuation, unit responses do not sporadically reappear during stimulus repetition. Sokolov (1960) has proposed that during habituation a model of the stimulus is formed. Each succeeding stimulus is compared with the model, and a match results in signal attenuation at the reticular level. A more parsimonious explanation is that in each input channel a "self-generated depression" results in a transmission decrement (Horn, 1967). The generality or specificity of the unit attenuation is a function of the number of its overlapping inputs which a new stimulus shares with an habituated stimulus. Intracellular recordings favor the latter view for, in the mesencephalon, the only observable change during habituation is an attenuation of postsynaptic potentials (Segundo, Takenaka, & Encabo, 1967). This suggests a process of presynaptic depression.

An outstanding difficulty in interpreting these studies is the lack of evidence that the attenuating units are related to behavioral plasticity. It remains to be shown that the recorded neurons actually control orienting behavior, that they are not themselves controlled by other habituating systems, but are the locus of plasticity. To classify a single unit as a novelty detector, for example, it is not sufficient to determine that it is maximally excited by novel stimuli; it must also be shown that its output is appropriately read by the next higher order neuron. Single units are ambiguous: what they mean depends, to some extent, on who listens to them.

Although obvious parallels can be drawn between single unit activity and animal behavior, the orienting response recovers more slowly than the single units purportedly controlling it. This disparity may result from the physical constraint of animals in the single unit studies we have reviewed. A closer correlation may be found by recording neurons in freely moving animals. However, single units recorded in the freely moving locust demonstrate that habituation may have less effect on behavior than other processes. Responsiveness is correlated with the general dispositional state of the animal, with no attenuation occurring in the aroused, active animal (Rowell, 1970).

G. Habituation and Brain Gross Potentials

A large electrode placed in virtually any cellular region of the vertebrate brain can detect both continuous rhythmic activity (1–30 per second) and complex waveforms elicited by discrete stimuli. Features of these potentials such as frequency, amplitude, and component waveshapes vary with arousal state, brain region, and characteristics of sensory input. These events are readily observed in chronically implanted, freely moving animals; hence, many experiments are concerned with the relations between these potentials and behavior. However, a price is paid. The ease of observing these events is a small reward for the arduous interpretive labors that can confront either experimental man or computer. To this point in our discussion, we have consistently asserted that the language of nervous systems consists primarily of graded potentials—excitatory or inhibitory, and action potentials. What then are the neuroelectric events observed with a large electrode whose spatial resolution is a large aggregate of nerve cells, fibers, and glial cells?

To understand what gross potentials are made of, most investigators have sought to establish their relation to cellular graded or spike events. An early suggestion that such potentials could be a summation of temporally dispersed spike discharges in a large population of neurons has consistently failed to find experimental confirmation. However, Fox (1970) has argued that the waveform of the gross evoked response may describe the probability of cell discharge in some collection of neurons whose size is unspecified. This suggestion is based on his observation of a close relation between the gross waveform elicited by light flashes and averaged poststimulus time histograms of cell discharge.

Most studies have pointed to synaptic potentials of nerve cells as the basic elements that generate gross potentials. Thus, gross cortical negative waves are said to represent postsynaptic depolarization of pyramidal cell apical dendrites, and biphasic positive-negative waves reflect postsynaptic depolarization near the cell body (e.g., Creutzfeld, 1966). The faster transients in evoked potential waveforms are often attributed to cell discharges or fiber spikes. Any gross potential waveform is a summation of spatially and temporally distributed synaptic activation of an ensemble whose size is rather indeterminate.

Clearly, gross potential analyses do not readily enable the description of the synaptic mechanisms and coding operations of particular neural circuit arrangements. The relatively unambiguous use of these neural indicants in studies of learning has been in relation to questions of where, that is, questions of site in nervous systems. For example, a problem posed in several evoked potential studies of habituation has been the determination of the differential sensitivity of sensory and nonsensory pathways to stimulus repetition. Further, within an afferent pathway, at what level can decremental processes be produced by the repetition of an appropriate stimulus? The earliest of these studies came along with a proposed mechanism for the gating of "inconsequential" or non-novel events. Notably, Hernandez-Peon's (1959) hypothesis of "afferent neuronal inhibition." He suggested that stimulus repetition led to the activation of an inhibitory mechanism which consisted of centrifugal pathways that acted at a sensory receptor level. Strong criticism of this view came from experimenters who argued that the data offered in support of this model, for example, evoked response amplitude decrements at the cochlear nucleus level, were unreliable or confounded with poorly controlled experimental conditions. And, so, there started a long series of experiments which dealt with the features of an experimental environment that might affect gross evoked responses such as room acoustics, the stimulus attenuation possibilities of the pupillary mechanism, external ear, and middle ear muscles. These problems are reviewed in detail by Worden (1966) and Horn (1965).

A well controlled, recent look at this problem has been provided by Wickelgren (1968a, b). Click evoked responses were recorded at various levels of the auditory pathway from cochlear nucleus to auditory cortex. Average evoked potentials at brain stem level (cochlear nucleus, superior olive, inferior colliculus) show no amplitude changes over the course of a series of click stimuli. The principal changes in evoked potentials related to stimulus repetition were noted at the thalamic relay (medial geniculate) and auditory cortex. The cortical change was limited to a significant decrement in the late surface negative component of the summated evoked potential. In other studies, the duration of this habituation effect is rather short, that is, spontaneous recovery can occur within one minute. A similar effect recorded in occipital cortex with light flashes has been described by Hall (1968). The translation of these events to the details of neural transactions poses some difficulties. Amplitude changes in gross sensory evoked potentials may arise from varied combinations of changes in synaptic potentials and numbers of activated neurons.

The anatomical themes across a large number of experiments dealing with the problem of gross neural place and habituation are rather consistent. These experiments generally emphasize the lability of sensory evoked potentials in nonclassical sensory pathways, for example, thalamic and mesencephalic reticular formation, and limbic system as contrasted with the less modifiable evoked responses within a classical sensory pathway.

H. Mechanisms of Habituation: A Summary and Assessment

The habituation paradigm has provided a model for the study of neuronal events mediating memory. Neurological explanations of response habituation have ranged from a cellular level to generalized block diagrams that ascribe particular analytic properties to specific brain regions. The requirements for an adequate cellular representation of this process include a characterization of transmission efficiency and the location of the plastic elements in a neuronal network. Attenuating single units must be shown to drive either a command system or the motoneurons responsible for the response. Further, any attenuating cell must be shown to be the locus of decrement rather than a reflection of a plastic process in other portions of a network. These specifications for a cellular depiction are met by a few of the systems we have described, most notably, the gill withdrawal reflex in *Aplysia*, some variants of invertebrate escape behavior, and the flexion reflex of spinal cat. Although these successful explanations have all involved presynaptic depression, we cannot ignore other plastic mechanisms. We shall therefore briefly review the possible forms of synaptic plasticity.

1. Synaptic Mechanisms

In the nervous system of some animals there are two forms of synaptic transmission, the familiar chemical type involving the release of a transmitter agent from a presynaptic terminal, and the less frequent electrical synapse, involving transmission across a narrow cleft by electrotonic conduction. All evidence favors the location of plasticity in chemical rather than electrical synapses. No electrical synapses have been found that show attenuation or facilitation with repetitive stimulation (Bennett, 1968). When both chemical and electrical synapses make contact with the same neuron [e.g., chick ciliary ganglion, Martin and Pilar (1963, 1964)], repetitive stimulation can potentiate the chemical synapse by as much as 800 percent with no change in the efficacy of the electrical synapse.

In all chemical synapses the presynaptic action potential elicits the release of a neurotransmitter which, in turn, acts upon a postsynaptic surface to produce a local change in conductance. The postsynaptic electrical sign of this process is either excitatory or inhibitory. At a synaptic level of analysis attenuating outputs can arise from either a diminution of excitatory postsynaptic potentials or the progressive increment in inhibitory postsynaptic potentials. If due to presynaptic depression, a decline in excitatory synaptic drive may involve either a change in the processes by which a neurotransmitter is synthesized, organized, and maintained in a form accessible to release, or a modification of the link between the presynaptic action potential and transmitter release. In addition to these mechanisms, synaptic efficiency may also decline if the postsynaptic membrane becomes less sensitive to the neurotransmitter. The current understanding of these processes—constituted more by hiatus than fact—must be applied to a consideration of the possible mechanisms mediating habituation.

a. Presynaptic Mechanisms. Transmitter molecules are thought to be contained in an "immediately available" form within the vesicles of the axon terminals. The vesicle contents, a quantum of transmitter molecules, are released in a packet form. If postsynaptic sensitivity is held constant, the magnitude of the postsynaptic potential indicates the quantity of released transmitter. The simplest possible synaptic mechanism of habituation is a depletion of neurotransmitter. However, a number of observations in adequately studied synapses militate against this possibility. Although a single nerve impulse may release several hundred quanta of neurotransmitter, the number of packets immediately available for release number in the hundreds of thousands. Several reports of a decrease in the number of vesicles following intense synaptic activation have not been confirmed. For example, most recently it has been shown that high frequency stimulation of the sympathetic ganglion does not produce a decrease in the number of presynaptic vesicles (Dolivo, 1970). Unfortunately, at present there are no electron microscopic methods for determining the amount of transmitter in a vesicle or its availability for release. Biochemical studies suggest a large margin of safety for the resynthesis and storage of transmitter substances. Thus, unreplaced transmitter loss is probably not the cause of a decline in synaptic transmission, although it may be a factor in small synapses.

Part of the presynaptic neurotransmitter is in a nonreleasable storage compartment (Eccles, 1964). The mobilization of stored transmitter, by its transfer to a releasable form, may be changed in synaptic plasticity. This mobilization may be independent of the actual amount of transmitter released. Bruner and Kehoe (1970) have shown that a decreased calcium ion concentration attenuates the neuromuscular end plate potential and hence presumably decreases the amount of transmitter released. Nevertheless, habituation of the endplate potential proceeds at its normal rate. Apparently, the amount of attenuation is a function of the number of presynaptic action potentials rather than the quantity of transmitter released.

The processes linking an axon terminal action potential and the ultimate release of neurotransmitter have not been elucidated. It has been shown that the hyperpolarization of a presynaptic ending increases the size of its elicited postsynaptic potential and the converse effect is noted with terminal depolarization. This raises the possibility that repetitive presynaptic action potentials produce a residual polarization of the axon ending which decreases the amount of released transmitter. Moreover, depolarization or hyperpolarization of a terminal by the activity of axo-axonal synapses offer a polysynaptic explanation of habituation and dishabituation. This theory of plasticity is not, however, confirmed at the neuromuscular junction, since during habituation no fall in the presynaptic membrane potential is observed (Miledi & Slater, 1966). Further, the amount of released transmitter can be changed by varying the calcium ion concentration of the bathing solution; but this effect occurs with no change in the amplitude of the action potential at the presynaptic ending.

b. Postsynaptic Mechanisms. The transmitter released from an axon terminal makes the postsynaptic membrane more permeable to particular ions. This process involves the combination of the transmitter molecule with a subsynaptic receptor site. Although a cholinergic receptor protein has recently been isolated (Changeaux, Kasai, & Chen-Yuan, 1970; Miledi, Molinoff, & Potter, 1971) its molecular structure and function are tantalizingly unknown. It has been observed that the same neurotransmitter (acetylcholine) can exert either an excitatory or inhibitory influence; hence, synaptic sign is apparently determined by the subsynaptic receptor complex. A progressive desensitization of this postsynaptic system might mediate transmission attenuation. By injecting neurotransmitter from a microelectrode, one can hold constant the amount of transmitter reaching the postsynaptic membrane and thus assess postsynaptic sensitivity by measuring the amplitude of the postsynaptic potential. In the vertebrate motor end plate, a pulse of neurotransmitter from a microelectrode or repetitive motor nerve stimulation produces an attenuation of the postsynaptic potential elicited by a pulse of constant size. The effect lasts up to 2 minutes (Katz & Thesleff, 1957; Thesleff, 1958). A similar brief pulse of transmitter delivered to certain neuron soma of invertebrates results in a postsynaptic desensitization for as long as 20 minutes (Tauc & Bruner, 1963). Thus, the attenuation of postsynaptic responsiveness must be considered as a possible mechanism of habituation.

Thus far we have assumed that the habituation mechanism is a decline in an excitatory synaptic process. Other candidates include a progressive potentiation of an inhibitory synapse (Blankenship, Wachtel, & Kandel, 1971) and the tonic hyperpolarization of a neuron by a barrage of inhibitory inputs (Holmgren & Frenck, 1961; Waziri, Kandel, & Frazier, 1969). The latter process, of course, presupposes control by a plastic mechanism located elsewhere.

A neuronal network using presynaptic attenuating mechanisms is probably more efficient than one using postsynaptic inhibitory mechanisms. Synaptic depression effects only those synapses which are activated, and, hence, in presynaptic networks the specificity of habituation is attained without interneurons exerting inhibitory control. Experimentally, habituation is produced without a general depression of the postsynaptic neuron, which thus remains able to respond to new, nonhabituated inputs.

   c. Synaptic Connections. Changes in the synaptic connections of cells, known to be affected by long periods of disuse or treatment, may occur rapidly enough to mediate behavioral change, and may themselves be produced by short functional alterations. In allergic encephalomyelitis, a decrease in synaptic function preceeds neuronal degeneration. And in botulinum toxin poisoning, a depression of excitatory postsynaptic potentials occurs before the subsequent sprouting of the presynaptic fibers. An observable decrease in the width of retinal synapses is noted within 3 minutes of placing dark-reared rats in light (Cragg, 1969). Thus, a change in synaptic connections may be caused by an altered tonic level of synaptic use. This could be due to a trophic effect of the neurotransmitter, or to an action of other substances released with the transmitter. Below we will discuss additional theories formulated to explain other types of learning, but which may also be applied to habituation.

2. Regional Mechanisms

   Is habituation a product of changes in particular brain regions? Clearly, the structural plan of the brain includes a spatial segregation of some functions, and one of the persistent missions of neuropsychology has been the demonstration of covariations of structural or areal differences and behavioral states. Studies concerned with the differences in the rate of habituation in various brain regions alert us to the importance of anatomical differentiations although one might argue that each region is wired to analyze different features of an experience and, hence, the attenuation in different regions may have different effects on behavioral habituation. One might also argue that just as synaptic transmission takes place at all levels of the brain, transmission attenuation is an equally ubiquitous phenomenon.

Various investigations indicate that the limbic system and reticular formation have a primary control of orienting behavior and the gating of sensory input. Hippocampal ablations produce in cats a syndrome of "unrestrained curiosity." Hippocampal theta is a prominent feature of responses to novel stimuli. Electrical stimulation of the hippocampus decreases the arousing effect of stimulation of the reticular formation, and increases the threshold for a cortical evoked response. Apparently the hippocampus exerts a tonic inhibitory effect on the reticular formation. Following a startling stimulus, a familiar stimulus evokes electroencephalographic responses in many previously habituated areas. The wide anatomical ramifications of the reticular system may mediate these global activating effects.

Sokolov (1960) has proposed that the reticular formation controls the amount of sensory input and the elicitation of the orienting response. During stimulus repetition the cerebral cortex elaborates a model of the stimulus and attempts to match incoming stimuli to it. If a novel stimulus produces a mismatch, the cortex activates the reticular modulating system, which increases the strength of incoming signals and initiates orienting behavior. This enhances the organism's ability to discriminate stimuli. It is known that sensory axons projecting to the sensory receiving areas in the thalamus also send axon collaterals into the recticular formation of the brain stem. The cortex also projects to the reticular formation, which, in turn, sends relatively slow conducting fibers to all areas of the brain. The anatomy is thus consistent with this model, for the cortex receives sensory information quickly and is involved in sensory discrimination. The reticular formation is in the proper anatomical position to be modulated by the cortex, and, in turn, to activate wide areas of the brain by its diffuse projection system.

Unfortunately, this theory does not specify the mechanism which matches incoming stimuli to a model. As we saw above, neuronal networks can be constructed in which changes in stimulus parameters result in the activation of different input channels. The habituation of the network can then be explained by postulating a self-generated depression in each channel. The "model" of a habituated stimulus is now the location of attenuated synapses in a neuronal network, and a mismatch occurs when a novel stimulus excites unattenuated channels. Thus, seemingly complex psychological concepts can be reduced to simple changes in a neuronal circuit (Horn, 1967).

Groves and Thompson (1970) have advanced a dual process theory to explain the biphasic response of the central nervous system to repetitive stimuli. They propose that during response habituation the sensory projection system, together with its linkages to the final common pathway producing that response, undergoes transmission attenuation. Dishabituation is produced by a second system, generally identified with the reticular formation, which is also responsible for sensitization (the increased responsiveness of an animal to any stimulus). The sensory projection system is independent of the reticular system and both influence some response command center. Groves and Thompson have provided good evidence for two independent systems having a joint influence on a habituated response. Although this properly controverts the notion of dishabituation as simply the release from habituation, the question is now where the two independent systems converge to form a common pathway mediating a response. In the sensory projection systems, the convergence could take place at the receptor neuron and at each subsequent neuron. Moreover, it is not even necessary that two independent mechanisms occupy different neurons, since we have seen that both inhibitory and facilitatory effects can be produced at the same synapse by varying the input frequency (Bruner & Kennedy, 1969). A similar biphasic effect at a single synapse depends on the summation of inhibitory and excitatory postsynaptic potentials, produced independently by the same neurotransmitter and apparently mediated by two receptor mechanisms on the postsynaptic membrand (Blankenship *et al.*, 1971; Wachtel & Kandel, 1971).

3. Systems Approach

Habituation can be seen from a broader perspective as one of many processes an organism uses to extract information from sensory input. Formally stated, the amount of information in any input is inversely related to the probability of its occurrence. In a spatial display, the transition between two different homogeneous areas has a higher information content than either area. By means of lateral inhibition neurons signalling the position of this transition inhibit surrounding neurons. Thus, only the most informative signals are sent to the brain. The simplest extraction of temporal information is the signalling of the occurrence and duration of an applied stimulus. A neuron could fire repetitively for the duration of the stimulus, but the information content of its firing is greatly increased if it fires only at the beginning and end of the stimulus. In fact, there are many "on" and "off" neurons at various levels of sensory systems and very few neurons which exhibit sustained firing during a stimulus. In the habituation paradigm, by definition, one stimulus has a high probability of occurrence, and hence a low information value. The net effect of habituation is to assess the information value of this stimulus: during its repetition the animal assigns it a high probability of occurrence and, thus, comes to regard it with the indifference shown low information events.

By the damping of investigatory behavior toward commonplace stimuli, habituation thus aids in detecting novel, high information events in the environment. In lower organisms this process may simply prevent fatigue induced by the repetitive elicitation of a species specific behavior. In higher animals it also interacts with other learning mechanisms. When a habituated stimulus is followed by punishment or reward, it again elicits orienting behavior. The previously neutral stimulus has acquired new information value (or, more properly speaking, significance) as an indicator of a biologically important event. An animal must adapt to a world in which only some stimuli are important. By eliminating responses to stimuli not biologically indicative, habituation prepares the organism to detect novel stimuli which are either themselves biologically important events, or are generally associated with such events. To learn one must learn to ignore.

III. ASSOCIATIVE LEARNING

Although some may quibble over whether habituation is a form of "true learning," very few experimenters offer any skeptical glances when one discusses the memory processes related to the application of classical or instrumental conditioning paradigms; indeed, for some these are the only forms of "Grade-A Certified Learning" (Miller, 1967). Clearly, from the standpoint of examining the biology of learning, these paradigms afford the comfort and safety of many years of careful descriptions of the rules governing behavioral modifications. Most of the studies described in this section have employed these paradigms in one fashion or another.

A. Ganglionic Learning: Operant Conditioning in Headless Insects

Several years ago, Horridge (1964) introduced a learning preparation which he suggested might provide a simplified system for detailed electrophysiological analysis of associative learning. His experiment took advantage of the fact that a locust or cockroach suspended by the thorax will occasionally make spontaneous metathoracic leg movements. This will also occur with headless animals. When the animal's leg falls a preset distance it touches a saline bath in which it receives an electrical shock producing immediate leg lifting. A yoked control animal receives a shock at the same time, although in this animal the shock is then not contingent on leg position. The clearest indication of the establishment of some associative process is observed during test sessions following a period of training. The "contingent" animal receives fewer shocks during this session than the animal that served in the yoked or noncontingent condition. This form of learning can be accomplished by a headless animal and can survive removal of the head following initial training. The establishment of a dynamic trace system at the level of the relevant thoracic ganglion is partially suggested by Horridge's observation (1964) that electrical stimulation of the ventral connective following training can abolish the learned response.

Extensions of this work have been provided by Hoyle (1965) who further simplified this preparation. In these experiments, the thoracic ganglion was isolated and the firing rate of the muscle related to the leg movement was monitored. Shocks to the leg were timed to follow spontaneous changes in muscle discharge rate. If shocks follow a decline in discharge rate the mean rate increases and can ultimately be "led" to a level which is three to four times the initial rate. Conditioned decreases in firing rate could also be established (Aranda & Luco, 1969).

B. Neuronal Analogs of Learning in the Abdominal Ganglion of Aplysia

1. Theoretical Models

Although the intact *Aplysia* can learn to withhold an appetitive response to proffered inedible objects (Lickey, 1968), it is not known if its isolated abdominal ganglion can mediate associative learning. Nevertheless, the strikingly large neurons of the abdominal ganglion have made it a favored preparation of some electrophysiologists. When employed as a neuronal model for learning, the ganglion has usually been isolated and the activity on one neuron, recorded intracellularly, taken as the response to be modified. Either natural stimuli or the electrical stimulation of nerve cells has been applied in a manner analogous to the patterning of stimuli in behavioral conditioning. Experiments have involved the pairing of two stimuli, a neuronal analog of classical conditioning, or have made a stimulus contingent on spontaneous neuronal activity, an operant analog. The parameters of these stimulus paradigms, as well as the paradigms themselves, have been adopted from a literature of animal conditioning based primarily on vertebrate species.

After the demonstration of neuronal plasticity, the goal of these experiments has been to simplify the underlying circuitry and thereby identify the synaptic or neuronal mechanisms responsible for altered activity. Methodologically, this is an attempt to find and elucidate general plastic mechanisms. The existence of such mechanisms in the ganglion does not imply that they mediate the acquisition of a learned response. However, once discovered, they do become candidates for any behavioral plasticity which can be found in this organism, and, by generalization, in other organisms.

A related rationale for looking at neuronal analogs of learning is the general hypothesis that behavioral plasticity is mediated by analogous neuronal plasticity. The theory explains how two appropriately paired stimuli produce a conditioned behavioral response by proposing that the excitation of two input channels will produce a conditioned response at an individual neuron. The conditioned neuron then drives a command or motorneuron producing the behavioral response. Although this explanation may have a prima facie appeal, there are a number of reasons why the behavior exhibited in learning paradigms places few constraints on the possible neuronal organization underlying it. In neuronal circuits with even a modicum of complexity, the properties of individual neurons are obscured in the operation of the system. Nor does the behavior of the system indicate the nature of its components or circuits.

Moreover, in proposing the analogy of neuron and behavior, the behavior of a conditioned animal has been theoretically interpreted as exhibiting stimulus substitution: the same unconditioned response coming to be elicited by the conditioned stimulus. Rarely, however, does the conditioned response have the same topology as the unconditioned response.

Because it imputes the interesting parameters of learning to the plastic properties of single neurons, this explanation reduces many properties of the neuronal circuit to the attributes of single neurons. It is therefore more easily tested than more complex theories of learning. For whatever the organization of its nervous system, if an animal displays learning, then on this explanation it must have neurons which display a process analogous to learning. If this approach can successfully explain behavioral plasticity, it will be hailed as revealing a basic similarity in the function of vastly different structures. If the approach fails, it will be condemned as a naively zoomorphic interpretation of neuronal circuits.

The crucial property of classical conditioning to be explained is temporal specificity: only the stimulus immediately preceding the unconditioned stimulus comes to elicit a conditioned response. Kupferman and Pinsker (1969) have provided schematic models at the neuronal level of proposed mechanisms that may meet the requirement for temporal specificity. The first approach uses the known properties of synapses, and interposes an interneuron which fires only when the CS and UCS inputs are simultaneously active. By requiring that the CS and UCS inputs must be simultaneously active to maximally excite the inter-neuron (INT), the CS comes to control the output of the circuit only if it is paired with the unconditioned stimulus.

The second way to obtain temporal specificity is by novel plastic processes which require, for their initiation, the simultaneous occurrence of two events in the same neuron. One such proposal is the "successful use" hypotheses (Hebb, 1949). The transmission of a synapse is proposed to be strengthened if it is activated together with the firing of the postsynaptic neuron. Attributing the recognition of simultaneity to the synapse or to the postsynaptic membrane permits a simple analog of conditioning. Another possible process is specific hetero-synaptic facilitation, in which simultaneous presynaptic and synaptic activation is required to increase synaptic efficiency (Kandel & Tauc, 1965a, b). This elegant mechanism also permits a simple circuit to produce temporal specificity in conditioning.

2. Experimental Findings

The successful use hypothesis has been tested in a number of neurons by pairing an EPSP with spike activity. Nerve stimulation was used to produce an EPSP below the cell's spike threshold, and this was paired with intracellular depolarization sufficient to cause the neuron to fire. When the test EPSP preceded cell firing by from 200 to 500 msec, repetitive pairing produced no change in the amplitude of the EPSP (Kandel & Tauc, 1965a, b). Nor is the amplitude of the EPSP changed by being induced after or simultaneously with an action potential (Wurtz, Castellucci, & Nusrula, 1967). Amplification is rarely produced when an individual spontaneous EPSP, recognized by its waveform, is followed by an induced action potential. When an EPSP does increase during this treatment, it is found that the EPSP of all other synapses also increases. The successful use hypothesis thus remains unverified.

Hetero-synaptic facilitation has been investigated in the abdominal ganglion by pairing the stimulation of two nerves afferent to the same neuron (Kandel & Tauc, 1965a, b). Parameters of stimulation were chosen so that a test stimulation produced only an EPSP, while the priming stimulus produced a burst of spikes. Pairs of stimuli were given once every ten seconds, with the test stimulus preceding the priming stimulus by 200 to 300 msec. In most cells tested, pairing had no effect on the amplitude of the test EPSP, but in the right giant cell (RGC) and a number of unidentified cells nearby the test EPSP increased and remained elevated for as long as 40 minutes after pairing. The increase in the efficacy of one nerve with the stimulation of a second nerve is called heterosynaptic facilitation. This is a descriptive and not an explanatory term. It can be asked whether hetero-synaptic facilitation is a result of post-tetanic potention or presynaptic facilitation. Also, it must be determined whether heterosynaptic facilitation can be specific: dependent on the temporal contiguity of the test and priming stimuli.

The right giant cell, reidentifiable in any *Aplysia* abdominal ganglion, has received the most scrutiny. It does not exhibit specific heterosynaptic facilitation, because the repetitive presentation of the priming stimulus alone can increase the amplitude of the test EPSP. This neuronal analog of pseudoconditioning can be quite dramatic, with an increase in the EPSP of from 100 to 700 percent, often sufficient to produce spikes in this normally quiet cell. Heterosynaptic facilitation may have physiological significance, for stroking the siphon also provides a good priming stimulus.

A number of experiments suggest that heterosynaptic facilitation in the RGC is due to long-term presynaptic facilitation. During heterosynaptic facilitation, there is no change in the membrane conductance of the RGC. Nor can facilitation be produced by the direct elicitation of spikes by intracellular depolarization, either alone, or paired with the test stimulus. Because the test EPSP retains the same waveform during facilitation, its amplification is apparently due to an increase in synaptic transmission.

The priming stimulus used in these experiments also excited the recorded neuron. Hence, facilitation could be explained by posttetanic potentiation if the priming stimulus also caused the test synapse to fire. Because the activity of the presynaptic terminal of the test nerve fiber could not be recorded directly, the possibility of posttetanic potentiation had to be disproven by indirect means. Heterosynaptic facilitation could be produced by priming the RGC when the test nerve fiber was functionally isolated to prevent its excitation by the priming stimulus (Tauc & Epstein, 1967; Epstein & Tauc, 1970). Also, posttetanic potentiation, produced by high frequency stimulation of one input nerve, has different parameters than heterosynaptic facilitation. Posttetanic potentiation produces maximal synaptic efficacy from 20 to 40 seconds after stimulation, and lasts from 1 to 4 minutes. Heterosynaptic facilitation requires 2 to 3 minutes to reach peak efficiency and may last from 10 to 30 minutes. A similar latency for heterosynaptic facilitation exists in the giant cell of the left pleural ganglion (Haigler & von Baumgarten, 1970). Moreover, heterosynaptic facilitation does occur at low temperatures and when sodium is replaced by lithium, conditions which abolish posttetanic potentiation (Epstein & Tauc, 1970).

The evidence thus favors the view that heterosynaptic facilitation in the RGC is due to long lasting presynaptic facilitation. Whether this is produced by a tonic hyperpolarization of the test presynaptic terminals or due to other and, perhaps, entirely new neuronal mechanisms, remains to be seen.

Specific heterosynaptic facilitation has been reported in a number of unidentified cells of the abdominal ganglion. In three cells, paired stimulation produced heterosynaptic facilitation, while unpaired priming had no effect on the test EPSP. In two tested cells, the pairing of one EPSP with the priming stimulus produced an increase in the amplitude of that EPSP but no change in a second unpaired EPSP (Kandel & Tauc, 1965a). Unfortunately, the presence of an interneuron cannot be ruled out, and thus unspecific heterosynaptic facilitation may account for the effect.

The specificity of heterosynaptic facilitation can be increased by decreasing the strength of the priming stimulus. By so doing, an increase due specifically to pairing can be demonstrated in addition to a nonspecific effect (von Baumgarten & Djahapawar, 1967). Both specific and nonspecific heterosynaptic facilitation may thus be present. In these unidentified neurons, the most efficient test-priming stimulus interval is 350 msec, which compares favorably, though perhaps spuriously, with the best CS-UCS interval in the classical conditioning of vertebrates (von Baumgarten & Hukuhara, 1969). Yet, until specific heterosynaptic facilitation has been demonstrated in identifiable neurons, and depicted in neuronal circuits, its description will remain intriguing anecdotage.

An operant analog which may restrict the experimentally induced changes to a single cell has involved attempts to modify the parameters of endogenously active cells. The *Aplysia* abdominal ganglion includes a number of large pacemaker neurons, which, in the absence of input, produce a fairly constant rhythmic cycle of a spike burst followed by a quiet period. The strong stimulation of an afferent nerve produced a nonspecific increase in the general spike frequency. With weaker stimulation, effects were specifically related to the contingency of the stimulus and endogenous response. Stimulation given soon after burst onset shortened the subsequent quiet period. If given later during the burst, or during the quiet period, the cycle was lengthened. The effect increased progressively and lasted a number of minutes (Frazier et al., 1965; Pinsker & Kandel, 1967).

The synaptic input of contingent stimulation can be eliminated by directly exciting a cell through intracellular depolarization. Some endogenous bursting neurons became entrained to the frequency of an imposed depolarization, and demonstrated the new rhythm briefly during extinction before returning to their normal rhythms. A pairing of a subthreshold depolarization followed by depolarization sufficient to fire the neuron produced weak conditioning. When only the subthreshold depolarization was subsequently presented, it elicited a spike with a latency comparable to the delay in the induced spike during conditioning (von Baumgarten, 1970). These experiments generally suggest that in addition to synaptic modifications, plasticity may involve changes in the nonsynaptic parameters of a cell, such as modification in the slow depolarization of a membrane or a change in spike threshold. Moreover, they provide a mechanism for modifying sustained neuronal oscillators, which may result in the tuning of neuronal aggregates.

The great utility of the *Aplysia* abdominal ganglion is further illustrated by studies indicating that the synaptic excitation of a neuron increases its rate of RNA synthesis. By stimulation of an afferent nerve, spikes were elicited in the giant neuron R2 in a ganglion bathed in a perfusion fluid containing radioactive RNA precursors. After electrical stimulation and recording, the R2 soma could be isolated and subjected to biochemical fractionation and radioactivity counting procedures. It was found that elicited spiking substantially increased RNA radioactivity (Berry, 1969; Peterson & Kernell, 1970). The effect is apparently dependent on synaptic activation, for when the same number of spikes are induced in R2 by either stimulation of a neuronal afferent or by direct intracellular depolarization, only synaptic activation significantly increases RNA labeling (Kernell & Peterson, 1970).

C. Analogs of Learning in Vertebrate Nervous Systems

Single unit analogs of behavioral learning have been demonstrated in vertebrates. In the operant conditioning paradigm, a reward was made contingent on a change in the ongoing behavior of a single unit. In the classical conditioning paradigm, the unconditioned stimulus was neuronal activity directly elicited by current passed through the recording microelectrode. Both peripheral and central stimulation has been employed as the conditioned stimulus. The general strategy is an attempt to delimit the locus of plasticity in the brain, either by locating units which can be brought under "voluntary" control, or by restricting the effect of the unconditioned stimulus to a small number of neurons.

Neuronal activity in many brain regions can be brought under operant control by arranging suitable reinforcement contingencies. In rats sedated with meprobamate, the frequency of bursts of spike activity can be increased by reinforcement with electrical stimulation of the medial forebrain bundle at sites known to cause self-stimulation (Olds & Olds, 1961). All units were chosen such that the random presentation of the reinforcer had no effect on their activity. Operant conditioning was successful within minutes in many paleocortical and subcortical neurons, but neocortical neurons rarely exhibited plasticity.

The operant conditioning of a neuron does not imply that it is near the locus of plasticity. Animals may have been reinforced for a movement of their musculature producing a feedback driving the recorded neuron. In fact, when single units did respond to operant conditioning, their activity was often accompanied by movements of the animal.

Therefore unit activity in freely moving rats was reinforced with food only if they remained motionless for 2 seconds (Olds, 1965). The frequency of bursts of eight or more spikes could be increased with reinforcement, but no conditioning occurred when either single spikes or the cessation of ongoing activity was rewarded. After initial operant conditioning, a discriminative stimulus was introduced; criterial unit activity was rewarded only when it occurred during a light-on period. Over a period of days, units in both the hippocampus and the pons showed an increase in the frequency of the rewarded bursting. During the discriminative stimulus, spike bursts usually occurred at least twice as often as during nonreinforced periods. Pontine units acquired the operant control more readily and were more resistant to extinction than hippocampal units.

This result also fails to show that the single neuron with altered activity has acquired a modified firing pattern in any way independent of the vast aggregate of neurons to which it is connected. The activity of most units in the pons and many units in the hippocampus covaries with the activity of the reinforced cell. Therefore, the recorded bursting in one cell is a sample from the activity of a large number of neurons altered by contingent reinforcement. Moreover, close behavioral observation revealed that many reinforced bursts in pontine units are accompanied by slight movements of the head, and hippocampal unit activity occurs together with twitches of the nose or whiskers. Thus, the experimenter defined task may have been the acquisition of a covert response. It is known that in humans the isolated contraction of a motor unit, perhaps involving a single anterior horn cell, can be brought under operant control (Basmajian, 1963). Even if the modified units are not driven by response produced feedback, the covariation of many units and the accompaniment of a response is not surprising. It may be that the only units subject to operant conditioning are part of large neuronal aggregates, driven as a system and responsible for basic movements of the animal. This is consonant with a rather old yet still lively idea that the brain is organized to produce general movements rather than discrete muscular contractions.

Single unit bursting activity in the precentral motor cortex of monkeys can also be controlled by food reinforcement (Fetz, 1969). In any one animal, the first few recorded units showed little conditioning, but the animal acquires the ability to quickly change the rate of bursting of any neuron isolated by the microelectrode. Random reinforcement produced no increase in unit activity. Here again, unit responses were often accompanied by obvious movements of the animal.

The most parsimonious explanation of these experiments is that movements are being conditioned. They do not demonstrate that the function of a solitary neuron is modified by reinforcement, nor do they indicate that with extended conditioning, the activity of the many unreinforced units would extinguish. It therefore does not appear that operant conditioning can be explained by the effect of feedback on the activity of many neurons in independent parallel circuits. It should be noted that learned responses do not develop from the successive shaping of random muscular contractions. Rather, most learning involves the selection from a small repertoire of fully coordinated responses (Bolles, 1970).

Localization of plasticity has been a recurrent problem in all physiological approaches to learning. An interesting method to assure that changes in the activity of an observed neuron are not caused by changes in distant plastic neurons is to deliver the unconditioned stimulus directly to the recorded neuron as current passed through the recording microelectrode. Weak DC anodal polarization of the cells at the electrode tip was preceded by either an acoustic (Bures & Buresova, 1967) or a tactile stimulus (Gerbrandt et al., 1968). With the parameters of stimulus employed, most units in the cortex, hippocampus, nonspecific thalamic nuclei, and reticular formation of curarized rats failed to show modification of the CS elicited activity. However, with the exception of the cortex, about 10 percent of neurons in each area exhibited an altered responsiveness to the CS during conditioning. These changes often lasted for a number of minutes during extinction, and could be reconditioned. An equal percentage of units could be conditioned to either the tactile or acoustic stimulus. Conditioning occurred when microelectrode current produced either excitation or inhibition, and the conditioned response did not always resemble the effect of polarization.

These changes may be due to the nonspecific activation of a unit caused by repetitive polarization. It is known that many originally unresponsive units can become entrained to peripheral stimuli during continuous microelectrode polarization (Bures & Buresova, 1965; Gerbrandt et al., 1968). However, there is some evidence that these changes are specific to the pairing of stimuli. The effects of polarization rarely last longer than the polarization itself, whereas many units continue to exhibit a conditioned response during extinction. The conditioning of a single unit occurs without a significant change in its spontaneous firing level, indicating that its general excitability has not been modified.

In addition to peripheral stimulation, the conditioned stimulus can be the passage of current through a second electrode located near the recording microelectrode (Bures & Buresova, 1970). As the current is increased to excite more cells, the number of units exhibiting plasticity increases to about 10 percent of all isolated units. The similar percentage of plastic units found with both peripheral and central stimulation may indicate that in the class of large and therefore recordable neurons, about one in ten have plastic properties.

D. Single Unit Plasticity in the Mammalian Central Nervous System

When an animal learns a new response, it must modify the activity of its muscles by changing the pattern of input to the motorneurons which innervate them. To explain these changes, researchers have attempted to find modifications in the activity of individual neurons in various regions of the central nervous system. The underlying presupposition has been predominately connectionistic, with the learning of a response equated either with a change in the efficiency of a connection or with the establishment of a new connection. The attempts to find neuronal alterations during learning have been all too successful, for one is embarrassed with a superfluity of neurons changing their activity. There are single units at all levels of the mammalian central nervous system that exhibit changes in activity concomitant with behavioral conditioning. Most of these units probably have nothing more to do with producing a changed behavior in the animal than the activity of the muscles themselves; they are simply following altered input. To identify the neurons initiating these changes, it must be shown that the output of a neuron is altered while its input remains constant. This criterion of primary neuronal change has not yet been satisfied. Therefore, indirect measures, such as the correlation of neuronal activity with the conditioned response, provide the only evidence of the behavioral relevance and primacy of single unit modification.

1. Advantages and Disadvantages of Mammalian Systems

There is presently a dilemma in the neurophysiology of associative learning. With few exceptions, the relatively simple neuronal systems that are amenable to the full use of electrophysiological techniques do not respond to conditioning with long-term changes in either behavior or neuronal activity. On the other hand, the organisms which readily learn have highly complex nervous systems.

Thus, the advantage in using mammalian preparations to investigate associative learning is that they do exhibit the phenomenon to be explained, and, despite their complexity, the mammalian central nervous system may obey general anatomical rules of organization, in terms of which the activity of single units can be interpreted. In cortical and many subcortical regions there are only a few anatomical types of neuron. Strict rules may govern the aborization of dendrites, the placement and functional significance of synapses, and, in general, the input and output of neuronal aggregates, thus producing a finite number of modes of organization. The bewildering complexity of these systems may thus be due not to the complexity of the individual circuits, but rather to the multiple occurrences of the same basic circuit. Although vertebrate single units are not reidentifiable, they may be identified as basic types, having a fixed place in a neuronal circuit. Such an analysis has been most successful in the cerebellum (Eccles, Ito, & Szentagothai, 1967).

Additional advantages of vertebrate preparations include the possibility of establishing the functional properties of single units. The input properties of sensory neurons can be determined, as well as the motor connections of some units. The highly plastic nature of much mammalian learning permits the use of various behavioral paradigms. Stimulus, motivation, and response can all be varied during learning to facilitate an analysis of how a unit's activity relates to the animal's behavior.

The disadvantages of using vertebrate (and most invertebrate) preparations in neuronal studies of learning include the difficulty in establishing the circuit depiction of a response. On the sensory side, this prevents a verification that the relevant input to a changing neuron remains constant during learning. On the motor side, it is manifest as an inability to link a neuron to the relevant response and, hence, to assess the significance of a change in neuronal parameters. Moreover, the activity of an individual neuron is neither necessary nor sufficient for any behavior. Even the most rudimentary response requires the simultaneous activity of a cluster of neurons (Phillips, 1966; Stoney, Thompson, & Asanuma, 1968). The long duration of electrical stimulation necessary to elicit a conscious sensation in humans suggest that rather complex neuronal aggregates must be organized (Libet, 1967).

To record vertebrate single units, a thicket of methodological problems must be faced and solved. Single units must be held for long periods of time. In interpreting the results, cognizance must be taken of the bias of a microelectrode, which samples from only the largest and perhaps the least plastic of neurons in any region (Towe and Harding, 1970). Experimenter bias is introduced with the inclusion of only those units having an initial response to the unconditioned stimulus. The stress and distraction caused by the paraphenalia of an electrophysiological experiment may produce animal bias, and may indeed be inimical to normal learning. Finally, a conditioning paradigm produces a number of conditioned responses. The pairing of a tone with shock to the paw, for example, produces not only a conditioned leg flexion, but also a conditioned heart rate response, a conditioned respiratory response, as well as conditioned arousal. Therefore, the plastic unit irrelevant to one response may be driving another response.

2. Steady State Unit Activity

In the steady stage paradigm, a population of neurons is sampled before and after conditioning. Because the same neuron is not observed at these two times, only general statements about changes in the average behavior of units are possible.

The classical conditioned eye blink of cats has been most thoroughly investigated (Woody, Vassilevsky, & Engel, 1970). Units responding to the click conditioned stimulus (CS) in the coronal-precruciate area, one of the cortical regions mediating eye blink, were recorded in the naive, conditioned, and extinguished animal. In conditioning, the click was followed by a glabellar tap eliciting an eye blink. After 500 trials, a conditioned eye blink was being elicited on 90 percent of the trials. During extinction, the pairing of stimuli was reversed. After the activity of each single unit was observed, it was classified as projecting to the eye if an arbitrary low current passed through the recording electrode elicited electromyographic activity in the *orbicularis oculi* muscle of the eye.

The threshold for elicited electromyographic activity in the eye muscle was generally lower in the conditioned than in the naive animal. Moreover, after conditioning there were significant changes in the number and the type of units responding to the click. In the naive animal, the click elicited equally small responses in both projective units. After conditioning, the click caused larger and longer increases in the activity of projective units. This activity follows the CS quickly enough to possibly mediate the behavioral response, the latency of cortical units being 8–16 msec, while the latency of eye muscle activity is 20 msec. After conditioning, many of the projective units had latencies 4 msec less than in the naive animal.

Thus the general responsiveness of many units paralleled the development of the conditioned response. However, the activity of the elicited activity in the recorded units was not significantly less when the conditioned stimulus failed to elicit a response. This lack of correlation may be explained by the many parallel cortical units controlling the eyeblink response, or it may indicate the effect of other brain regions. It was also found that projective units with spontaneous frequencies of less than 5 spikes per second showed a greater conditioned increase in evoked activity than units with higher spontaneous activity. In the naive animal, low activity units are not responsive to a click. During conditioning, therefore, either units with high activity are depressed, or low activity units become responsive to the CS.

An attempt has been made to map the brain in terms of units responsive to two conditioned stimuli having a different significance (Travis & Sparks, 1967).

Monkeys were conditioned by pairing one tone with automatic delivery of food, and pairing a tone of another frequency with shock. In the cortex and basal ganglia, single units were selected which were not related to gross movements of the animal. Of these units, 31 percent were changed in some way by one of the conditioned stimuli, exhibiting facilitation, inhibition, or more complex responses. The majority of responsive units gave differential responses to the two stimuli. In the anterior commissure, cingulate cortex, sensorimotor cortex, and the globus pallidus, about one half of the tested units were responsive to the stimuli. No responsive units could be found in the caudate, the interior capsule, or the putamen.

The operant conditioning paradigm also changes the activity of many neurons. In a pioneering study, monkeys were trained to flex an arm to avoid a shock to the hand (Jasper, Ricci, & Doane, 1960). The discriminative stimulus was a flickering light presented 5 seconds before the shock. Single unit activity and the surface EEG were recorded from the cortex. In the naive animal, the unpaired light flicker elicited unit responses in all parts of the cortex, and this activity was generally correlated with electroencephalographic desynchronication elicited by the novel CS. With repetition the CS gradually failed to elicit activity in most units. After an avoidance response had been conditioned, the activity of many units in the arm area of the motor cortex was correlated with the response. Units responded quickly to the CS with either a tonic facilitation or inhibition which preceded and was held past the behavioral response. The same units did not respond to the flicker of a higher frequency not preceding shock. The unit activity was correlated with the occurrence of the response, being generally absent when the animal failed to respond to the CS.

In the arm area of the sensory cortex, units in the conditioned animal responded to the CS with a latency longer than that of the behavioral response. These units may simply have been driven by proprioceptive feedback from the response itself. Single units in the parietal area may play a larger role in the animal's discrimination of a significant conditioned stimulus. Thirty percent of parietal units respond to the stimulus preceding shock, often following at the same frequency as the flicker, and are inhibited by the unreinforced stimulus. Moreover, when the unreinforced stimulus is first presented to a conditioned animal, it elicits leg flexion as well as unit activity following its higher frequency. With repetition, this stimulus progressively fails to elicit the avoidance response as single units come to be inhibited rather than excited by its presentation. Neurons in the parietal cortex may thus mediate an animal's discrimination of stimuli relevant to a response.

In a more complex paradigm, the responsiveness of units may be related to the previous conditioning of the animal (Travis, Houten, & Sparks, 1968; Travis & Sparks, 1968; Travis, Sparks, & Houten, 1968). In the globus pallidus of a monkey trained to lever press for food, about 30 percent of recorded single units are inhibited during various components of the response sequence by which an animal obtains and consumes the familiar reward. Units are inhibited during either the lever press, the search in the food hopper, the grasping of food, or the consummatory response. Moreover, these units are not inhibited when the animal is grasping unfamiliar or inedible objects, or when unfamiliar food is being ingested. These units could serve as the neuronal homologues of secondary reinforcement, or as the intermediates in the chaining of stimulus response sequences. Clearly, more behavioral paradigms must be run to establish the psychological correlates of these interesting units.

3. Single Unit Modification during Conditioning

In the steady state experiments it is not possible to specify the functional properties of single neurons which undergo change during learning. A preferable approach is to record from one neuron during the entire time an animal learns a response. Due to the exigencies of holding single units for any length of time, such experiments have used curarized animals and intertrial intervals of from 5–30 seconds. Stimuli to be conditioned have included a flash, click, or brief somatic stimulation. The unconditioned stimulus, which initially elicited activity in the neurons selected by the experimenter for observation, was either a shock to the skin or the stimulation of the sciatic nerve. Units have been recorded in the ponto-bulbar reticular formation (Buresova & Bures, 1965), the pontine reticular formation (Yoshii & Ogura, 1960), the nonspecific thalamus (Kamikawa, McIlwain, & Adey, 1964), the sensorimotor cortex (Adam, Adey, & Porter, 1966), and the motor cortex (O'Brien & Fox, 1969a, b). Although it was not demonstrated that the training paradigm actually produces a conditioned response, it is known that the classical conditioning of a curarized animal can facilitate the acquisition of a conditioned reflex in a subsequent unparalyzed state (Buchwald, Standish, Eldred, & Halas, 1964), and similar conditioning of unparalyzed animals produces a conditioned response within 75 to 100 trials.

During the repetitive presentation of the unpaired conditioned stimulus to the naive animal, few units habituate. In the motor cortex most units show a stable response during 90 trials. About 85 percent of the units in the reticular formation do not habituate to click, flash, or somatic stimulation with the intertrial intervals employed.

In many brain regions, the unit activity elicited by the CS undergoes progressive modification during conditioning. In the reticular formation, about 50 percent of the units responding to the unconditioned stimulus (UCS) can be conditioned. An equally large number of modifiable units exist in the nonspecific thalamic nuclei, and about 30 percent of the appropriate units in the sensorimotor cortex show conditioning.

Units in caudal brain structures can be most rapidly modified. The fastest conditioning usually occurs in the reticular formation, with most modifiable units entrained to the conditioned stimulus within 25 trials; however, some units in the dorsal hippocampus develop a conditioned response within 10 trials. Fifty trials is sufficient for plastic units of the nonspecific thalamic nuclei. In the cortex, 100 to 150 trials are required, although units in previously conditioned animals exhibit substantial savings, usually exhibiting a conditioned response within 30 to 60 trials. Conditioned unit responses do not appear during pseudo-conditioning.

Although a large percentage of units in all areas are conditioned to the CS, most extinguish rapidly. Many units are not even stable during extended conditioning, and either decline and stabilize at a reduced level of responsiveness, or disappear altogether. The units which do give a stable conditioned response following conditioning have not been shown to have unique electrophysiological properties.

The patterns of activity elicited by the CS are diverse. In all brain regions, the conditioned unit response can be either facilitation or inhibition of ongoing activity. It need not be similar either to the unconditioned response or to the response elicited by the CS before pairing with the unconditioned stimulus. Reticular formation neurons respond to the UCS with either excitation or inhibition, which, sign usually unchanged, comes to be elicited by the CS. Similarly, in areas of the diffuse thalamic nuclei, most sciatic nerve stimuli produce an inhibition of the ongoing activity which moves forward in time during conditioning. In the motor cortex, where the patterning of the CR has been most carefully investigated, two types of response can be distinguished. An excitatory conditioned response occurs at a fixed time after the CS, while an inhibitory conditioned response occurs at a fixed time before the US.

During extinction, when the CS is presented unpaired at the same intertrial interval as during conditioning, the conditioned unit response quickly wanes. The conditioned response is extinguished within a few trials in both the reticular formation and the diffuse thalamic nuclei. In the motor cortex, although the inhibitory conditioned response extinguishes rapidly, an excitatory response may persist for 15 to 30 trials. Together with the differential patterning of excitatory and inhibitory units, this suggests that two plastic processes are present in the motor cortex. Following extinction, units in all areas can usually be reconditioned and show savings, although the responsiveness of many diffuse thalamic neurons declines with repeated conditioning. Units not exhibiting plasticity under original conditioning do not become plastic during a second conditioning series.

During successful conditioning, a unit becomes functionally multimodal; it is driven by both the somatic UCS and the visual, or auditory, CS. This may result from the strengthening of existing multimodal connections, or the switching in of new lines. In both the reticular formation and the diffuse thalamic nuclei, originally unresponsive units can be entrained by the conditioned stimulus. However, because the level of habituation was not controlled in these experiments, an initial lack of responsiveness to the CS need not mean an absence of CS modality input. In the motor cortex, where little habituation occurs with the parameters of stimulation employed, only units originally responsive to the CS develop conditioned responses. It thus appears that in the motor cortex, conditioning involves the modification of existing pathways.

In addition to single units recordings from well-defined neurons, multiunit recordings have been made during classical and instrumental conditioning. The multiunit "hash" probably records the action potentials of both cell bodies and fibers located within 1.0 mm of the electrode tip (Halas & Beardsley, 1968). The spikes can be integrated over short time periods to give a running measure of multiunit activity, the amplitude of which is correlated with the size of the surrounding cell bodies (Grover & Buchwald, 1970), and is often independent of the slow wave activity recorded through the same electrode (Buchwald, Halas, & Schramm, 1966). The low impedance of multiunit electrodes permits chronic implantation and recording in freely moving animals.

Observations during conditioning have shown that multiunit activity in the reticular formation is quite similar to single unit activity, and have demonstrated a surprising amount of plasticity in the sensory projection system of the conditioned stimulus (Buchwald et al., 1966; Halas, Beardsley, & Sandlie, 1970). During the repetitive presentation of a tone, most electrodes in the auditory projection system record an evoked increase in multiunit activity which habituates. With prolonged habituation, an evoked inhibition of activity is seen in the medial geniculate body and the auditory cortex. When the tone is paired with foot shock in either unparalyzed or curarized cats, the first detectable conditioned response occurs within 20 to 30 trials in the reticular formation, the diffuse thalamus nuclei, and the cochlear nucleus. With continued pairing, conditioned multiunit activity appears in the higher brain structures of the auditory system. In the sensory projection system of the unconditioned stimulus, conditioned activity appears late in training and has the same latency as leg flexion, suggesting that this pathway merely registers feedback from the behavioral response.

A similar rostral sequential development in multiunit responsiveness occurs during the conditioning of a shock avoidance response. The greater number of trials to the first occurrence of a conditioned response in the instrumental paradigm is consonant with the greater difficulty of learning this task. In these two basic behavioral paradigms, then, conditioning of multiunit activity occurs in the reticular formation and the sensory system of the conditioned stimulus. Detectable entrainment occurs first in the lower brainstem, and with further training is found in more rostral structures.

Only one experimenter has attempted to record the activity of a single neuron for days at a time—long enough to study its behavior during an animal's acquisition of a difficult discrimination and response (Ito & Olds, 1970). A chronically implanted electrode was used to record multiunit activity in freely moving rats. An automatic system was programmed to single out and recognize the spike of one neuron by the parameters of its waveform. The accuracy of this system, however, is less than one employing standard microelectrode techniques. There is some doubt that a reidentified spike was actually generated by the same neuron throughout the experiment, and that the spike emanated from a cell body rather than a fiber.

Animals were rewarded with food on a variable interval schedule only if they remained motionless during the presentation of a one-second auditory stimulus. In a number of brain regions, excitatory unit responses to the conditioned stimulus were increased while decremental responses were attenuated, with the greatest changes taking place in the hippocampus and thalamus (Olds & Hirano, 1969). In discrimination training, one auditory stimulus was followed by the delivery of food, while a second stimulus predicted no food. The activity of purported single units was followed through habituation, conditioning, and extinction (Hirano, Best, & Olds, 1970). In habituation, when both stimuli were not paired with food, they elicited an equal response in the unit activity of the midbrain reticular formation. During 300 conditioning trials, the two stimuli came to elicit slightly different responses; this difference vanished during extinction. Hippocampal unit activity exhibited little decrement during habituation. Conditioning quickly increased the elicited unit responses, with a greater sustained pattern of activity occurring during the food reinforced stimulus. This differential responsiveness to two stimuli having different predictive significance was quite stable, persisting during 150 extinction trials.

In a second series of experiments, rats were trained to hold down a pedal for 2 seconds (Olds, Mink, & Best, 1969). Originally, two pedals were present, responses to one pedal being reinforced with food, while the second pedal delivered water. A number of units in the reticular formation were active during the later portion of the two-second waiting period. There is evidence that their activity depended on the relevance of the expected reward to the animal's ongoing motivation. The response of these units was usually higher when animals were working for food, for which they had higher motivation. When food drive was decreased by making food constantly available, the facilitation pattern of unit activity occurred only during the pedal press delivering water. Animals were then presented with only one pedal which had to be held down for 2 seconds to obtain any reward (Phillips & Olds, 1969). During the pedal press, one of three tones signalled whether food, water, or no reward would be forthcoming. With time, an excitatory response was present only during the CS signalling food reward. When the pairing of the stimuli was changed, the unit response changed accordingly, coming to occur only during the new stimulus signalling food. Also, when food was given spontaneously, the unit response gradually shifted to occur only during the CS signalling water. These units, therefore, do not differentiate between the stimulus properties of the CS, nor do they differentiate between the signalling properties of the CS. Rather, they seem to be of a higher order, responding to the motivational appropriateness of what the CS is signalling. It is as if they respond when the expected outcome is what the animal desires.

During the same series of experiments, single units in the hippocampus were also monitored. Some showed activity somewhat similar to neurons in the reticular formation. Other units, mostly located in the CA3 region, showed differential responsiveness to the conditioned stimuli. They were apparently conditioned to the type of reward which would follow the conditioned stimulus.

REFERENCES

Adam, G., Adey, W. R., & Porter, R. W. Interoceptive conditional responses in cortical neurons. *Nature*, 1966, Vol. 209, 920-921.

Adey, W. R. Neural information processing: Windows without and the citadel within. In L. D. Proctor (Ed.), *The proceedings of an international symposium on boicybernetics of the central nervous system*. Boston, Massachusetts: Little, Brown, 1969. Pp. 1-27.

Altman, J. Autoradiographic examination of behaviorally induced changes in the protein and nucleic acid metabolism of the brain. In J. Gaito (Ed.), *Macromolecules and behavior*. New York: Appleton-Century-Crofts, 1966. Pp. 103-126.

Aranda, L. C., & Luco, J. V. Further studies on an electric correlate of learning. Experiments in an isolated insect ganglion. *Physiology and Behavior*. 1969, Vol. 4, 133-137.

Basmajian, J. V. Control and training of individual motor units. *Science*, 1963, Vol. 141, 440-441.

Bell, C., Sierra, B., Buendia, N., & Segundo, J. P. Sensory properties of neurons in the mesencephalic reticular formation. *Journal of Neurophysiology*, 1964, Vol. 27, 961-987.

Bennett, M. V. L. Similarities between chemically and electrically mediated transmission. In F. D. Carlson (Ed.), *Physiological and biochemical aspects of nervous integration*. Englewood Cliffs, New Jersey: Prentice-Hall, 1968. Pp. 73-128.

Berry, R. W. Ribonucleic acid metabolism of a single neuron: correlation with electrical activity. *Science*, 1969, Vol. 166, 1021-1023.

Blankenship, J. E., Wachtel, H., & Kandel, E. R. Ionic mechanisms of excitatory and inhibitory and dual synaptic actions mediated by an identified interneuron in abdominal ganglion of Aplysia. *Journal of Neurophysiology*, 1971, Vol. 34, 76-92.

Bolles, R. Species-specific defense reactions and avoidance learning. *Psychological Review*, 1970, Vol. 77, 32-48.

Bruner, J., & Kennedy, D. Habituation: Occurrence at a neuromuscular junction. *Science*, 1970, Vol. 169, 92-94.

Bruner, J., & Kehoe, J. Long term decrements in the efficacy of synaptic transmission in molluscs and crustaceans. in G. Horn and R. A. Hinde (Eds.), *Short-term changes in neural activity and behaviour*. London & New York: Cambridge University Press, 1970. Pp. 323-359.

Bruner, J., & Tauc, L. Long-lasting phenomena in the molluscan nervous system. *Symposia of the Society for Experimental Biology*, 1966, Vol. 20, 457-475.

Buchwald, J. S., Halas, E. S., & Schramm, S. Relationships of neuronal spike populations and EEG activity in chronic cats. *Electroencephalography & Clinical Neurophysiology*, 1966, Vol. 21, 227-238.

Buchwald, J. S., Halas, E. S., & Schramm, S. Changes in cortical and subcortical unit activity during behavioral conditioning. *Physiology & Behavior.* 1966, Vol. 1, 11-22.

Buchwald, J. S., Standish, M., Eldred, E., & Halas, E. S. Contribution of muscle spindle circuits to learning as suggested by training under Flaxedil. *Electroenchepalography & Clinical Neurophysiology,* 1964, Vol. 16, 582-594.

Bures, J., & Buresova, O. Relationship between spontaneous and evoked activity in the inferior colliculus of rats. *Journal of Neurophysiology,* 1965, Vol. 28, 641-654.

Bures, J., & Buresova, O. Plastic changes of unit activity based on reinforcing properties of extracellular stimulation of single neurons. *Journal of Neurophysiology,* 1967, Vol. 30, 98-113.

Bures, J., & Buresova, O. Plasticity in single neurons and neural populations. In G. Horn and R. A. Hinde (Eds.), *Short-term changes in neural activity and behavior.* London and New York: Cambridge University Press, 1970.

Buresova, O., & Bures, J. Classical conditioning and reticular units. *Acta Physiologica Hungry,* 1965, Vol. 26, 53-57.

Burke, W. Neuronal models for conditioned reflexes. *Nature,* 1966, Vol. 210, 269-271.

Castellucci, V., Kupfermann, I., Pinsker, H., & Kandel, E. R. Neuronal mechanisms of habituation and dishabituation of the gill withdrawal reflex in *Aplysia. Science,* 1970, Vol. 167, 1745-1748.

Changeux, J. P., Kasai, M., & Lee, C. Y. Use of snake venom toxin to characterize the cholinergic receptor protein. *Proceedings of the National Academy of Science,* 1970, Vol. 67, 1241-1247.

Chow, K. L., and Leiman, A. L. The photo-sensitive organs of crayfish and brightness learning. *Behavior Biology.* 1972, Vol. 7, 25-35.

Cragg, B. G. Are there structural alterations in synapses related to functioning? *Proceedings of the Royal Society (Series B),* 1968, Vol. 171, 319-323.

Creutzfeld, O. D., Watanabe, S., & Lux, H. D. Relations between EEG phenomena and potentials of single cells.I. Evoked responses after thalamic and epicortical stimulation. *Electroencephalography & Clinical Neurophysiology,* 1966, Vol. 20, 1-18.

Dagan, D. & Parnas, I. Giant fibre and small fibre pathways involved in the evasive response of the cockroach. Periplaneta americana. *Journal of Experimental Biology,* 1970, Vol. 52, 312-324.

Dawkins, R. Selective neuron death as a possible memory mechanism. *Nature,* 1971, Vol. 229, 118-119.

Dolivo, M., & Rouiller, C. Changes in ultrastructure and synaptic transmission in the sympathetic ganglion during various metabolic conditions. *Progress in Brain Research,* 1969, Vol. 31, 111-123.

Ebbecke, U. *Die Kortikalon Erregingen.* Leipzig: Barth, 1919.

Eccles, J. C. *The neurophysiological basis of mind.* London & New York: Oxford University Press (Claredon), 1953.

Eccles, J. C. *The physiology of synapses.* Berlin: Springer-Verlag, 1964.

Eccles, J. C., Ito, M., & Szentagothai, J. *The cerebellum as a neuronal machine.* New York: Springer-Verlag, 1967.

Epstein, R., & Tauc, L. Heterosynaptic facilitation and posttetanic potentiation in *Aplysia* nervous system. *Journal of Physiology,* 1970, Vol 209, 1-23.

Fetz, E. E. Operant conditioning of cortical unit activity. *Science,* 1969, Vol. 163, 955-958.

Fox, S. Evoked potential, coding, and behaviour. In F. O. Schmitt (Ed.), *The Neurosciences: Second study program.* New York: Rockefeller University Press, 1970. Pp. 243-259.

Frazier, W. T., Kandel, E. R., Kupfermann, I., Waziri, R., & Coggeshall, R. E. Morphological and functional properties of identified cells in the abdominal ganglion of *Aplysia californica*. *Journal of Neurophysics*, 1967, Vol. 30, 1288-1335.

Frazier, W. T., Waziri, R., & Kandel, E. Alterations in the frequency of spontaneous activity in *aplysia* neurons with contingent and noncontingent nerve stimulation. *Federation Proceedings*, 1965, Vol. 24, 522.

Galambos, R. A *glia-neural* theory of brain function. *Proceeding of the National Academy of Science*, 1961, Vol. 47, 129-136.

Gerbrandt, L. K., Skrebitsky, V. G., Buresova, O., & Bures, J. Plastic changes of unit activity induced by tactile stimuli followed by electrical stimulation of single hippocampal and reticular neurons. *Neuropsychologia*, 1968, Vol. 6, 3-10.

Griffin, J. P. Neurophysiological studies into habituation. In G. Horn and R. A. Hinde (Eds.), *Short-term changes in neural activity and behaviour*. London and New York: Cambridge University Press, 1970. Pp. 141-180.

Grover, F. S., & Buchwald, J. S. Correlation of cell size with amplitude of background fast activity in specific brain nuclei. *Journal of Neurophysiology*, 1970, Vol. 33, 160-171.

Groves, P. M., & Thompson, R. F. Habituation: A dual-process theory. *Psychological Review*, 1970, Vol. 77, 419-450.

Gwilliam, G. F. Electrical responses to photic stimulation in the eyes and nervous system of nereid polychaetes. *Biological Bulletin*, 1969, Vol. 136, 385-397.

Haigler, H. J., & von Baumgarten, R. J. The minimum latency of heterosynaptic facilitation in *Aplysia*. *Federation Proceedings*, 1970, Vol. 29, 589.

Halas, E. S., & Beardsley, J. V. Specificity of multiple unit activity in the sensory nuclei of cats. *Physiology & Behavior*, 1968, Vol. 3, 275-279.

Halas, E. S., Beardsley, J. V., & Sandlie, M. E. Conditioned neuronal responses at various levels in conditioning paradigms. *Electroencephalography & Clinical Neurophysiology*, 1970, Vol. 28, 468-477.

Hall, R. D. Habituation of evoked potentials in the rat under conditions of behavioral control. *Electroencephalography and Clinical Neurophysiology*, 1968, Vol. 24, 155-165.

Hamlyn, L. H. The fine structure of the mossy fiber endings in the hippocampus of the rabbit. *Journal of Anatomy*, 1962, Vol. 96, 112-120.

Harris, J. D. Habituatory response decrement in the intact organism. *Psychological Bulletin*, 1943, Vol. 40, 385-422.

Hebb, D. O. *The organization of behavior*. New York: Wiley, 1949.

Hernandez-Peon, R. Neurophysiological correlates of habituation and other manifestations of plastic inhibition (internal inhibition). *Electroencephalography & Clinical Neurophysiology, Supplement* 1960, Vol. 13, 101-114.

Hirano, T. , Best, P., & Olds, J. Units during habituation, discrimination learning, and extinction. *Electroencephalography & Clinical Neurophysiology*, 1970, Vol. 28, 127-135.

Holmgren, B., & Frenk, S. Inhibitory phenomena and "habituation" at the neuronal level. *Nature*, 1961, Vol. 192, 1294-1295.

Horn, G. Neuronal mechanisms of habituation. *Nature*, 1967, Vol. 215, 707-711.

Horn, G., & Hill, R. M. Responsiveness to sensory stimulation of units in the superior colliculus and subjacent tectotegmental regions of the rabbit. *Experimental Neurology*, 1966, Vol. 14, 199-224.

Horn, G., & Hinde, R. A. (Eds.) *Short-term changes in neural activity and behavior*. London & New York: Cambridge University Press, 1970.

Horn, G., & Rowell, C. H. F. Medium and long term changes in the behaviour of visual neurons in the tritocerebrum of locusts. *Journal of Experimental Biology*, 1968, Vol. 49, 143-169.

Horn, G., & Wright, M. J. Characteristics of transmission failure in the squid stellate ganglion: A study of a simple habituating system. *Journal of Experimental Biology*, 1970, Vol. 51, 217-231.

Horridge, G. A. The electrophysiological approach to learning in isolatable ganglia. In W. H. Thorpe & D. Davenport (Ed.), *Learning & associated phenomena in invertebrates*. Pp. 163-182. *Animal Behavior Supplement* No. 1, 1964.

Horridge, G. A., Scholes, J. H., Shaw, S., & Tunstall, J. Extracellular recordings from single neurons in the optic lobe and brain of the locust. In J. E. Treherne & J. W. L. Beament (Eds.), *The physiology of the insect central nervous system*. New York.: Academic Press, 1965. Pp. 165-203.

Horridge, G. Analysis of the rapid response of Nereis and Harmothoe (Annelida). *Proceedings of the Royal Society (Series B)*, 1959, Vol. 150, 245-262.

Hoyle, G. Neurophysiological studies on "learning" in headless insects. In J. E. Treherne & J. W. L. Beament, (Eds.), *The physiology of the insect central nervous system*. Academic Press, New York, 1965, 203-232.

Huber, F. Brain controlled behaviour in Orthopterans. In J. E. Treherne & J. W. L. Beament (Eds.), *The physiology of the insect central nervous system*. London & New York: Academic Press, 1965.

Hughes, G. M. Neuronal pathways in the insect nervous system. In J. E. Treherne & J. W. L. Beament (Eds.), *The physiology of the insect central nervous system*. New York: Academic Press, 1965. Pp. 79-112.

Ito, M., & Olds, J. Changes in unitary discharges of cortical and subcortical neurons during self stimulation. *Federation Proceedings*, 1970, Vol. 29, A590.

Jasper, H. H., Ricci, G., & Doane, B. Microelectrode analysis of cortical cell discharge during avoidance conditioning in the monkey. *Electroencephalography & Clinical Neurophysiology*, 1960, Vol. 13, (Supplement), 137-155.

Jennings, H. S. *Behavior of the lower organisms*. New York: Macmillan, 1906.

John, E. R. Higher nervous system functions: brain functions & learning. *Annual Review of Physiology*, 1961, Vol. 23, 451-484.

John, E. R. *Mechanisms of memory*, Academic Press, New York, 1967.

Kamikawa, K. J., McIlwain, T., & Adey, W. R. Response patterns of thalamic neurons during classical conditioning. *Electroencephalography & Clinical Neurophysiology*, 1964, Vol. 17, 485-496.

Kandel, E. R., & Spencer, W. A. Cellular neurophysiological approaches in the study of learning. *Physiological Review*, 1968, Vol. 48, 65-134.

Kandel, E. R., & Tauc, L. Heterosynaptic facilitation in neurons of the abdominal ganglion of *Aplysia depilans*. *Journal of Physiology (London)*, 1965, Vol. 181, 1-27. (a)

Kandel, E. R., & Tauc, L. Mechanism of heterosynaptic facilitation in the giant cell of the abdominal ganglion of *Aplysia depilans*. *Journal of Physiology (London)*, 1965, Vol. 181, 28-47. (b)

Kappers, C. U. & Ariens, --. --., Further contributions on neurobiotaxis IX. *Journal of Comparative Neurology*, 1917, Vol. 27, 261-298.

Katz, B., & Thesleff, S. On the factors which determine the amplitude of the "miniature end-plate potential." *Journal of Physiology*, 1957, Vol. 137, 267-278.

Kernell, D., & Peterson, R. P. The effect of spike activity versus synaptic activation on the metabolism of ribonucleic acid in a molluscan giant neuron. *Journal of Neurochemistry*, 1970, Vol. 17, 1087-1094.

Kozak, W. & Westerman, R. Basic patterns of plastic change in the mammalian nervous system. *Society of Experimental Biology*, 1966, Vol. 20, 509-543.

Krasne, F. B. Excitation and habituation of the crayfish escape reflex: The depolarizing response in lateral giant fibres of the isolated abdomen. *Journal of Experimental Biology*, 1969, Vol. 50, 29-46.

Krasne, F. & Woodsmall, K. S. Waning of the crayfish escape response as a result of repeated stimulation. *Animal Behavior*, 1969, Vol. 17, 416-424.

Kupferman, I., Pinsker, H., Castellucci, W. & Kandel, E. R. Neuronal correlates of habituation and dishabituation of the gill withdrawal reflex in *Aplysia*. *Science*, 1970, Vol. 167, 1743-1745.

Kupferman, I. & Pinsker, H. Plasticity in *Aplysia* neurons and some simple neuronal models of learning. In J. T. Tapp (Ed.), *Reinforcement and behavior*. New York: Academic Press, 1969. Pp. 356-386.

Landauer, T. K. Two hypotheses concerning the biochemical basis of memory. *Psychological Review*, 1964, Vol. 71, 167-179.

Lashley, K. S. The Mechanism of Vision. *Journal of Comparative Neurology*, 1934, Vol. 59, (3), 341-374.

Lashley, K. S. In search of the engram. *Symposia for the Society of Experimental Biology*, 1950, Vol. 4, 454-482.

Libet, B. Long latent periods and further analysis of slow synaptic responses in sympathetic ganglia, *Journal of Neurophysiology*, 1967, Vol. 30, 494-514.

Lickey, M. E. Learned Behavior in *Aplysia Vaccaria*. *Journal of Comparative, & Physiological Psychology*, 1968, Vol. 66, 712-718.

Loeb, J. *The mechanistic conception of life*, Chicago, Illinois: University of Chicago Press, 1912. Cambridge, Massachusetts: Harvard University Press, 1964.

Martin, A. R., & Pilar, G. Dual mode of synaptic transmission in the avian ciliary ganglion. *Journal of Physiology (London)*, 1963, Vol. 168, 443-463.

Martin, A. R., & Pilar, G. An analysis of electrical coupling at synapses in the avian ciliary ganglion, *Journal of Physiology*, 1964, Vol. 171, 454-475.

Morrell, F. Electrophysiological contributions to the neural basis of learning. *Physiological Review*, 1961, Vol. 41, 443-494.

Miledi, R., Molinoff, P., & Potter, L. T. Isolation of cholinergic receptor protein of tropedo electric tissue. *Nature*, 1971, Vol. 229, 554-557.

Miledi, R., & Slater, C. R. The action of calcium on neuronal synapses in the squid. *Journal of Physiology (London)*, 1966, Vol. 184, 473-498.

Miller, N. E. Certain facts of learning relevant to the search for its physical basis. In G. C. Quarton, T. Melnechuk, & F. O. Schmitt (Eds.), *The neurosciences: a study program*, New York: Rockefeller University Press, 1967. Pp. 643-652.

O'Brien, J. H., & Fox, S. S. Single-cell activity in cat motor cortex. I. Modifications during classical conditioning procedures. *Journal of Neurophysiology*, 1969, Vol. 32, 267-284. (a)

O'Brien, J. H., & Fox, S. S. Single-cell activity in cat motor cortex. II. Functional characteristics of the cell related to conditioning changes. *Journal of Neurophusiology*, 1969, Vol. 32, 285-296. (b)

Olds, J. Operant conditioning of single unit responses. *Proceedings of the 23rd International Congress of Physiological Science, Tokyo*, 1965, Vol. 4, 372-380.

Olds, J., & Hirano, T. Conditioned responses of hippocampal and other neurons. *Electroencephalography & Clinical Neurophysiology*, 1969, Vol. 26, 159-66.

Olds, J., Mink, W. D., & Best, P. J. Single unit patterns during anticipatory behavior. *Electroencephalography & Clinical Neurophysiology*, 1969, Vol. 26, 144-58.

Olds, J., & Olds, M. E. Interference & learning in paleocortical systems. In J. F. Delafresnaye (Ed.), *Brain mechanisms and learning*. Oxford: Blackwell, 1961. Pp. 153-88.

Peterson, R. P., & Kernell, D. Effects of nerve stimulation on the metabolism of ribonucleic acid in a molluscan giant neuron. *Journal of Neurochemistry*, 1970, (in press).

Phillips, C. G. Changing concepts of precentral motor area. In J. C. Eccles, *Brain and conscious experience*. New York: Springer-Verlag, 1966. Pp. 389-421.

Phillips, M. I., & Olds, J. Unit activity: Motivation-dependent responses from midbrain neurons. *Science (Washington)*, 1969, Vol. 165, 1269-1271.

Pinsker, H., Kupferman, I., Castellucci, V., & Kandel, E. Habitutation and Dishabituation of Gill-Withdrawal reflex in *aplysia. Science*, 1970, Vol. 167, 1740-1742.

Pribram, K. H. Some dimensions of remembering: steps toward a neuropsychological model of memory. In J. Gaito (Ed.), *Macromolecules and behavior*. New York: Appleton-Century-Crofts, 1966. Pp. 165-186.

Prosser, C., Ladd, --., & Hunter, W. S. The extinction of startle responses and spinal reflexes in the white rat. *American Journal of Physiology*, 1936, Vol. 117, 609-618.

Purpura, D. P. Comparative physiology of dendrites. In G. C. Quarton, T. Melneckuk, & F. O. Schmitt (Eds.), *The neurosciences: a study program*. New York: The Rockefeller University Press, 1967, Pp. 372-393.

Roberts, M. B. V. The giant fibre reflex of the earthworm, *Lumbricus terrestris*. I. The rapid response. *Journal of Experimental Biology*, 1962, Vol. 39, 219-228. (a)

Roberts, M. B. V. The giant fibre reflex of the earthworm, *Lumbricus terrestris*. II. Fatigue. *Journal of Experimental Biology*, 1962, Vol. 39, 229-237. (b)

Roberts, E. Models for correlative thinking about brain, behavior and biochemistry. *Brain Research*, 1966, Vol. 2, 109-144.

Roeder, K. D. *Nerve cells and insect behaviour*. Cambridge, Massachusetts: Harvard University Press, 1963.

Rowell, C. H. Fraser, Central Control of an Insect Segmental Reflex II. Analysis of the Inhibitory Input from the Metathoracic Ganglion. *Journal of Experimental Biology*, 1969, Vol. 50, 191-201.

Rowell, C. H., Fraser, ., & Horn, G. Response characteristics of neurons in an insect brain. *Nature (London)*, 1967, Vol. 216, 702-703.

Scheibel, M. E., & Scheibel, A. B. The response of reticular units to repetitive stimuli. *Archives Italian Biology*, 1965, Vol. 103, 279-299.

Scheibel, M. E., & Scheibel, A. B. Anatomical basis of attention mechanisms in vertebrate brains. In G. C. Quarton, T. Melnechuk, & F. O. Schmitt (Eds.), *The neurosciences: A study program*. New York: The Rockefeller University Press, 1967, Pp. 577-602.

Segundo, J. P., Takenaka, T., & Encabo, H. Electrophysiology of bulbar reticular neurons. *Journal of Neurophysiology*, 1967, Vol. 30, 1194-1220.

Sharpless, S. K. Reorganization of function in the nervous system—use and disuse. *Annual Review of Physiology*, 1964, Vol. 26, 357-388.

Sherrington, C. S. *The integrative action of the nervous system*. New Haven, Connecticut: Yale University Press, 1906.

Sokolov, E. N. Neuronal models and the orienting influence. In M. A. B. Brazier (Ed.), *Central nervous system and behavior*. New York: Josiah Macey, Jr. Foundation, 1960. Pp. 187-239.

Spencer, W. A., Thompson, R. F., & Neilsen, D. R., Jr. Response decrement of the flexion reflex in the acute spinal cat and transient restoration by strong stimuli. *Journal of Neurophysiology*, 1966. Vol. 29, 221-239. (a)

Spencer, W. A., Thompson, R. F., & Neilsen, D. R., Jr. Alterations in responsiveness of ascending and reflex pathways activated by iterated cutaneous afferent volleys. *Journal of Neurophysiology*, 1966. Vol. 29, 240-252. (b)

Spencer, W. A., Thompson, R. F., & Neilson, D. R. Jr. Decrement of ventral root electrotonus and intracellularly recorded PSP's produced by iterated curaneous afferent volleys, *Journal of Neurophysiology*, 1966, Vol. 29, 253-273. (c)

Spira, M. E., Parnas, I., & Bergmann, F. Organization of the giant axons of the cockroach *Periplaneta Americana. Journal of Experimental Biology*, 1969, Vol. 50, 615-627.

Stoney, S. D., Jr., Thompson, W. D., & Asanuma, H. Excitation of pyramidal tract cells by intracortical microstimulation: Effective extent of stimulating current. *Journal of Neurophysiology*, 1968, Vol. 31, 659-669.

Tauc, L., & Bruner, J. "Desensitization" of cholinergic receptors by acetylcholine in molluscan central neurons. *Nature,* 1963, Vol. 198, 33-34.

Tauc, L., & Epstein, R. Heterosynaptic facilitation as a distinct mechanism in *Aplysia. Nature (London)*, 1967, Vol. 214, 724-725.

Thesleff, S. A study of the interaction between neuromuscular blocking agents and acetylocholine at the mammalian motor end-plate, *Acta Anaesthesiologica Scandinavica*, 1958, Vol. 2, 69-79.

Thompson, R. F., & Spencer, W. A. Habituation: a model phenomenon for the study of neuronal substrates of behavior. *Psychological Review*, 1966, Vol. 173, 16-43.

Towe, A. L., & Tyner, C. F. Cortical Circuitry underlying mixed receptive fields of certain pyramidal tract neurons. *Experimental Neurology*, 1971, Vol. 31, 239.

Travis, R. P., Jr., Hooten, T. F., & Sparks, D. L. Single unit activity related to behavior motivated by food reward. *Physiology and Behavior*, 1968, Vol. 3, 309-318.

Travis, R. P., Jr., & Sparks, D. L. Changes in unit activity during stimuli associated with food and shock reinforcement. *Physiology and Behavior*, 1967, Vol. 2, 171-177.

Travis, R. P., Jr., Sparks, D. L., & Hooten, T. F. Single unit response related to sequences of food motivated behavior. *Brain Research*, 1968, Vol. 7, 455-458.

Vinogradova, O. S. Dynamic classification of the reaction of hippocampal neurons to sensory stimulation. *Zhurnal Vysskei Nervnoi Deyatel' Nosti imeni I. P. Pavlova*, 1965, Vol. 15, 500; *Federation Proceedings, Translation Supplement*, 1966, Vol. 25, T397-T403.

Vinogradova, O. S. Investigation of habituations in the single neurons of caudate nucleus. *Journal of Higher Nervous Activity*, 1968, Vol. 8, 671-680.

von Baumgarten, R. J. Plasticity in the nervous system at the unitary level. In F. O. Schmitt (Ed.), *The Neurosciences: Second study program*. New York: Rockefeller University Press. 1970. Pp. 260-271.

von Baumgarten, R. J., & Djahnparwar, B. Time course of repetitive heterosynaptic facilitation in *Aplysia Californica. Brain Research*, 1967, Vol. 4, 295-297.

von Baumgarten, R. J., & Hukuhara, T. The role of the interstimulus interval in heterosynaptic facilitation in *Aplysia californica. Brain Research*, 1969, Vol. 16, 369-381.

Wachtel, H., & Kandel, E. R. Conversion of synaptic excitation to inhibition at a dual chemical synapse. *Journal of Neurophysiology*, 1971, Vol. 34, 56-68.

Wall, P. D. Sensory role of impulses travelling in dorsal columns towards cerebral cortex. *Brain*, 1970, Vol. 93, 505.

Waziri, R., Kandel, E. R., & Frazier, W. T. Organization of inhibition in abdominal ganglion of *Aplysia.* II. Post-tetanic potentiation, heterosynaptic depression and increments in frequency of inhibitory postsynaptic potentials. *Journal of Neurophysiology*, 1969, Vol. 32, 509-519.

Wickelgren, B. G. Habituation of spinal motoneurons. *Journal of Neurophysiology*, 1967, Vol. 30, 1404-1423. (a)

Wickelgren, B. G. Habituation of spinal interneurons. *Journal of Neurophysiology*, 1967, Vol. 30, 1424-1438. (b)

Wickelgren, W. A. Effect of state of arousal on click-evoked responses in cats. *Journal of Neurophysiology*, 1968, Vol. 31, 757-768. (a)

Wickelgren, W. A. Effects of walking and flash stimulation on click-evoked responses in cats. *Journal of Neurophysiology*, 1968, Vol. 31, 769-777. (b)

Wood, D. C. Parametric studies of the response decrement produced by mechanical stimuli in the protozoan *Stentor coeruleus. Journal of Neurobiology*, 1970, Vol. 1 (3), 345-360. (a)

Wood, D. C. Electrophysiological studies of the protozoan *Stentor coeruleus. Journal of Neurobiology*, 1970, Vol. 1 (4), 363-377. (b)

Wood, D. C. Electrophysiological correlates of the response decrement produced by mechanical stimuli in the protozoan, *Stentor coeruleus. Journal of Neurobiology*, 1970, Vol. 2 (1), 1-11. (c)

Woody, C. D., Vassilevsky, N. N., & Engel, J. Conditioned eye blink-unit: activity at coronalprecruiciate cortex of cat. *Journal of Neurophysiology*, 1970, Vol. 33, 838.

Worden, F. G. Attention and Auditory electrophysiology. In Eliot Stellar and James M. Sprague (Eds.), *Progress in Physiological Psychology*, 1966, Vol. 1, 45-116.

Wurtz, R. H., Castellucci, V. F., & Nusrula, J. M. Synaptic plasticity-effect of action potential in post-synaptic neuron. *Experimental Neurology*, 1967, Vol. 18, 350-368.

Yoshii, N., & Ogura, H. Studies on the unit discharge of brainstem reticular formation in the cat. I. Changes of reticular unit discharge following conditioning procedure. *Medical Journal of Osaka University*, 1960, Vol. 11, 1-17.

Young, J. Z. *The memory system of the brain*. Berkeley, California: University of California Press, 1966.

CHAPTER

7

SELF-STIMULATION: THE NEUROPHYSIOLOGY OF REWARD AND MOTIVATION

C. R. GALLISTEL[1]

[1] I wish to thank Drs. Frank Irwin, Martin Seligman, and Peter Van Sommers for reading and criticizing parts of early drafts. Their suggestions have been extremely helpful. The editor, J. A. Deutsch, also read the manuscript and made numerous valuable suggestions, for which I am grateful. Particular thanks go to my wife, Rochel, for invaluable, painstaking criticism of every draft. The writing of this chapter and much of the author's research reported in it were supported by NIH grant No. 13628.

I. INTRODUCTION

In 1954 Olds and Milner reported that rats would learn to seek out electrical stimulation of certain areas of the brain, much as rats will learn to seek out food. That is, whenever a behavior such as pressing a lever or running a runway produced electrical stimulation of the appropriate area of the brain, the rat would repeat that behavior pattern with increasing frequency. The same phenomenon was soon observed in many other species. Since brain stimulation in certain areas has an effect on behavior similar to the effect of natural rewards, experiments on the self-stimulation phenomenon may lead to a better understanding of the way in which natural rewards affect the central nervous system.

A self-stimulation electrode may be viewed as a voltage probe that permits activation of a neural circuit at a central point in such a way as to mimic the effect of offering an animal a reward. Just as with complex electrical circuits, the use of a central probe should help to reveal the structure and organization of the neural tissue. Inputs delivered via the central probe can be used to test certain hypotheses about the structure of the neural circuit that would not be readily testable with external inputs. For example, in electronics a central probe is helpful in deciding whether the output of a black box amplifier is direct or AC coupled. This review examines the data from self-stimulation experiments to see if they give similarly helpful insights into the structure of the neuronal circuits that mediate the effects of rewards such as food and water.

The review focuses on "homeostatic" rewards, such as food and water, because electrodes which sustain self-stimulation will often elicit stimulation-bound eating, drinking, and other components of homeostatic or quasi-homeostatic behaviors. The neural circuits mediating the effects of other reinforcing events, such as "escape-from-pain" or "opportunity-to-explore," may or may not be similar to the circuits mediating homeostatic reinforcers. It is not clear that it is reasonable to seek a general and unitary theory of reinforcement that explains all the instances in which the term is currently employed.

In order to facilitate the use of self-stimulation data to test theories of homeostatic reward mechanisms, the theories have been organized and presented within a single framework—the framework provided by control theory. The use of this framework was dictated by the close association between self-stimulation and homeostatic consummatory behaviors. Control theory provides a flexible framework for elaborating theories about feedback systems. Feedback system (e.g., homeostats) are systems in which the output (e.g., eating) affects the input (e.g., hunger).

Another advantage of control theory is that it provides a common set of conventions for describing various models (see legends to Figs. 7-1 and 7-2). The review makes frequent use of the terms drive, reward, and incentive. These terms have figured in most theories that sought to explain simple food-rewarded learning. Since there have been many theories, the terms have acquired a variety of meanings. When the terms are used without reference to a framework, their meanings are necessarily vague. In order to clarify the various meanings of these common terms, the review begins by schematizing, within the framework of control theory, the fundamental aspects of some well known theories of learning.

The schemata are intended only to clarify the usage of the terms drive, reward, and incentive in the discussion of self-stimulation. The schemata are oversimplified because they were created to represent the common theories of learning only insofar as these theories have been or might be applied to self-stimulation. Hopefully, the schemata adequately represent the models that have been developed specifically to account for self-stimulation. They necessarily do the more general theories an injustice in that these oversimplified schemata do not address themselves to many matters dealt with by the general theories. However, they adequately represent the general theories of learning in the following limited sense: If one applies the schemata to a body of data relevant to the relation between drive and reward in which, say, Hull's (1943) theory and Spence's (1956) theory have been thought to disagree, then the schema attributed to Spence predicts what Spence predicted and the schema attributed to Hull predicts what Hull predicted.

The schematization of the well-known theories of learning deliberately avoids the question of how new behavior patterns are organized. That is, the schemata do not explain what the mechanism is that restructures itself in such a way that the animal becomes capable of successfully executing a previously novel sequence of movements, such as the sequence required in pressing a lever or negotiating a maze. It is assumed that the mechanisms underlying the execution of behavior patterns, new or old, can be separated from the mechanism whereby the behavior patterns are brought under the control of motivational states. That is, the mechanism underlying the actual sequence of movements a rat makes in pressing a lever can be separated from the mechanism which leads the rat to "call-up" that sequence and related sequences when, and only when, the rat is hungry.

A. Drive, Reward, and Incentive

Drive usually refers to the effects that internal conditions such as tissue needs and hormone levels have on the direction and avidity of behavior. When we deprive a rat of food for 48 hours, the rate at which it runs an alley for food increases. This effect on the avidity of runway performance is attributed to the higher level of the hunger drive. When we deprive a rat of water but not food, it chooses an alley that leads to water in preference to an alley that leads to food. This effect on the direction of behavior is attributed to the higher level of the thirst drive.

Drive, then, is conceived of as something that energizes or potentiates patterns of behavior. "Potentiates" is perhaps more precise than "energizes," because "energizes" would imply that drive could activate behavior patterns even in the absence of the appropriate external stimulus conditions. Sometimes this does appear to occur. Lorenz (1937), for example, describes a starling which "killed" and "ate" nonexistent insects. Lorenz termed this a Leerlaufreaktion (vacuum behavior). In general, however, most theorists, including Lorenz, have treated drive as something that "potentiates" behavior, that is, increases the likelihood that a behavior will occur given the appropriate stimulus conditions. This usage seems to capture the Hullian idea, shared by Morgan (1957), that drive facilitates the manifestation of S-R connections, and the related idea of Stellar (1960, p. 1502) that drives can determine "whether or not external stimuli will be effective." "Potentiates" also compasses Deutsch's (1960) treatment of drive. In general, theorists since Lashley (1938) and Lorenz (1937) have regarded drive as something that facilitates the emergence of specific types of behavior.

Reward usually refers to the effects of goal attainment on the direction and avidity of behavior. When we increase the amount of food a hungry rat receives for running an alley, the rat's running speed increases. This effect on the avidity of performance is attributed to the new reward level. When we increase the amount of food in one arm of a T maze, the rat will begin to choose that arm in preference to the arm with a smaller food reward. This effect on the direction of behavior is attributed to the relative levels of reward.

Incentive usually refers to the potentiating or behavior-heightening effects of reward. If we change the partial reinforcement schedule in a Skinner box, so that a rat suddenly receives many more rewards than it previously was receiving, the rat's rate of pressing shows a temporarily exaggerated increase, before settling down to the rate characteristic of the new schedule. This temporary overshoot (positive contrast) is usually attributed to incentive. There is, however, more diversity in the use of the term incentive than in the use of the other two terms. Incentive is sometimes used to refer to the combined effect of drive and reward. Using incentive in this broader fashion allows one to speak of the incentive of a food reward waxing and waning as a function of hours of food deprivation. The models underlying this broader usage are seldom precisely spelled out.

Sometimes incentive is used as a general term that refers to the mechanism (hypothetical construct) by which rewards or reinforcements influence performance (see Logan, 1960, Introduction). When incentive is used in this way, any effect of reward on performance is necessarily an incentive effect. Thus, what we here call the reward or reinforcement components of the various models would be called the incentive components by other theorists. In other words, reward and incentive do not necessarily refer to different theoretical concepts. Reward can be used to refer to the actual goal that an animal's response produces, while incentive is used to refer to some or all of the theoretical processes that occur in the animal as a result of the reward. Most typically, incentive does not refer to all of these theoretical processes, but rather only to a behavior potentiating process whose effects are similar to the effects of drive (e.g., Bindra, 1968; Logan, 1960; Spence, 1956; Trowill, Panksepp, & Gandelman, 1969).

In some theories (e.g., Deutsch, 1960; Hull, 1943), reward does not potentiate behavior in the sense in which drives potentiate behavior. These purely homeostatic schemata are considered first.

B. Learning Models

1. The Pure Homeostat Schema

The first class of models (Fig. 7-1) treat drive as a source of behavioral potentiation and reinforcement as an adjustment of the parameter that transfers potentiation from the drive system to the behavior pattern that produced reward. For each behavior pattern in an animal's repertoire there is a parameter which determines how much drive potentiation is transferred from the source (the drive center or central drive state) to the behavior pattern. Under equally favorable external stimulus conditions the behavior pattern receiving the most potentiation prevails. When a particular behavior pattern is followed by a reward, the reinforcement system adjusts the drive-transfer parameters so that the behavior pattern will receive more of whatever drive potentiation is available. Once adjusted, drive-transfer parameters remain fixed until there is a change in the reward contingencies.

In this schema, a behavior pattern does not appear just because it has been rewarded. In addition to the appropriate stimuli, there must be suprathreshold drive potentiation in order for a behavior pattern to appear. However, given a fixed drive and constant stimulus conditions, the size and number of previous rewards determine which pattern will appear and how avidly the pattern will be executed. The relation between drive and reward embodied in this schema has frequently been termed the multiplicative relation between drive and habit strength (Kimble, 1961, p. 408).

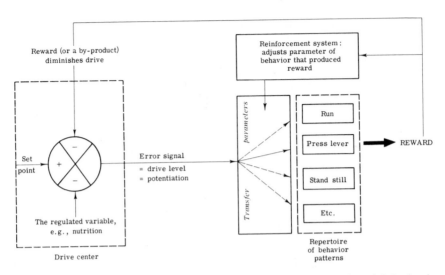

Fig. 7-1. Schematization of the relation between drive, reward, and behavior in purely homeostatic models. It is assumed, for the sake of example, that lever pressing is being rewarded and all other patterns are not being rewarded. The parameter changing effect of the reward is indicated by the solid arrow pointing to the Press lever behavior pattern. The broken arrows pointing to the other behavior patterns indicate that no parameter change has occurred for these patterns because these patterns have not produced an appropriate reward. The changing of a drive-transfer parameter can also be thought of as the establishment of a connection between the drive center and the behavior pattern that produced reward. In this diagram and subsequent diagrams certain control-theory conventions are followed. Solid lines forming rectangles, circles, and triangles indicate points where signals are integrated and/or transformed. Such points are referred to as transfer functions. Arrows indicate the direction of signal flow between transfer functions. Singnals which act to change the parameters (i.e., operating characteristics) of earlier transfer functions are referred to as parameter forcing feedback signals. They are indicated with arrows that penetrate into the transfer function boxes. Signals which do not alter the parameters of the transfer functions but simply serve as inputs that are operated on by the transfer functions are indicated by arrows that do not penetrate into the transfer functions. Whenever there is a comparator, that is, a transfer function which compares one variable, for example, the actual level of nutrition, against another variable, for example, the level of nutrition which the system is trying to maintain (the set point), this transfer function is indicated by a circle partitioned into four or more wedges. The signs in the wedges indicate which variables are compared against which. All positive variables are compared against all negative variables. If the result is not equal to zero, an error signal appears at the output from the comparator. When the minuses and pluses exactly cancel out, the comparator is said to be in balance.

2. The Pure Incentive Schema

A second class of models, hedonic or incentive models, is schematized in Fig. 7-2. These models (e.g., Olds & Olds, 1965; Stein, 1964) assume that the consequences of a behavior pattern, that is, the reward it produces, are responsible for potentiating repetition of the behavior. Reward, in other words, operates through a positive feedback amplifier.

It is not always made clear in models of this type why the output of the positive feedback amplifier potentiates only the rewarded behavior rather than potentiating all behaviors indiscriminately. In the schema shown in Fig. 7-2, reward is assumed to have an additional effect—a parameter adjusting effect similar to one of the effects which reward has in the homeostatic models. This additional assumption enables the positive feedback from reward to selectively potentiate rewarded behaviors. It is, however, possible to dispense with this assumption (see caption to Fig. 7-14, Section III, B).

Positive feedback models confront two difficulties: (1) They must explain why positively rewarded behavior ever ceases once it has begun. If water reward, for example, feeds back to potentiate even more of the behavior that produces water reward, it is not clear why such water-producing behavior should not continue indefinitely. (2) They must explain why rewarded behavior that has once ceased ever resumes. Once water-producing behavior ceases, there soon is no more water to potentiate resumption of the behavior in the future. The latter difficulty is generally resolved by the assumption that stimuli in the environment where a behavior has been rewarded acquire the properties of the reward. For example, the stimuli in a Skinner box where an animal has been rewarded with water acquire the ability to arouse lever pressing. The former difficulty is frequently ignored. Sometimes it is assumed that the operation of factors extrinsic to the model, for example, fatigue, or aversion to the cumulative effects of repeated reward, eventually outweigh the positive feedback. For example, an animal might keep drinking until the discomfort in its stomach overrode the positive feedback from the water reward.

3. Mixed Theories

The third class of models (e.g., Hull, 1952; Spence, 1956; Trowill *et al.*, 1969) combines the two previous classes. Reward is assumed to have both drive enhancing (K in the Hull-Spence system) and drive reducing effects. The drive enhancing effects are frequently called arousal effects. These models are schematized in Fig. 7-3. In these models, reward can either potentiate behavior or reduce the potential for behavior, depending on the balance between the drive reducing effects of the reward and the arousal effects of the reward. Hence, changes in the parametric assumptions can convert these models from positive feedback systems to negative feedback systems, and vice versa.

As in the second class of models, these models generally assume that the stimuli in the environment in which the behavior has been rewarded acquire the arousing properties of the reward. This explains why, when the animal is reintroduced into the experimental situation, it will show signs of arousal prior to the receipt of its reward.

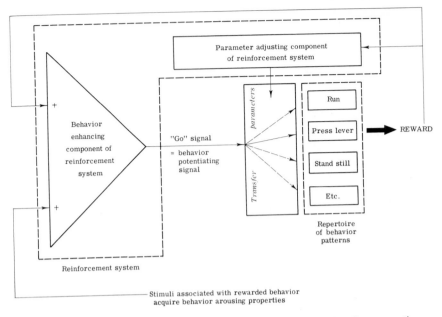

Fig. 7-2. Schematization of pure hedonic or incentive theories. By convention, a triangle indicates the amplifier.

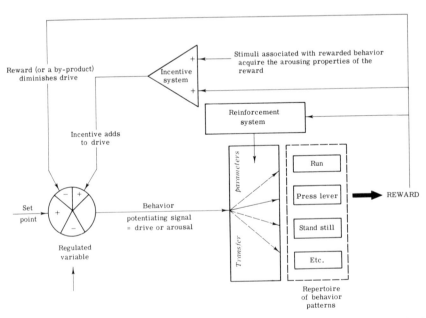

Fig. 7-3. Schematization of the relation between drive, reward, and behavior in mixed models, that is, models with both homeostatic (negative feedback) and hedonic (positive feedback) assumptions.

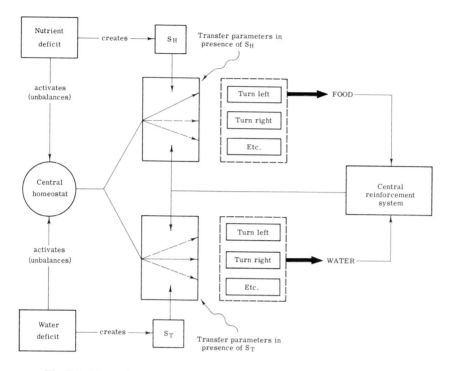

Fig. 7-4. Schematization of the mechanism by which different drives direct behavior in single homeostat models of the type favored by Hull and Spence. As in Fig. 7-1, reward also feeds back to reduce the activity of the central homeostat. However, for the sake of graphic simplicity, these loops are not shown.

4. Single Homeostat Theories

The schemata in Figs. 7-1, 7-2, and 7-3 do not deal with the directing or behavior selecting effects of different drive states. An animal familiar with a T maze in which food is always found on the right and water on the left will turn right when hungry and left when thirsty. There are two classes of models for dealing with this behavior-directing effect of drives—single homeostat models and multiple homeostat models.

The single homeostat models (e.g., Hull, 1952; Spence, 1956) have a single drive system that can be unbalanced by different factors, for example, water deprivation or food deprivation. These different factors, in addition to their common activating effect on the central homeostat, produce different internal sensations (drive stimuli), which act as discriminative cues. These cues become conditioned to different response patterns. Thus, the drive transfer parameters of behavior patterns differ depending on which drive stimulus is present. This is schematized in Fig. 7-4.

The single homeostat theories have difficulty accounting for certain behavioral data (e.g., Kendler, 1946). The difficulty arises from the assumption of a unitary reinforcement system, activated by diverse rewards (e.g., both food and water). When a rat is trained, while simultaneously hungry and thirsty, in a T maze with food on the left and water on the right, the rat, on subsequent testing, goes immediately to the left if hungry and immediately to the right if thirsty. In other words, the response of going to the left becomes connected to the hunger drive, and the response of going to the right becomes connected to the thirst drive, even when both responses are reinforced in the presence of both drives. The assumption of a single reinforcement system activated by diverse rewards makes it difficult for single homeostat models to explain these drive-specific effects of food and water rewards.

5. Multiple Homeostat Theories

Multiple homeostat models (e.g., Deutsch, 1960; Grossman, 1966; Morgan, 1957; Stellar, 1960; Tolman, 1937)[2] are not prey to the difficulty raised by the Kendler experiment since they assume (or imply) a separate reinforcement system for each homeostat. These models are schematized in Fig. 7-5. They assume that there are several homeostats, each homeostat regulating something different (e.g., one regulates body temperature, another regulates water balance). When a behavior produces a reward that tends (or would normally tend) to rebalance one of the homeostats, that behavior becomes connected to that homeostat. Should that homeostat again become unbalanced, it will potentiate the behaviors to which it has become connected. Because each homeostat has its own reinforcement mechanism, water reward selectively connects responses to the thirst drive state and food reward selectively connects responses to the hunger drive state.

II. SELF-STIMULATION: SALIENT CHARACTERISTICS

A survey of the literature on self-stimulation yields certain general conclusions about the phenomenon, viz., the primary locus of the stimulating electrodes, the effect of lesions in various structures, the physiological concomitants of rewarding stimulation, the peculiarities of self-stimulation behavior, and the effects of parametric variation in the stimulation. It is useful to have these conclusions in mind before approaching the more theoretical conclusions motivated by self-stimulation data.

---

[2] Grossman, Stellar, and Morgan have emphasized that external stimuli, as well as hormones and other internal stimuli, play an important role in exciting the central motive state, that is, the drive center.

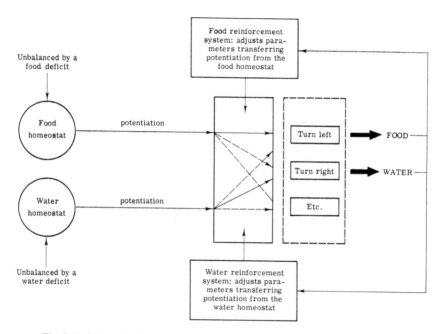

Fig. 7-5. Schematization of the mechanism by which drives direct behavior in multiple homeostat models of the type suggested by theorists, such as Lashley, Morgan, Stellar, Deutsch, and Grossman. For the sake of graphic simplicity, the loops from the rewards back to the homeostats are not shown.

A. Locus

1. Electrode Sites

It has proved difficult to construct a map of the rat brain which precisely delimits the diverse areas where electrical excitation will sustain self-stimulation behavior. Even less progress has been made in mapping the brains of other species. As Wetzel (1968) has pointed out, the main obstacles to the attainment of more precise maps are the wide variety of behavioral techniques used to screen for self-stimulation and a general tendency to publish inadequate reproductions of the histology.

Nonetheless, there is agreement that the medial forebrain bundle (MFB) is the principal locus of self-stimulation in the rat (Olds & Olds, 1965; Valenstein, 1966). The course of this tract through the basolateral diencephalon is depicted in Fig. 7-6. The rostral end of this diffuse tract is in the ventrum of the anterior forebrain. The tract exchanges fibers with the diagonal band of Broca (DBB) and with the nuclei of the lateral hypothalamus. The caudal end of the tract is the ventral tegmental area of Tsai and the limbic midbrain area of Nauta. The tract carries both ascending and descending fibers. Self-stimulation sites have been

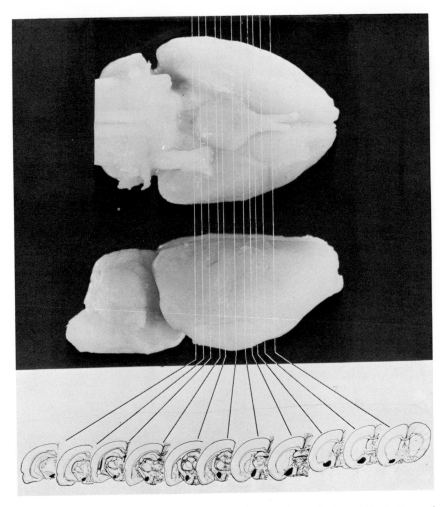

Fig. 7-6. The medial forebrain bundle (MFB) in the rat brain. At the bottom of the figure is a series of drawings of cross-sections through the rat brain, on which the MFB has been blacked out (lower, middle-left part of each drawing). The region of the brain through which each cross-section is made is indicated on the side view (middle of figure) and bottom view (top of figure) of the intact brain. Drawings from Konig and Klippel (1963); reproduced by permission of the Williams & Wilkins Company.

reported by numerous investigators all along the MFB from the diagonal band of Broca to the ventral tegmentum. The extreme rostral end of the MFB—the part anterior to the DBB—has not been systematically studied.

Although the MFB is clearly the principal locus of self-stimulation electrodes, electrodes in a wide variety of other telencephalic and diencephalic structures have sustained self-stimulation-like behavior. A complete survey would be beyond the scope of this review, but a brief survey will indicate the anatomical diversity of self-stimulation sites.

In the rat, self-stimulation has been reported for electrodes in the amygdala (Hodos, 1965; Valenstein & Valenstein, 1964; Wurtz & Olds, 1963), hippocampus (Ursin, Ursin, & Olds, 1966), entorhinal, retrosplenial, and cingulate juxtallocortex (Brady & Conrad, 1960; Stein & Ray, 1959), caudate (Olds, 1960), thalamic reticular system and central gray (Cooper & Taylor, 1967), and in the olfactory bulbs (Phillips & Mogenson, 1969).

The phenomenon is difficult to produce and usually rather weak in the cat (Justesen, Sharp, & Porter, 1963). However, self-stimulation electrodes have been reported in the caudate (Justesen *et al.*, 1963) as well as in the MFB (Roberts, 1958).

In the monkey, self-stimulation electrodes have been reported in the amygdala, caudate, and putamen (Brady, 1960; Brady & Conrad, 1960), the thalamus (Lilly, 1960), the basal tegmentum (Porter, Conrad, & Brady, 1959), and the reticular formation (Brady, 1960) as well as the MFB (Brodie, Malis, Moreno, & Boren, 1960).

The self-stimulation phenomenon has been reported in a much wider variety of species, including dogs (Stark & Boyd, 1963), dolphins (Lilly, 1962), and man (Bishop, Elder, & Heath, 1963; Sem-Jacobsen & Torkildsen, 1960). In most reports the MFB was the most frequent site for positive electrodes.

It has repeatedly been suggested that self-stimulation sites fall predominantly within the limbic system (Albino & Lucas, 1962; Brady & Conrad, 1960; Olds, 1958a; Zeigler, 1957). It is difficult to establish the truth or falsity of this proposition. If one reads the limbic system literature and lists the structures included in one or another working definition of the limbic system, the list soon includes nearly every structure between the neocortex and the caudal mesencephalon. Three expansions of the limbic system are indicated in Fig. 7-7. The first (Fig. 7-7A) is the purely telencephalic "limbic lobe" of the anatomists (as elaborated by Pribram & Kruger, 1954). Largely on the basis of clinical evidence, Papez (1937) added some diencephalic structures to the telencephalic limbic system (Fig. 7-7B). And, finally, Nauta (1960) used anatomical data to add several more diencephalic and mesencephalic areas to the limbic system (Fig. 7-7C). If one limits the definition of the limbic system to the structures described by Nauta, Papez, and Pribram and Kruger (see composite, Fig. 7-7D), then self-stimulation sites show little correlation with the limbic system (Gallistel, unpublished review). If one considers still further expansions of the limbic system, then self-stimulation sites will no doubt fall predominantly within the limbic system, insofar as the further expansions make the limbic system coextensive with the rhinencephalon cum subcortical telencephalon cum diencephalon cum mesencephalon.

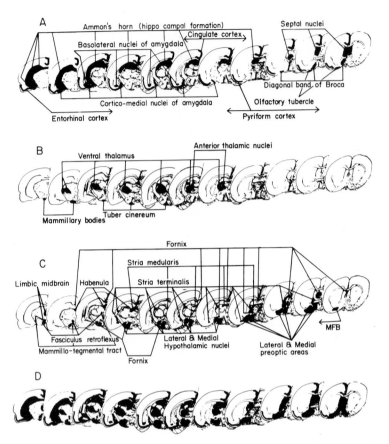

Fig. 7-7. A. The limbic lobe of the telencephalon, as described by Pribram and Kruger (1954), is indicated by the blacked out portions on a series of cross-sections through the brain of the rat. B. Papez's (1937) diencephalic additions to the limbic lobe. C. Projections of the limbic system, described by Nauta (1960). D. The composite limbic system. Drawings from Konig and Klippel (1963); reproduced by permission of the Williams & Wilkins Company.

The MFB, which is the principal locus of self-stimulation sites, is one of the two secondary projections (and also one of the three tertiary projections) of the limbic system, as outlined by Nauta (1960). Whether this relation is significant is a moot point. There is no correlation between self-stimulation sites and the other secondary and tertiary projections of the limbic system that were described by Nauta. The MFB is also one of the main afferent and efferent tracts for the lateral hypothalamic nuclei known to be concerned with regulatory (homeostatic) behavior. This latter relation may be more important for an understanding of self-stimulation than is the relation to the limbic system.

2. Lesion Studies

Extensive lesions of limbic system structures—hippocampus, amygdala, fornix, dorsal thalamus, septum, the limbic midbrain area of Nauta, and the mesencephalic gray—do not have large effects on self-stimulation (Asdourian, Stutz, & Rocklin, 1966; Valenstein, 1966; Ward, 1960, 1961).

Despite the fact that the MFB is the main locus of electrodes producing self-stimulation, it is not necessary for this tract to be intact either. Valenstein (1966) and his co-workers have shown that extensive lesions in the MFB rostral to, or caudal to, the stimulating electrode do not disrupt self-stimulation. Lorens (1966) has shown that simultaneous lesions both rostral and caudal to the electrode produce only minor changes in self-stimulation performance, a result slightly at variance with earlier findings by Morgane (1961). Boyd and Gardner (1967) found that small lesions would sometimes produce a large decrement in performance during the first few days after the lesion, but performance improved as the animals recovered. Reid and Porter (1965) found no consistent effect from cortical lesions. Valenstein (1966) concluded that the pathways mediating self-stimulation must be extremely diffuse and that no single area would prove essential to the manifestation of self-stimulation—a conclusion at odds with the conclusion reached by Olds and Olds (1965, 1969).

The disagreement as to the severity of the disruption produced by lesions is traceable chiefly to differences in length of the post-lesion recovery time allowed prior to testing. The longer the recovery, the less the disruption. However, Olds and Olds (1969) have recently shown that lesions in the MFB caudal to sites of MFB stimulation can cause substantial decrements in the rate of self-stimulation even after an eight-week recovery period. These results were apparently not an artifact of a general disability, since lesions midway in the MFB affected the rate of self-stimulation on electrodes rostral to the lesion, while not affecting the rate on electrodes caudal to the lesion.

In summary, the MFB is clearly the principal locus of self-stimulation electrodes. Nonetheless, lesions in this tract have surprisingly little effect. There is, however, some recent evidence that lesions caudal to the electrode can have an effect.

B. Physiological Concomitants

1. Cardiovascular

The physiological effects of brain stimulation reward (BSR) have not been extensively studied. Only two of the many possibilities—cardiovascular effects and EEG effects—have been explored with any thoroughness. Malmo (1961) reported that transitory decreases in heart rate occurred in rats self-stimulating on septal placements. Perez-Cruet, Black, and Brady (1963) reported that the opposite was true for lateral hypothalamic placements in the rat. Meyers,

Valenstein, and Lacey (1963) reported that, under appropriate conditions, both septal self-stimulation and lateral hypothalamic self-stimulation produced a biphasic heart rate response—a brief acceleration followed by a longer depression. However, rates of bar pressing for lateral hypothalamic stimulation were so rapid that the next stimulation could prevent the appearance of the depression, unless stimulations were spaced out by the use of a partial reinforcement schedule.

Perez-Cruet, McIntire, and Pliskoff (1965) showed that lateral hypothalamic self-stimulation increased heart rate and blood pressure in dogs. However, the injection of an adrenergic blocking agent (dibenzyline) eliminated the cardiovascular effects without affecting self-stimulation, indicating (1) that the effects were probably mediated via the sympathetic nervous system, and (2) that the effects were epiphenomena.

2. EEG

Porter *et al.* (1959) reported that seizure-like activity frequently appeared in the EEG during self-stimulation. Similar findings were made by Newman and Feldman (1964). However, Bogacz, St. Laurent, and Olds (1965) reported that self-stimulation on posterior hypothalamic and mesencephalic electrodes was not accompanied by seizure discharges in the EEG. Reid, Gibson, Gledhill, and Porter (1964) found that anticonvulsant drugs, which reduced seizure activity, enhanced self-stimulation. They concluded that the seizure effects, like the cardiovascular effects, were epiphenomena.

3. Other Variables

Prescott (1967) found that the rate of self-stimulation varied with the rat's diurnal activity cycle. Terman and Terman (1970) have further shown that the rate of self-stimulation rises and falls in a circadian rhythm even when external pace-making stimuli are eliminated.

Routtenberg and Huang (1968) found that stimulation at rewarding posterior hypothalamic areas usually drove single units in the brainstem; whereas stimulation at rewarding septal areas did not.

Ward and Hester (1969) found that MFB self-stimulation in cats was unimpaired by bilateral surgical removal of the sympathetic chain and bilateral sectioning of the vagus and the pelvic splanchnics. This finding reinforces the conclusions about the epiphenomenal nature of cardiovascular effects reached by Perez-Cruet *et al.*. It strongly suggests that autonomic effects are not of causal importance in self-stimulation.

C. Characteristics of Self-Stimulation Behavior

Behavior sustained by electrical reward has a number of characteristics that have attracted experimental and theoretical attention. Most of these characteristics can be viewed as manifestations of the "positive feedback" quality of self-stimulation behavior. Self-stimulation resembles the behavior of a system that has positive feedback in that self-stimulation, once initiated, is extremely intense and persistent; if, however, the self-stimulation is interrupted for a length of time, it is slow to resume.

1. Persistence

Olds (1958b) reported that, in the rat, behavior sustained by *continuously available* brain stimulation reward (BSR) was unusually persistent. Lilly (1958) reported that the same was true in the monkey. Since then there have been many reports that rats would self-stimulate at high rates hour after hour (Olds, 1958c; Ray, Hine, & Bivens, 1968) and even day after day (Valenstein & Beer, 1964) to the exclusion of other rewarded activities (Falk, 1961; Spies, 1965) until exhaustion set in. Generally, the higher the rate of self-stimulation, the longer it will persist (Ray *et al.,* 1968).

With some placements, self-stimulation tapers off after four to eight hours (Olds, 1958c). However, it is difficult to find a natural reward that will sustain continuously rewarded responding for even that long a period. Valenstein, Cox, and Kakolewski (1967) have reported one such natural reward—a mixture of saccharin and extremely dilute sucrose. Like BSR this reward produced little satiation.

2. Spontaneous Extinction

Olds (1955) noted that behavior sustained by BSR extinguished unusually rapidly under most circumstances. This was convincingly demonstrated by Seward, Uyeda, and Olds (1959). These authors let rats bar press for BSR fifteen minutes every day for fifteen to twenty days. The rats made roughly 10,000 reinforced responses. The day after the final day of training the rats were replaced in the box to begin extinction. Extinction was extremely rapid. In fact, the published data indicate no extinction curve. The response frequency on the first two days of extinction was only slightly above the pretraining operant level. It showed no significant decline over the fourteen subsequent days of extinction. In other words, in the Seward *et al.* data, it appears as though extinction had occurred spontaneously without any unreinforced responding.

Howarth and Deutsch (1962) showed that, under normal conditions, the extinction of a BSR sustained habit was a function not of the number of unreinforced responses but, rather, of the time elapsed since the last BSR. This demonstration of the temporal dependency of spontaneous extinction has since been replicated by Pliskoff and Hawkins (1963) and by Quartermain and Webster (1968). The latter further showed that the effect did not occur in thirsty rats trained for water.

3. Overnight Decrements

Spontaneous extinction is only one of several manifestations of the fact that interrupting self-stimulation behavior by a length of time greatly weakens the rat's tendency to engage in the behavior. Overnight (i.e., between sessions) decrements in self-stimulation performance provide another instance of the behavior-weakening effect of a temporal interruption. Olds and Milner (1954) noted that some rats did not resume lever pressing at the beginning of each day's session, but could be induced to do so by a few free stimulations administered by the experimenter. This same observation was made by Elder, Montgomery, and Rye (1965), Valenstein (1966, some rats), and Wetzel (1963). It is not characteristic of performance sustained by food reward (Skinner, 1950, p. 200).

Overnight decrements are also found in runway behavior maintained by BSR. Olds (1956) found that rats ran slower on the first trial of each day than on succeeding trials. This observation has since been made by Wetzel (1963), by Panksepp, Gandelman, and Trowill (1968), and by Wasden, Reid, and Porter (1965), although the last cited report emphasizes that this effect was not seen in every rat.

The overnight decrement phenomenon appears to be peculiar to self-stimulation. Slight overnight decrements sometimes occur in hungry rats running for food (Logan, 1960, pp. 62-64). However, the magnitude of the effect, when it occurs, is not as great as with BSR. In those studies which compared BSR groups with food reinforced groups run in the same test situation, the food reinforced groups showed no overnight decrement (Olds, 1956; Wetzel, 1963).

4. Poor Performance After Long Intertrial Intervals

The overnight decrement in runway performance can be viewed as the effect of interposing a long intertrial interval (ITI) between the last trial of one day's session and the first trial of the next day. Viewed in this way, it is consistent with a number of studies reporting that much smaller increases in the ITI also lead to a decrement in performance (Gallistel, 1966, 1967; Johnson, 1968; Newman, 1961; Panksepp et al., 1968; Seward et al., 1960; Spear, 1962; Wetzel, 1963). As long as the ITI is on the order of five seconds, performance is good, but when it is increased by as little as ten seconds, performance deteriorates. With ITI's of several minutes some rats will not perform (see Fig. 7-8).

Again, the deleterious effect of lengthening the ITI is peculiar to self-stimulation. The ITI does not affect the performance of thirsty rats running for a water reward, even when care is taken to make the administration of the water reward resemble, as closely as possible, the administration of BSR (Gallistel, 1967). The ITI does not affect the performance of hungry rats running for food in the same experimental apparatus in which rats running for BSR show an effect of ITI (Newman, 1961; Wetzel, 1963). More generally, the effect of ITI on learning for natural rewards is the opposite of its effect on learning for BSR. With natural rewards, the longer the ITI, the more rapid the learning and the faster the final performance (Lashley, 1918; Mayer & Stone, 1931; Ulrich, 1915); whereas with BSR, the longer the ITI, the more retarded the learning and the slower the final performance.

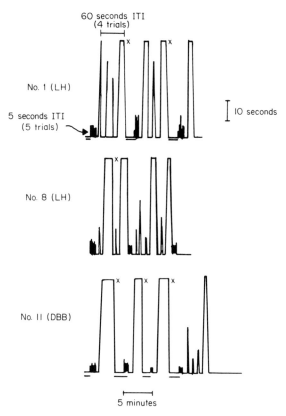

Fig. 7-8. Records from three rats, showing a strong effect of ITI on running time to a brain stimulation reward. Trials with a 5-second ITI appear as short, fused together black bars. Trials with a 60-second ITI appear as tall, tapering bars. The height of each bar is proportional to the running time on that trial. The tall, flat-topped bars indicate trials on which the running time substantially exceeded 1 minute. An X at the upper right hand corner of such bars indicates that the rat was finally placed on the goal lever by the experimenter. The short lines below the upper and lower records indicate periods when the rats were allowed continuously rewarded lever pressing. Redrawn from Gallistel (1966); reproduced by permission of the American Psychological Association.

The effect of ITI on runway performance appears with electrodes any-where in the MFB from the septum to the tegmentum and persists when rats are trained to asymptotic levels of performance (Gallistel, 1967). This effect of ITI is one of the clearest and simplest demonstrations of the effect of temporal interruptions on self-stimulation behavior.

The effect of ITI could be taken as showing that spaced BSR is less reinforcing than massed BSR (Seward *et al.*, 1960). However, Gallistel (1967), in a study replicated by Panksepp *et al.*, (1968), showed that the deterioration in performance produced by lengthening the ITI, and the improvement produced by shortening the ITI, occurred on the first trial after the change in ITI. That is, the change in performance occurred before the rats had experienced a reinforcement under the new conditions. Thus, the effect could not be ascribed to any differential reinforcement efficacy of massed versus spaced BSR, because it appeared before differential reinforcement would have had opportunity to exert its influence.

5. *Poor Performance on Partial Reinforcement Schedules*

Long temporal intervals between runway trials weaken runway performance whether these intervals occur within sessions ("the effect of ITI") or between sessions ("overnight decrements"). Similarly, in Skinner box behavior there is a within-session phenomenon that parallels the between-session (overnight decrement) phenomenon. All species so far studied with BSR have shown a poor tolerance for partial reinforcement schedules that impose a substantial time interval between successive rewards. Sidman, Brady, Conrad, and Schulman (1955), Brady (1960), and Brodie, Moreno, Malis, and Boren (1960) found it difficult to train rats or monkeys to respond for BSR on schedules that imposed an interval of more than a minute or two between successive rewards. Brady (1958) also reported that monkeys performed poorly for BSR on a DRL schedule (differential reinforcement of low rates); whereas the same animals performed well for a food reward on this same schedule. Like other partial reinforcement schedules, the DRL schedule imposes an interval between rewards. Keesey and Goldstein (1968) found that they could not get responding beyond FR 30 (30 responses per reinforcement) even with intense stimulating currents (see also Elder *et al.*, 1965; Hodos, 1965). Their procedure was modelled on one developed by Hodos and Kalman (1963). Hodos and Kalman, using hungry rats responding for sugared milk, obtained performance on FR 120 to FR 200, even at the smallest reward magnitude (0.025 ml). Keesey and Goldstein, on the other hand, observed that self-stimulation performance deteriorated whenever the FR schedule elicited post-reinforcement pauses of longer than fifteen seconds (see also Elder *et al.*, 1965). This contrasts with the Hodos and Kalman records, which show frequent post-reinforcement pauses of more than sixty seconds, without disruptive effect, in rats responding for a natural reward.

Culbertson, Kling, and Berkley (1966) reported that rats responding on FR 10 worked more slowly for BSR than rats working for food. The opposite was true on continuous reinforcement schedules. In general, rats and monkeys will not perform as well on "poor" partial reinforcement schedules when rewarded with brain stimulation as when rewarded with natural rewards. These findings indicate that temporal interruption of the reinforcing stimulation is the important variable, not temporal interruption of the reinforced behavior.

6. The Effect of Priming

Just as the overnight decrement in Skinner box performance can be overcome by the administration of a few "priming" stimulations, similar priming stimulation given to rats before the start of a runway trial eliminates the effect of a long ITI, even when this priming is administered to the rat in a waiting box outside the runway or T maze (Deutsch, Adams, & Metzner, 1964; Gallistel, 1969a,b; Wetzel, 1963).

Priming with BSR does not facilitate performance for food reward (Wetzel, 1963), and priming leads thirsty rats to prefer BSR over water (Deutsch et al., 1964). Thus, the priming effect is apparently not a simple arousal effect, since its effects are selective and directive.

As one would expect, the priming effect decays as a function of time since priming (Deutsch et al., 1964). The longer the time elapsed since priming, the slower the rat runs and the less likely it is to choose BSR in preference to another reward.

Prefeeding, in various amounts, hungry rats about to run an alley or maze for food has an effect opposite the effect of priming—it reduces overall running speed (Bruce, 1938; Morgan & Fields, 1938), although in small amounts it can increase speed in the early segments of the runway (Morgan & Fields, 1938). Bruce (1937, 1938) claimed to show that small prewaterings enhanced the speed of rats running for water, but his data, on close inspection, do not bear this out. It is, in other words, difficult to find priming-like effects in the literature on natural rewards.

7. Contradictory Results

These various effects—spontaneous "extinction" as a function of time since the last rewarding stimulation, overnight decrements in Skinner box and runway performance, deterioration in performance when an interval between rewards is imposed in the runway or the Skinner box, the elimination of such decrements by the administration of priming, and the decay of the priming effect as a function of time since priming—these effects demonstrate that the time elapsed since the last stimulation is an important variable in BSR sustained performance. The theoretical implications of these phenomena are discussed later, but it must first be noted that under certain conditions many of these effects disappear or become much less pronounced.

When rats responding for BSR are kept on a food or water deprivation schedule, they take longer to extinguish (Deutsch & DiCara, 1967; Gibson, Reid, Sokai, & Porter, 1965; Olds, 1956). In some hungry rats, runway performance is not strongly affected by long ITI's, although in other rats hunger does not have this counteracting effect (Wetzel, 1963). Hungry rats also perform much better on partial reinforcement schedules and will tolerate higher FR's (Elder et al., 1965). The tendency for natural drives to eliminate the behavior-weakening effects of temporal interruptions has implications for theories of self-stimulation. It suggests that the effects of temporal interruption might be ascribed to the decay of drive-like aftereffects of rewarding brain stimulation.

Scott (1967) observed no overnight decrement in the later stages of runway training. However, he used a fifteen-minute ITI. It is likely that the within session decrement in his control comparison was large enough to prevent his observing a further decrement between sessions. Wasden *et al.* (1965) reported no overnight decrement in half their rats, using a one-minute ITI. Again, a shorter ITI (e.g., five seconds) would have provided a more convincing control comparison.

Kornblith and Olds (1968) had difficulty inducing many rats to perform for BSR in a standard two-choice discrimination maze. When they switched to a maze with a large "open-field" start area, they found that the performance of their rats improved with training, even though they used a 24-hour ITI. Apparently, performance for BSR after long ITI's is not so slow if one adopts a procedure that discourages rats' remaining in the start box. However, such procedures will probably erase most differences in speed of performance. Hence, the implications of the results obtained by such procedures are unclear.

Pliskoff, Wright, and Hawkins (1965) and Pliskoff and Hawkins (1967) have shown that rats will respond on partial reinforcement schedules with interreward intervals of fifteen minutes and more, if each reward consists of 10-100 trains of BSR, instead of the single train used in most experiments. It is not clear whether the effect of multitrain rewards should be attributed to the enhancement of reward value or to the prolongation of drive-like aftereffects (see Section III, A, 1).

Kent and Grossman (1969) have recently reported that some rats show none of the temporal decay phenomena, whereas other rats show all of the phenomena. Their "nonprimer" rats did not require priming to begin lever pressing at the start of a session, did not run more slowly as the ITI in a runway was lengthened from five seconds to five minutes, did not take longer to return to a withdrawn and returned lever as the period of withdrawal was lengthened, and did not extinguish so rapidly. There was some indication that electrodes of the nonprimers were more centrally located in the MFB than were the electrodes of the primers. Kent and Grossman's findings are consistent with several other reports of wide individual differences in the effects of temporal interruptions (Valenstein, 1966; Wasden *et al.*, 1965; Wetzel, 1963). Any truly satisfactory theory of self-stimulation will have to account for this wide range of individual differences.

D. Varying the Parameters of Stimulation

1. The Electrical Stimulation of the CNS

a. Definition of Terms. Before discussing the effects which varying the parameters of stimulation have on animals' choice behavior and rate of responding, it will help to explain the terms that are used to describe the parameters of stimulation.

The total period of stimulation produced by one activation of the stimulating circuit (e.g., one lever press) is called the *train duration*. Sometimes this parameter is predetermined by the experimenter. Sometimes it is under the animal's control, that is, stimulation initiated by some act of the animal persists until the animal performs another act that terminates stimulation (e.g., takes its paw off the lever).

The stimulation current (or stimulation voltage) during a single train of stimulation is never steady. Thus, one must give additional parameters that describe the variation in current (or voltage) during a train. The variation in current during a train assumes one of two basic forms: sinusoidal variation about zero, or pulsatile variation. When sinusoidal variation is used, only two parameters need be specified in addition to train duration—the *frequency of variation* (usually 60 cycles per second) and the *current intensity* [usually the peak current reached during the cycle; sometimes the root mean square (rms) of the current].

When pulsatile variation is used, it may be either *biphasic* (the pulses alternate from positive to negative) or *monophasic* (the pulses are always positive or always negative, usually the latter). Three parameters must be specified in addition to train duration—the *pulse duration* (or pulse width), the *pulse frequency* (pulses per second), and the current intensity during the pulse. Since the animal introduces capacitance into the stimulating circuit, rectangular pulses are not truly rectangular unless a cathode follower or high impedance, constant current circuit is used. In other words, the current through the animal is not constant during a pulse; rather, the pulses are rectangles with exponentially relaxing overshoot at onset and offset. The current intensity of such pulses is usually measured from some point in the later part of the pulse, where the onset-overshoot has disappeared.

b. The Theory of Stimulation. It is also difficult to discuss the effects of parametric variations without giving, as background, some indication of how voltages applied through an indwelling electrode excite neurons in the brain.

Neurons have an electrical charge across the membrane which constitutes their outer wall, the outside being positive with regard to the inside. Anything that sufficiently depolarizes the neuron, that is, reduces the difference in electrical potential between the outside and the inside, will cause the neuron to "fire," that is, transmit a neural impulse. If a negative electrical potential suddenly appears at an electrode tip near the neuron, this negative (cathodal) potential will drain away some of the positive potential outside the neuronal membrane. As the positive potential outside the neuron drains away, the difference in potential between the outside and the inside of the neuron is reduced. If this reduction (depolarization) is sufficiently large and rapid, the neuron will fire.

It is also possible to excite neurons using positive (anodal) voltages. To understand how this happens requires a more elaborate discussion of neuron theory. Briefly, the effect of any electrical stimulus depends mostly on two characteristics of the neuronal membrane (Hill, 1936). The first characteristic is the rate at which a subthreshold depolarization decays. This is the rate at which the difference in potential across the neuronal membrane returns to its normal level, after the difference in potential has been only partially reduced—that is, not reduced enough to fire the neuron. This rate of decay of subthreshold depolarization is probably determined by simple physical properties of the membrane, *viz.*, its resistance and capacitance. The second characteristic on which the electrical excitation of neurons depends is the rate of accommodation. Whenever a prolonged potential difference is imposed across a neuronal membrane, the membrane accommodates to the imposed difference. Roughly speaking, this means that the neuron comes to behave as though the imposed difference in potential were the true or normal (i.e., "resting") potential difference. When positive electrical potential appears at the tip of an electrode near the neuron, this positive potential adds to the positive potential that already exists on the outside of the neuron, thereby increasing the difference in potential between the outside and the inside of the neuron. If the positive potential added by the electrode is very strong, or if it persists for some time (one to several milliseconds), then the neuronal membrane will accommodate to the new and greater difference in potential. When the positive potential from the electrode abruptly ceases (at the end of the stimulus pulse), there is a sudden drop in the amount of positive potential on the outside of the neuron. As a result, the difference in potential between the outside and the inside of the neuron is rapidly reduced (the neuron is depolarized). This rapid depolarization fires the neuron—even though the "depolarization" in this case is merely a return to what would normally be the resting difference in potential. Accommodation, in other words, is an adjustment in what constitutes the threshold level of depolarization. During a positive pulse this adjustment can be great enough so that the threshold level of depolarization is crossed when the difference in potential returns to normal at the end of the stimulus pulse.

The excitatory effect of brief (0.1 msec) cathodal stimulation is less complicated and more readily interpreted than the excitatory effect of any other kind of stimulation, because brief cathodal pulses do not produce much accommodation. Accommodation is necessarily involved in excitation produced by anodal stimulation, and accommodation is a relevant factor when cathodal pulses of long duration are used. As would be expected from Hill's analysis of the electrical excitation of neurons, given above, we have found that the threshold of self-stimulation is much lower for cathodal stimulus pulses than for anodal stimulus pulses. Wetzel, Howell, and Bearie (1969) and Deutsch (personal communication) report similar findings.

c. Electrode Configurations. In order to deliver only cathodal stimulus pulses to brain tissue an experimenter must use a *monopolar* configuration for the stimulating electrodes. In a monopolar configuration one electrode, insulated everywhere but at its tip, is lowered into the brain. Current flows between the tip of this "stimulating" electrode and the "indifferent" electrode, which lies on the skull. If one employs biphasic stimulation with a monopolar electrode configuration, then the stimulating electrode serves as a cathode during one phase of the cycle (i.e., during the negative phase) and as an anode during the other phase (i.e., the positive phase). Since cathodal pulses are more effective than anodal pulses, most of the neuronal excitation caused by the stimulation must arise during the negative phase. Biphasic stimulation, although common, should be avoided unless nonpolarizable platinum electrodes are used. The anodal stimulation that occurs during one phase of biphasic stimulation causes harmful metallic deposits in the tissue when stainless steel electrodes are used (Wetzel *et al.*, 1969).

For simplicity of interpretation and in order to avoid tissue damage a *bipolar* electrode configuration should not be used. In a bipolar configuration two stimulating electrodes, insulated except at their tips, are lowered into the brain in close proximity to one another. Current flows between the two tips. As is expected from the analysis of neuron excitation given above, it has been found that the locus of most effective stimulation in a bipolar configuration is at the electrode which serves as the cathode (Stein, 1962; Valenstein & Beer, 1961). When monophasic stimulation is used in conjunction with a bipolar configuration, then one electrode serves always as the cathode while the other serves always as the anode. Harmful metallic deposits accumulate at the tip of the anode, unless the electrode is made of a nonpolarizable metal such as platinum (Wetzel *et al.*, 1969). When biphasic stimulation is used in conjunction with a bipolar configuration, each electrode serves as a cathode during one phase and as an anode during the other. Harmful deposits accumulate at both tips (Wetzel *et al.*, 1969). Also, the locus of excitation no doubt shifts from one electrode to the other during each phase reversal.

It can be seen that brief pulsatile cathodal stimulation from a monopolar electrode configuration is the simplest and least harmful form of stimulation. This form of stimulation is now used in many labs. Hopefully it will come into even wider use.

2. Choice and Rate of Response

a. Current Intensity and Pulse Duration. Parametric variations can be divided into those which vary the population of neurons being fired by the stimulation and those which vary the number of times a population of neurons fires. Increasing the strength of the pulses in a train will increase the number of neurons fired by the stimulation. On the other hand, increasing the number of

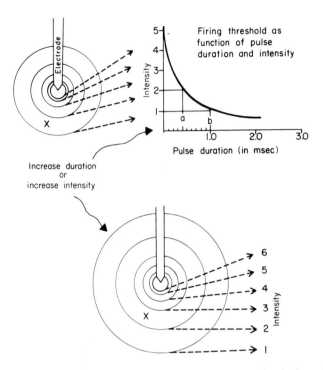

Fig. 7-9. Diagram of the trade-off between pulse duration and pulse intensity. In the upper right hand corner is a typical time-intensity function. This function shows the pulse intensity (in arbitrary units) required to just fire a neuron, as a function of the duration of the pulse. The shorter the pulse duration, the more intense the pulse must be in order to fire the neuron. In the upper left hand corner is a representation of the spread of potential away from an electrode tip. Each circle represents a line of iso-potentiality; the farther away from the tip, the lower the intensity of the stimulation. At the stimulus intensity shown in this diagram, a neuron at point X would not be fired by a pulse of duration 0.4 msec. This can be seen by reference to the time-intensity graph. The line marked *a* has been drawn at 0.4 msec. Note that at this duration, the intensity of the stimulus pulse in the region of neuron X would have to be greater than 2 in order to excite neuron X. The stimulus pulse would excite neuron X if the duration of the pulse were increased to 1.0 msec (line *b* on the time-intensity graph), or if the intensity of the stimulus were increased enough to raise the intensity at X above 2 (bottom diagram).

pulses in a train increases the number of neuron firings produced by the train but does not increase the population of neurons being fired.

There are two ways to increase the strength of a stimulus pulse—increase its intensity, or increase its duration. It is probable that both methods of increasing the strength of a stimulus pulse have the same effect, that is, both methods increase the population of neurons fired by the pulse. This equivalence arises from the fact that in the electrical stimulation of neurons, as in the

stimulation of biological systems in general, there is a reciprocal relation between time and intensity, provided very short stimulation pulses are used. The
trade-off is illustrated in Fig. 7-9.

Generally speaking, the effects of increasing either current intensity or
pulse duration are monotonic. When animals are responding on a partial reinforcement schedule, increasing the current steadily increases the rate of responding, even up to very high levels of current (Beer, Hodos, & Matthews, 1964;
Hawkins & Pliskoff, 1964; Keesey, 1962), from most but not all self-stimulation
electrodes (McIntire & Wright, 1965). Increasing the pulse duration (from 0.25
to 2.75 msec) also increases the rate of response (Keesey, 1962). These findings
of monotonicity in the relation between rate of response and pulse strength are
consistent with the further finding that when rats are given control of current
intensity they set it very high (Stein & Ray, 1959). Furthermore, when rats may
choose between two intensities of BSR, or between BSR and another reward,
the more intense the BSR the more likely it is to be chosen (Hodos &
Valenstein, 1962; Valenstein & Beer, 1962).

However, when rats are responding on a continuous reinforcement schedule, there are many electrode placements that do not yield a monotonic relation
between current intensity and rate of response (Olds, 1958b, 1960; Reynolds,
1958). As Keesey (1962) and Valenstein (1964; see also Valenstein & Beer,
1962) have pointed out, this can most reasonably be attributed to motoric and
seizure-like side effects of intense stimulation. These side effects, which impede
rapid lever pressing, vary greatly at different loci of stimulation. The performance hindering artifacts introduced by these side effects have the greatest
effect on the rate of response when a continuous reinforcement schedule is used.
Hence, rate of pressing on a continuous reinforcement schedule should not be
the method of choice for assessing the potency of rewarding brain stimulation.

b. *Train Duration and Pulse Frequency.* Interestingly, manipulations
which increase the number of times neurons are fired without increasing the
population of neurons being fired have the same effect as the manipulations
which increase the population of neurons being fired without increasing the
number of times the neurons are fired. That is, increasing train duration (from
0.25 to 2.0 seconds) and increasing pulse frequency (from 20 to 140 pulses per
second) both produce monotonic increases in the rate of responding on a partial
reinforcement schedule, just as do increases in pulse intensity and duration
(Keesey, 1962, 1964). McIntire and Wright (1965) found that increasing train
duration sometimes led to a decrease in rate of response. However, the low fixed
ratio schedule they employed (FR 5) may not have been sufficient to eliminate
the rate suppressing influence of motoric side effects, which also become more
pronounced as train duration increases.

When rats are allowed to regulate duration, the duration they set depends
on the current intensity—the higher the intensity, the shorter the duration

selected (McIntire & Wright, 1965; Hodos, 1965) on most, but not all placements (Stein, 1962). However, the duration the rat selects can vary by an order
of magnitude, depending on whether the rat terminates the stimulation by
merely releasing the bar or by pressing another bar (Keesey, 1964; Valenstein,
1964). Somewhat paradoxically, the train duration the rat selects is not the train
duration that produces a maximal rate of responding on a partial reinforcement
schedule. Train durations substantially longer than those selected by the rat
produce a higher rate of responding (Keesey, 1964). This paradox is resolved if
one assumes that the rate of responding reflects primarily a drive-like aftereffect
of BSR; whereas the selection of a preferred train duration reflects primarily the
reinforcing effect of BSR (see Section III; A, 1).

In sum, the effects of varying the parameters of current intensity, train
duration, pulse duration, and pulse frequency are consistent with the assumption
that the system, or part of the system, whose excitation produces self-stimulation, integrates action potentials both over time and over the population of
functionally homogeneous neurons. It appears that, for most placements, efficacy is a monotonic function of this integral. Nonmonotonic data probably
result from the intrusive effects of other systems also activated by the stimulation.

3. Reward Magnitude

In reviewing the studies on parametric variation we avoided conclusions as
to the magnitude of the reward produced by manipulating the parameters of
BSR. Valenstein (1964) has given a cogent discussion of the difficulties encountered in trying to gauge the reinforcement efficacy of BSR. That this is not a
straightforward matter is apparent from the following: At high current levels rats
select rather short train durations (0.5–1.0 second). When, however, the experimenter removes control of the train duration from the rat, it is found that
increasing the duration well beyond the level selected by the rat continues to
increase both the response rate on a variable interval (VI) schedule (Keesey,
1964) and the number of responses the rat will emit on a progressively increasing
ratio schedule (Hodos, 1965). In a somewhat different vein, rats with lateral
hypothalamic placements prefer BSR to food reward to the point of starvation
(Routtenberg & Lindy, 1965), yet on a partial reinforcement schedule performance is better for food than for BSR.

The importance of determining the reward magnitude of BSR (and the
disagreement that still exists) can be seen from the fact that Pliskoff and
Hawkins have recently (1967) assumed that single trains of BSR constitute a
small reward while Gandelman and Trowill have even more recently (1968)
assumed that single trains constituted a very large reward—a conclusion also
reached by Kling and Matsumiya (1962), for almost opposite reasons.

In addition to the many difficulties discussed by Valenstein (1964), there
are some conceptual difficulties that have not been generally appreciated. It

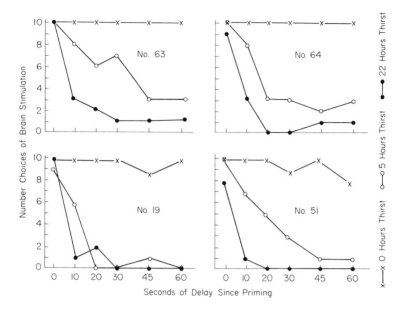

Fig. 7-10. Choice behavior of four rats as a function of degree of water deprivation and time since priming with BSR. The more thirsty the rats and the longer the time elapsed since priming, the more likely the rats were to choose water reward in preference to BSR. Conversely, the more recent the priming and the less the thirst, the more likely rats were to choose BSR in preference to water. Reproduced from Deutsch, Adams, & Metzner (1964); reproduced by permission of the American Psychological Association.

would be desirable to know how much BSR is required to produce a reward whose magnitude is roughly equal to that of a typical food reward (one to ten 47 mg Noyes pellets). However, qualitatively different rewards, that is, rewards that are relevant to different homeostats (e.g., food and water), are not strictly commensurable (although in Hullian theory they are assumed to be). To a hungry rat, no amount of water is equivalent to one Noyes pellet (Gallistel, 1969b).

We know that consideration of the drive type and drive intensity is important in estimating the reward value of BSR because Deutsch *et al.* (1964) have shown that rats' preference, when offered a choice between BSR and water, varies as a function of hours of water deprivation and recency of priming (see Fig. 7-10). Since we do not know what homeostat, if any, BSR is relevant to, we cannot assess its reward magnitude with a choice procedure that allows the animal to choose between BSR and some natural reward.

Nor can we in any straightforward manner use the avidity (bar pressing rate, runway speed) of BSR sustained behavior to estimate reward magnitude. With BSR, the avidity of behavior is a function not only of the reward which the behavior produces but also of the recency and magnitude of the BSR that precedes the behavior (Gallistel, 1969a). And with natural rewards, the avidity of behavior is a function not only of the reward but also of the drive level (Kimble, 1961).

We have used a runway procedure that circumvented these difficulties, enabling us to describe the growth of reward magnitude as a function of increasing stimulation (Gallistel, 1969a).

Crespi (1942) determined the function relating the runway speed of 24-hour hungry rats to the amount of food reward they received. He found that running speed increased rapidly as the reward increased from 0.020 gram to 1 gram. Between 1 gram and 5 grams, running speed did not increase as rapidly. This is intelligible on the basis of the rat's normal feeding habits. On an ad lib diet, rats eat about 2 grams per meal (Le Magnen & Tallon, 1966). It appears that the running speed versus reward magnitude function approaches asymptote as the amount of food approaches the size of an average meal. The leveling off point of the speed versus reward function is a useful index of reward magnitude because it (unlike absolute speed) is unaffected by drive level. Reynolds and Pavlik (1960), using three levels of food deprivation (3, 22, and 44 hours) and three levels of food (0.1g, 1g, and 2g) found no interaction between drive and reward level. Thus, provided one holds drive at some constant albeit unknown level, the leveling off point in the speed versus reward function should indicate a nearly maximal reward.

As was brought out above, BSR has a temporary aftereffect that influences the avidity of subsequent responses; the more recent and intense the BSR that precedes a response the more rapid the response. This phenomenon created a variable that had to be controlled for; as one varied the magnitude of the BSR given as a reward for each run, one would necessarily also be varying the magnitude of the BSR that preceded the next response. To control for this we gave rats ten trains of BSR just before each run. These ten priming trains represented an order of magnitude greater and more recent BSR than the BSR received as a reward on the preceding run. Thus, the influence on running speed of any variation in the aftereffects of preceding rewards was rendered negligible.

We used pulsatile BSR and varied the train duration (from 0.04 to 0.32 second), the pulse frequency (100–200 pulses per second), and the number of trains in the reward. In Fig. 7-11, the running speeds of several rats with different placements are plotted against the total number of pulses (0.1 msec wide, negative going) in the reward. Every function levels off at or before a reward of 64 pulses. We concluded that a 0.32 second train of BSR at 200 pulses per second, with current intensity 150–300 percent above the threshold for bar pressing, was in most instances a nearly maximal reward. For some placements, much smaller amounts of BSR were still enough to sustain asymptotic running speeds.

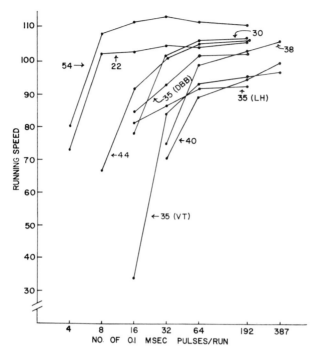

Fig. 7-11. Running speed versus reward magnitude functions for nine placements in seven rats. Reproduced from Gallistel (1969a); reproduced by permission of the American Psychological Association.

We obtained incidental confirmation of this conclusion in a later T-maze study (Gallistel, 1969b). In this later study we were attempting to get primed rats to choose the right and left arms equally often. The rats were reinforced in one arm on the priming electrode and in the other arm on another electrode. Whenever a rat began always to choose one arm, we reduced the number of pulses of BSR the rat received in that arm. It was always necessary to reduce the number of pulses to between 8 and 44 before a rat would begin to sample the other arm again.

These results do not, of course, establish any direct equivalence between the magnitude of BSR and the magnitude of a natural reward. As has already been pointed out, such an equivalence can only be established if the two rewards in question are appropriate to the same drive state. If they are not, they are incommensurable. It does not make sense to ask whether a given amount of food has a reward magnitude equal to a given amount of water. When rewards are qualitatively different, only the products of drive and reward can be compared. One can only ask, for example, whether 1 gram of food is equal to 1 ml of water for a rat that is 6 hours food deprived and 24 hours water deprived. Since the nature of the drive state appropriate to BSR remains unknown, the magnitude of BSR cannot be compared to the magnitude of a food or water reward. However, in many cases, the asymptotic running speed of the rats in the present experiment appeared to be close to the rat's physical limits. Thus, one may say that these small amounts of BSR, in combination with an intense priming-aroused drive-like state, produced running speeds that compare with those produced by sizeable food rewards in combination with intense hunger.

4. Duration of Aftereffect

While establishing the parameters of BSR necessary to produce a maximal reward, we also attempted to gain an idea of the parameters governing the aftereffect of BSR. The running behavior of three rats in the above study was particularly suitable for this second purpose. Although, when primed, these rats would run very rapidly for a reward of 32 pulses or less, these rats would run little, if at all, for the same amount of BSR when they had not been primed. This was true even when these rats were run on massed trials, such that only 3-5 seconds elapsed between the reward for one run and the start of the next run. We interpreted this to mean that for these rats small amounts of BSR had an adequate reward effect but a negligible aftereffect—an aftereffect so small that it dissipated in a few seconds.

This characteristic enabled us to study the time course of the aftereffect produced by larger amounts of BSR: We primed a rat with varying amounts of BSR and then ran it on a series of massed trials (to the small reward), making a point plot of the rat's gradually decreasing running speed. We found that, although there was a considerable difference in the magnitude of the effect in different rats, increasing the amount of "priming" from 1 or 3 trains to 10 or 20 trains (64 pulses per train) considerably increased and prolonged rapid performance in the subsequent series of massed trials. The data from the rat in which this effect was most pronounced are presented in Fig. 7-12. After one train this rat would only run for about 30 seconds; after 20 trains rapid running persisted for 10–15 minutes.

This result is consistent with the results of Keesey (1964) discussed above. Keesey found that the response rate on a VI schedule continued to increase as train duration was increased to 10 seconds. From his data, we concluded that some part of the system responsible for self-stimulation integrated neuron firing over a period of at least 10 seconds. The priming trains in the study just reported were 0.32 seconds long and delivered at 1 train per second. Ten trains were delivered in 10 seconds; 20 trains in 20 seconds. These results yield an estimate of the integration interval similar to the estimate derived from Keesey's data. The present results further suggest that this long-term integration occurs in the part of the system that mediates the aftereffect of BSR. Deutsch and Howarth

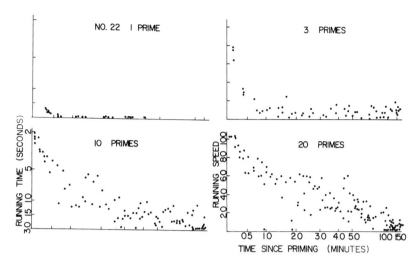

Fig. 7-12. Massed trial runway performance (for a 16 pulse reward) as a function of time since priming and number of priming trains (64 pulses per train). Priming occurred at the outset of a series of massed trials. Reproduced from Gallistel (1969a); reproduced by permission of the American Psychological Association.

(1963) have also demonstrated that it takes several trains of BSR to produce a maximal aftereffect.

This completes the review of the general aspects of the self-stimulation phenomenon. Subsequent sections give theoretical interpretations of these data and review data generated by experiments designed to test particular models of the self-stimulation system. The models for self-stimulation should be judged by how well they explain the following salient aspects of the phenomena.

The principal locus of rewarding electrodes is the MFB. However, successful placements are occasionally found in a wide variety of other brain structures. Self-stimulation is not seriously disrupted by lesions anywhere in the brain, with the possible exception of the caudal MFB.

Self-stimulation behavior has a positive feedback quality, that is, it continues intensely unless there are temporal interruptions, in which case the behavior becomes relatively slow and weak. The disruptive effects of temporal interruptions must be attributed to a temporally decaying excitatory aftereffect of BSR. The aftereffect of BSR influences both the avidity and the direction of behavior, that is, it affects both rate of performance and reward preference. In many cases, the decay effect disappears when a natural drive state is induced by deprivation of food or water, suggesting that the aftereffect is related to natural drives. However, the magnitude of the decay effect varies greatly from rat to rat. Some rats, in fact, show no evidence of a decaying aftereffect.

Varying those parameters of the stimulation that affect the size of the population of firing neurons has the same effect as varying the parameters that affect the amount of firing in a fixed population—intensity of self-stimulation is a monotonically increasing function in either case. The interchangeability of stimulation parameters suggests that the self-stimulation system employs a primitive code, in which only the total amount of firing is relevant. Obviously, this can only be true within some limits. What these limits are has not been determined.

It appears that a nearly maximal rewarding effect of BSR is produced by stimulation at roughly the following parameters: pulse duration, 0.1 msec; pulse intensity, 250–700 μA; pulse frequency, 100 pulses per second; train duration, 0.5 second. On the other hand, it requires 10 to 20 times as much stimulation for the aftereffect of BSR to reach its maximum.

III. THEORETICAL INTERPRETATIONS

A. Homeostatic Models

1. The Deutsch Model

The most systematically developed interpretation of self-stimulation has been presented by Deutsch (1960, 1963a; Deutsch & Howarth, 1963). Deutsch's model for self-stimulation derives from his more general model for simple homeostatic learning (Deutsch, 1960). The more general model belongs to the class of theories schematized in Fig. 7-1 (Section I, B, 1) and Fig. 7-5 (Section I, B, 5). The general model assumes a number of distinct homeostatic systems. Each of these systems has a drive component which provides a drive signal (potentiation) when the variable it is regulating (e.g., osmotic pressure) deviates from the desired level (the set point). Each homeostatic system has, in addition, a reinforcement component. Whenever a behavior pattern produces a reward that is appropriate to a given homeostat (e.g., water), then that reward activates the reinforcement system. The reinforcement system in turn sends out a signal which adjusts the drive-transfer parameter for the behavior pattern that produced the reward. This adjustment remains fixed unless some future instance of the behavior pattern produces a degree of activation of the reinforcement system which does not match the value at which the parameter has previously been set. As a result of this parameter change, any future drive signal will selectively potentiate the behavior pattern that produced reward. The general model, in other words, makes the assumptions discussed in Sections II, B, 1 and II, B, 5.

The model for self-stimulation further assumes that the self-stimulation electrode is exciting one or more of these homeostatic systems at two points— one point on the reinforcement side of the system(s), and one point on the drive side of the system(s), as shown in Fig. 7-13.

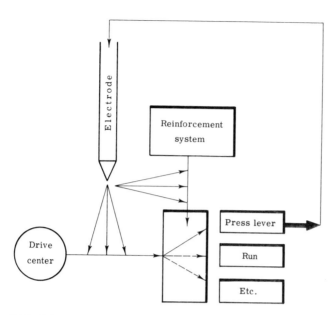

Fig. 7-13. Schematization of Deutsch's model for the relation between the self-stimulation electrode and the neural tissue mediating drive and reward. Note that the electrode is assumed to directly excite two components of a homestatic system. The parameter changing effect of excitation in the reinforcement loop is indicated by the solid arrow pointing to the Press Lever behavior pattern.

The excitation of the reinforcement loop adjusts the drive-transfer parameter of the behavior pattern that produced reward. This parameter change will channel any incoming drive potentiation toward the reward-producing response.

The excitation in the drive component of the homeostat behaves like a natural drive signal. It is channeled by the drive-transfer parameters toward reward-producing behavior patterns. It potentiates these behavior patterns, that is, makes them more likely to occur. Of course, the potentiation lasts only as long as the drive signal. As the drive signal dissipates, so does the potentiation of reward-producing behavior patterns.

Under normal circumstances, a drive signal is maintained as long as the discrepancy between the values of set point and the regulated variable persists. In self-stimulation, however, the drive signal is artificially produced by the electrical stimulation. It is assumed that, in this case, the drive signal will disappear shortly after the cessation of the stimulation which creates it, unless, of course, there is already a naturally arising drive signal in the system (e.g., the animal is thirsty).

Another way of putting the theory is to say that it assumes that self-stimulation electrodes excite what is normally a negative feedback (homeostatic) system in such a way that it behaves as a positive feedback system. Each response that produces BSR not only excites a reinforcement function, it also excites an appropriate drive function and, thereby, it potentiates a repetition of the response. The continual repotentiating of stimulation-producing behavior explains the lack of satiation in self-stimulation. Positive feedback loops, by their very nature, do not show satiation unless something intervenes to interrupt the feedback. In self-stimulation, the imposition of a time interval between successive stimulations constitutes such an interruption because it allows the drive signal excited by the stimulation to decay. When the animal is again permitted to perform, little or no drive signal remains to potentiate resumption of the BSR-producing behavior pattern. This explains the large body of data showing the behavior weakening effects of temporal interruptions in self-stimulation (Section II, C).

Interestingly enough, the theory, without any further assumptions, also explains much of the data on rats whose self-stimulation behavior did not show a strong effect of temporal interruption. If the drive component of a system excited by a self-stimulation electrode is already carrying a strong naturally arising drive signal, then the drive effect of BSR will have much less effect on self-stimulation behavior, for when the drive signal deriving from the artificial stimulation has dissipated, the naturally arising drive signal will still remain to potentiate the behavior pattern reinforced by the BSR.

Following the above line of reasoning to the effect that a natural drive should, under appropriate circumstances, eliminate drive decay effects in self-stimulation, Deutsch and DiCara (1967) compared extinction rates when rats trained for BSR were either hungry or satiated. Most of the rats took much longer to extinguish when hungry. That is, hunger did counteract the drive decay effect.

The theory also explains why hunger may fail to counteract the drive decay effect in some rats. If the self-stimulation electrode is so placed that it does not excite the reinforcement component of the nutrient homeostat, then a naturally arising hunger signal will not potentiate the BSR-producing behavior pattern because there will not have been a parameter change capable of conveying the hunger drive signal toward the response which produces the BSR. In the Deutsch model, the drive-transfer parameters that channel the hunger signal can only be adjusted by the reinforcement component of the nutrient homeostat. The drive-transfer parameters adjusted by the reinforcement component of another homeostat (e.g., the water homeostat) can only convey the drive signals originating in that homeostat (e.g., thirst signals). This can be seen by reference to Fig. 7-5, Section II, B, 5.

The data from several other experiments can readily be given the same interpretation which Deutsch and DiCara gave their data. In studies by Gibson *et al.* (1965), Olds (1956), Reid and Porter (1965), and Wetzel (1963), hunger was a variable that may well have influenced the data. In an experiment by Scott (1967), the sex drive may have had an influence (cf. the placements of Caggiula & Hoebel, 1966).

Another attraction of the theory suggested by Deutsch is its ability to explain otherwise paradoxical results. For example, in Section II, D, 3 evidence was presented to show that single trains of BSR produce a nearly maximal reinforcing effect. Yet, Pliskoff *et al.* (1965) found that increasing the number of trains per "reward" greatly improved performance on partial reinforcement schedules. They concluded that single trains of BSR were a poor reward. This apparent paradox is resolved if one assumes, as in the Deutsch model, that rats perform poorly for BSR on partial reinforcement schedules not because single trains of BSR are poor reinforcers but rather because the drive-like aftereffect of BSR decays in the interval between stimulations. This assumption puts the Pliskoff *et al.* data in a new light. In Section II, D, 4 evidence was presented to show that this drive-like aftereffect continues to build up over successive trains of BSR. After several trains it lasts much longer than after single trains. Hence, a multi-train reward would provide more drive potentiation during the subsequent interval of a partial reinforcement schedule.

Another apparent paradox is Keesey's (1964) finding that rats select fairly short train durations when the intensity of the BSR is high, yet the performance of these rats on a VI schedule can be improved by extending the train duration well beyond the duration the rats selected. Again this paradox is resolved if one assumes that the train duration selected by a rat is determined by the rewarding effect of BSR which rapidly reaches an asymptote (and may even begin to adapt out); whereas the rate of performance on a VI schedule is determined by the drive effect which takes much longer to reach asymptote.

The independence of drive and reinforcement, as postulated by Deutsch, can also explain Keesey's (1966) finding that the rate of responding maintained by BSR failed to predict the effects of BSR as a reinforcer in discrimination learning. Rate of responding would reflect primarily the drive effect of BSR, whereas performance in a discrimination task would reflect only the reinforcement effect. Since the two effects are assumed to be independent, they need not be correlated (see the discussion of the runway experiment, Section IV, C).

2. Objections to the Deutsch Model

There have been two sorts of objections to the Deutsch model, the first being that many of the drive decay effects do not occur (Kent & Grossman, 1970; Kornblith & Olds, 1968; Scott, 1967; Wasden, Reid & Porter, 1965), at least in some rats.

Many presumably satiated rats will show BSR directed behavior after sizeable intervals have elapsed since the last BSR, whereas the model implies that they should not. As Kent and Grossman (1970) have shown, some rats will resume pressing at the start of a day's session without any encouragement, and the nature of a rat's previous training will affect its performance after long intervals have elapsed since the last stimulation (Pliskoff & Hawkins, 1963; Stutz, Lewin, & Rocklin, 1965); whereas the model implies that there should be no performance, and, hence, no effect of previous training.

In earlier expositions of the model (e.g., Gallistel, 1964) it was assumed that when an animal had been trained under a drive, such as hunger, and then satiated on food, the animal would no longer perform the responses that had been rewarded with food. A perusal of the literature on performance under conditions of "zero" drive, that is, apparent satiation, has shown that this is not usually the case (see Bruce, 1938; Mandler, 1964; Timberlake, 1967; Zeaman & House, 1950). Kimble (1951), for example, trained hungry rats to push back a panel to obtain food. When the rats were thoroughly sated on food and replaced in the test situation, their first panel press occurred with a median latency of 0.2 seconds. It has also been noted that the type of partial reinforcement schedule used in initial training affects the performance of satiated pigeons (Holz & Azrin, 1963), and that extensive training on VI schedules reduces the performance decrement produced by satiation (Ferster & Skinner, 1957, pp. 370-371). Sidman and Stebbens (1954) showed that when animals had been trained on FR schedules, satiation affected only the probability of initiating a response burst—not the probability of completing the burst, nor the rate of pressing during the burst. The probability of initiating a burst did not go to zero after a half hour of prewatering.

There are two possibilities for reconciling the homeostatic model with the data showing performance after long intervals since the last stimulation. On the one hand, Deutsch (1963b) has argued that the model's basic prediction is that performance for BSR after a long interval since the last stimulation will closely resemble the performance of satiated animals previously trained for a natural reward. In other words, the performance for BSR will decline to some asymptote. The fact that satiated animals will show some performance, whether for BSR or a natural reward, is treated by Deutsch as a phenomenon lying outside the scope of his model, which is a model for behavior under homeostatic control. Deutsch's treatment of these data is similar to those earlier treatments of performance in satiated rats that regarded such performance as "functionally autonomous" (see Webb, 1952, for review). Seward et al. (1959) and Segal (1962), among others, have shown that well trained responses become partially independent of both drive and reward. Trowill et al. (1969) have also stressed the need to compare BSR performance with the performance of satiated animals responding for natural rewards.

Another approach to these data takes note of the difficulty of arriving at a satisfactory operational definition of zero drive, or complete satiation. One can argue that physiological homeostats are seldom completely balanced. There is, in other words, usually some low level of drive to potentiate well-trained responses. In the absence of an agreed upon operational definition of zero drive, this argument is untestable. That it may, however, have some merit can be seen from the fact that, in an experiment by Hodos and Kalman (1963), rats which were sated on water and lab chow performed rather well for a sugared milk reward. This performance was nonetheless under homeostatic control—when sated on the sugared milk solution, the rats would no longer respond. In other words, negative feedback from the reward eventually reduced drive potentiation to the point where even eating a highly palatable reward no longer occurred. With rats, as with humans, the degree of satiation (negative feedback) required to abolish homeostatically regulated performance depends in part on the quality of the reward. If BSR is equivalent to a highly palatable reward, and if some electrodes stimulate the food homeostat in the manner postulated by Deutsch, one would expect some rats, sated on lab chow, to perform for BSR at the start of a session, just as they would perform for any other highly palatable reward.

The second sort of objection to the Deutsch model has been that some of the phenomena, such as rapid extinction, that have been cited in support of it, are in fact attributable to other causes. The possible sources of artifact most frequently mentioned are the unusual temporal and spatial conditions surrounding the receipt of BSR and the fact that BSR frequently has mildly aversive side effects. Gibson et al. (1965) trained two groups of hungry rats to respond for a sugar-water reward. One group had only to lick a dipper containing sugar-water to obtain the reward; the other group had to first press a lever and then collect the reward from the dipper. In addition, two groups of hungry rats were trained to respond for BSR. One group had only to lick a dry dipper in order to produce BSR, whereas the other group had to first press a lever and then collect the BSR by licking the dipper. All four groups were then extinguished. The only differences in rate of extinction were between, on the one hand, the two groups which made a single component response and, on the other hand, the two groups that made a two component response. The nature of the reward did not affect rate of extinction. Gibson et al. suggested that the rapid extinction of BSR sustained responses and other peculiarities of BSR sustained performance were artifacts of the unusual conditions surrounding the administration of BSR in previous studies (see, however, Panksepp & Trowill, 1967a). In a similar vein, Wasden et al. (1965) and Kent and Grossman (1969) have suggested that the overnight decrement seen in some rats is an artifact of the aversive side effects of BSR (see, however, Scott, 1967).

Is is unlikely that the artifactual causes cited by Gibson et al., Wasden et al., and Kent and Grossman can account for most of the decay phenomena. First, there is little evidence that any arrangement of the reinforcement conditions will produce "spontaneous" extinction of a naturally rewarded response.[3] Quartermain and Webster (1968) have shown that when most of the factors mentioned by Gibson *et al.* are equated, rats rewarded with BSR still show spontaneous extinction, whereas rats rewarded with water do not. Second, the brain stimulation rewarded rats in the Gibson *et al.* study were hungry. These data can therefore, be interpreted as supporting the Deutsch model (cf., Deutsch & DiCara, 1967). Third, Gallistel (1967) found that arranging the presentation of a water reward so as to mimic the presentation of BSR did not induce a performance decrement after longer intertrial intervals. The water reward was short, immediate, and had an aversive accompaniment.

Nonetheless, it is beyond dispute that many factors other than drive will influence animal behavior, particularly the behavior of satiated animals. Trowill *et al.* (1969) have discussed a number of these factors. And Kavanau (1969) has given many cautionary examples of the degree to which behavior in constricting environments can be independent of homeostatic considerations.

Data causing considerable difficulty for the model come from the secondary reinforcement studies by Stein (1958) and Knott and Clayton (1966). Stein placed implanted rats in a Skinner box with two levers, one of which produced a tone. After recording the operant rate of pressing for 6 days, he withdrew the levers and presented a hundred pairings of the tone and brain stimulation. When the levers were returned, the brain-stimulation-positive group preferred the tone lever and increased their absolute rate of pressing. The brain-stimulation-negative group showed neither effect. Knott and Clayton replicated this study and added a partial reinforcement group—a group for which the BSR was only intermittently paired with the tone. The greatest secondary reinforcement effect was in this last group. The secondary reinforcement tests were conducted some time after the last BSR, and, hence, it is surprising, from the standpoint of Deutsch's model, to find that rats showed new learning. According to Deutsch's theory, the level of drive potentiation should have been low and it should have been difficult to induce the rats to perform the newly learned, secondarily reinforced habit. In neither case was there a group tested under similar circumstances with a natural reward as the primary reinforcement, so it is difficult to assess the relative magnitude of the effect. The secondary reinforcement effect with BSR appears somewhat fragile, since Mogenson (1965) was unable to replicate Stein's (1958) findings despite extensive efforts to do so. Other attempts to demonstrate secondary reinforcement with BSR have been similarly unsuccessful (Seward *et al.*, 1959). A possible explanation for this discord can be found in

---

[3] Panksepp and Trowill (1967b) claimed to have demonstrated such an effect in satiated rats responding for a chocolate milk reward. The claim, however, rested on a questionable use of inferential statistics, viz., a failure to reject the null hypothesis when comparing two samples, one of which contained only three observations.

Deutsch's (1963a) discussion of the conditions which will enhance or reduce manifestations of drive decay.

The findings by Kent and Grossman (1969) that a substantial proportion of rats show no drive decay effects also cause difficulty for the Deutsch model. Kent and Grossman suggest that decay effects appear only when stimulation has mixed rewarding and aversive qualities, in other words, only when there is an approach-avoidance conflict. It is, however, not clear why this conflict should become more pronounced simply as a function of time since last stimulation. As suggested in Section III, A, 1, another way to explain individual differences in the magnitude of the decay effect is to assume that rats who show no decay effects have electrodes in systems which maintain chronically elevated drive levels (e.g., sex).

Data from refractory period studies (discussed below) strongly support some aspects of Deutsch's model, while data from double electrode priming experiments (also discussed below) are not clearly consistent with other aspects of the model. Whatever the final verdict on Deutsch's model, it is clear that the model is sufficiently successful to make it highly likely that many of its important structural assumptions will appear in whatever models replace it.

B. Hedonic Models

Olds and Olds (1965) and Stein (1964) have suggested models for self-stimulation that closely resemble each other. Their models belong to the class schematized in Fig. 7-2, Section I, B, 2. The models assume that in self-stimulation the electrode is exciting one point in a positive feedback system, as indicated in Fig. 7-14. The models differ with regard to the details of the

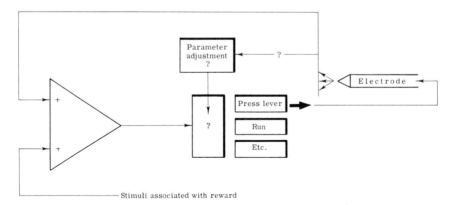

Fig. 7-14. Schematization of the relation between the self-stimulation electrode and the behavior-reward system in the Olds and Stein models. Note that the electrode excites the system at one point only.

interaction assumed to occur between the system responsible for self-stimulation and the system that controls aversive behavior.

In Fig. 7-14, there are question marks in the feedback loop leading through the parameter adjusting transfer function because it is not clear whether Olds and Stein wish to assume such a loop. It is not clear in their models why the positive feedback from reward selectively potentiates rewarded behavior in preference to other behavior patterns.

Stein (1964) suggests that rewarded behavior gives rise to stimuli that have been associated with reward. These stimuli produce positive feedback, which enhances the ongoing behavior (i.e., the rewarded behavior). Behavior that has not been rewarded gives rise to stimuli that have not been associated with reward. These stimuli do not feed back to further enhance the ongoing (unrewarded) behavior. Thus, only the rewarded behavior receives positive feedback from the stimuli it gives rise to. This suggestion could explain the selective potentiation of rewarded behavior without assuming a parameter-adjusting feedback loop.

The Olds and Stein models give a more straightforward account of those data which created difficulties for the Deutsch model, namely, the data showing BSR directed behavior occurring after long intervals since the last stimulation. In such instances, the stimuli associated with the reward, that is, the stimuli in the test environment, are assumed to excite the behavior enhancing system, thereby potentiating BSR directed behavior. These models do not account for the data showing performance decrements as a consequence of time elapsed since the last stimulation. Or, rather, they do not explain why the time variable is important in BSR sustained behavior but not in behavior sustained by natural rewards.

The general objections to hedonic models mentioned in Section II, B, 2 apply here. If the system underlying positively reinforced behavior is designed on the positive feedback principle, it is not clear why positively reinforced behavior ever ceases. Olds (1958c) has suggested that only the relative paucity of some rewards in the rat's natural environment counteracts this unfortunate tendency. That is, rats may persist until there is no more reward left to potentiate further responding. This suggestion is not consistent with a large body of data showing that rats accurately regulate their intake of food and water reward, even when there is unlimited supply.[4]

Trowill *et al.* (1969) have suggested a model of the kind outlined in Fig. 7-3, Section I, B, 3. Like Olds and Stein, they assume that the electrode excites

---

[4] P. Milner (1970, Chapter 18) has recently proposed a model similar to the Olds and Stein models but with the addition of a drive-controlled gate in the positive feedback loop. When there is no drive, the gate blocks the positive feedback from reward and the stimuli associated with reward. Thus, rewarded behavior is not indefinitely self-potentiating. This assumption of a negative feedback gate in the positive feedback loop remedies a serious deficiency in most previous positive feedback models.

only the reward part of the system, and that the reward system can arouse behavior. However, Trowill *et al.* postulate a further interaction between reward and drive. They assume that activating the reward system arouses behavior most strongly when the animal is satiated and the reward is of high quality.

As with Olds and Stein, Trowill *et al.* further assume that the environmental stimuli associated with the reward eventually acquire its arousing properties. Put more anthropomorphically, this is the assumption which is central to all hedonic models, that the stimuli of the test environment arouse in the rat the expectation of reward, and this expectation elicits behavior.

We have conducted an experiment to test this assumption (Gallistel, 1966). Four rats were trained to run two runways. The runways pointed in opposite directions; and one was painted black, the other white. The trials alternated between the two runways. A rat always ran in the white runway immediately after collecting a reward in the black runway, and vice versa. From time to time, the runways were converted to a T maze by joining them at their start areas and adding a stem. On the T maze trials, the rats were free to choose runways. After initial training with equal amounts of BSR in both runways, the current intensity of the BSR in one runway was significantly increased. This induced all four rats to run faster in the opposite runway. That is, they ran faster to the less intense BSR. This occurred despite the fact that, when they could choose, two rats showed a significant preference for the runway with the more intense BSR and two showed no preference. Thus, the choice data indicated that two rats had associated the stimuli in the high current runway with the greater reward, yet these rats ran more rapidly to the smaller reward. The choice data further indicated that the other two rats did not associate either runway with larger reward, yet these two rats also ran faster to the less intense BSR.

These data create difficulties for the expectancy assumption in the Olds, Stein, and Trowill *et al.*, models. It is not clear how these models explain a rat's running faster in a runway where it expects less reward. On the other hand, the data can be explained by the Deutsch model, which assumes that the expectation of reward (i.e., the state of the drive-transfer parameters) is independent of the desire for reward (i.e., the drive signal). Given that the reward effects of both the more intense and less intense BSR were large, the avidity of behavior would be controlled primarily by the relative intensities of the drive-like aftereffects. The experiment was so arranged that the drive effect resulting from the BSR received in the white runway was operating while a rat was running in the black runway, and vice versa.

C. Rebound Models

Ball (1967) has proposed a model along the lines of an early suggestion by Miller (1961). Ball's model is unique in that it does not assume that the electrode is exciting tissue having any direct relation to natural reinforcement processes (see, also, Ball & Adams, 1965). Ball's model resembles the traditional analysis of drug addiction. It is assumed that BSR excites a system which inhibits some or all sensory inputs. When the stimulating train ceases, this inhibition is suddenly removed. This leads to a postinhibitory rebound in the previously inhibited sensory channels. This rebound is aversive. The rat learns to reinitiate stimulation in order to suppress the aversive sensory input that follows stimulation.

This model accounts for the decay data in much the same way as the Deutsch model; only, in this model, it is the decay of a postinhibitory rebound, rather than the decay of a drive, that accounts for the declining avidity of behavior. This model has more difficulty than the Deutsch model in explaining the data showing performance after long intervals. It is not clear why a rat would reinitiate a generally aversive vicious circle, once the rat had escaped from the circle.[5]

Konorski (1967, p. 399) has suggested an explanation of self-stimulation, which, like Ball's explanation, assumes that the drive effect derives from a postinhibitory rebound. However, he has recently revised the model (personal communication). Konorski now assumes that the drive effect derives from the direct excitation of a separate component of his system. The schematization of his current model is similar in basic structure to the schematization of the Deutsch model.

IV. THE STRUCTURE AND NEUROPHYSIOLOGY OF THE SELF-STIMULATION SYSTEM

The various models for the structure of the self-stimulation system have generated a number of experiments designed to test their structural assumptions. These experiments in turn have led to experiments on the neurophysiology of the hypothetical structures.

A. One Component, Or Two?

Rebound and hedonic models have one structural feature in common: they assume that self-stimulation arises from the stimulation of a single, functionally homogeneous population of neurons. In the rebound models, the relevant function of this population is the inhibition of some other system. In the hedonic models, the function of this population is to mediate the positive feedback effects of natural rewards. In Deutsch's homeostatic model, on the other hand, self-stimulation is assumed to arise only when the electrode excites two neuronal populations with distinct functions. The function of one popu-

---

[5] Deutsch's model does not assume that the drive state is aversive.

lation is to mediate the reinforcing effects of some natural reward; the function of the other population is to mediate the potentiating effects of one or more natural drives.

We have recently conducted some behavioral and electro-physiological experiments that explored the implications of these contrasting assumptions. These experiments, in turn, have led to some preliminary investigations of the neurophysiology of the self-stimulation system.

The starting point for these experiments was an ingenious approach developed by Deutsch (1964). Deutsch realized that the paired-pulses stimulation technique, which produced much of our knowledge about the electrophysiology of peripheral nerve systems, could equally as well be applied to the physiology of the central neural systems. Before reviewing the way in which this technique has been used to decide between the alternative suggestions for the structure of the self-stimulation system, it will help make the rationale underlying the technique clearer if we review the history of its application to the peripheral nervous system.

As with many other techniques, the history of the paired-pulse technique begins with Helmholtz. In 1854, du Bois-Reymond sponsored a paper by Helmholtz at the annual meeting of the Berlin Academy. The paper reported on experiments involving stimulation of a nerve-muscle preparation from the frog. A muscle was connected to a kymograph to make a record of the time course and amplitude of the twitches evoked in the muscle by electric shocks applied to the attached nerve (Fig. 7-15A). Helmholtz then used pairs of shocks to stimulate the nerve. When the two shocks in a pair were separated from each other by more than a few tenths of a second, they evoked two twitches of similar time course and amplitude (Fig. 7-15B). When the shocks were close together, they evoked a single twitch. This single twitch, however, had a greater amplitude than the maximum twitch that could be evoked by a single shock (Fig. 7-15C). However, Helmholtz also noted that: "... two shocks (were) no more effective than one shock *when the interval between (was less than) ... roughly 1/600 second (1.6 msec)*." (See Fig. 7-15D.) "If, however, the shocks (were) so weak that, acting singly, they did not produce a maximal twitch, then they (reinforced) each other even at the shortest intershock intervals [p. 331]." (See Fig. 7-15E; present author's translation; italics added.)

Although it was 50 years before it was fully appreciated, what Helmholtz had demonstrated in the two sentences just quoted was the refractory period of neurons, and latent temporal addition in neurons stimulated by a shock below the threshold for firing.

The absolute refractory period of a neuron is the period following one suprathreshold stimulus during which a second stimulus, no matter how intense, cannot fire the neuron. In Helmholtz' preparation, when two strong shocks were sufficiently close, the second shock fell within the refractory period created by

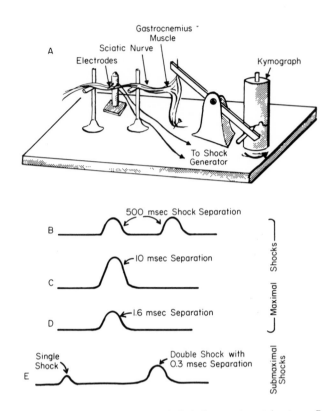

Fig. 7-15. A. Schematic sketch of Helmholtz's experimental set up. B., C., and D. Results using shocks sufficiently intense to produce a maximal twitch when acting singly (see text). E. Results using shocks too weak to produce a maximal twitch when acting singly.

the first shock. Hence, the second shock did not fire the nerve. As a result, only one set of neuronal impulses, instead of two, arrived at the neuro-muscular junction, and the muscle twitch had the same amplitude as would have been produced by the first shock alone.

Latent temporal addition refers to the fact that a subthreshold depolarization of a neuron, such as is produced by a weak stimulus pulse, takes time to decay. Hence, if a second stimulus pulse follows shortly after the first, the depolarization produced by the second pulse will add to the residual depolarization from the first pulse. The resulting sum is frequently sufficient to fire the neuron. Thus, when Helmholtz used weak shocks, some neurons in the nerve bundle were not fired by the first shock. However, these neurons did undergo subthreshold depolarization. Thus, when the second shock came, the depolarization it produced summed with the depolarization remaining from the first shock to produce a suprathreshold depolarization which fired the neurons left unfired by the first shock. The two shocks reinforced each other to produce a greater twitch, because together they fired a greater number of neurons than either shock could fire acting singly.

The interpretation of Helmholz' experiment became clear when Gotch and Burch (1899), using a capillary electrometer, demonstrated the neural refractory period by direct electrophysiological recording of the compound action potential in the nerve. Boycott (1899), a student in their lab, repeated Helmholtz' experiment and showed that the neuronal refractory period revealed by Gotch and Burch's electrophysiological technique was equally as well revealed by the contractile behavior of the muscle to which the nerve led. Bramwell and Lucas (1911) again validated the nerve-muscle preparation by showing that it yielded the same refractory period value as did electrophysiological recording.

In the next 35 years a variety of studies, particularly those of Lucas (e.g., 1906) and Adrian and Lucas (1912), used the contractile behavior of the innervated muscle to reveal, and precisely measure, the characteristics of the response of a neuron to electrical stimulation (see Hill, 1936 for references). The findings have since been confirmed by electrophysiological recordings from the same preparations (for references, see Furshpan, 1959; Grundfest, 1940; Tasaki, 1959).

The most elegant refinements of this technique were made by Lucas. In a paper published after his death in an airplane crash, Lucas (1917) showed that the adductor muscle of the claw of Astacus was innervated by two populations of neurons with different functions. His only index of neuron excitation was the contractile behavior of the muscle, yet he was able to show that, among other differences, the two neuron populations had different characteristic refractory periods (and different chronaxies as well).

The paired-pulses technique enables one to use the behavior of a muscle, or other effector system, to study the properties of neurons whose excitation produces a response in the effector system. If one arranges the preparation so that the effect of pairs of stimulus pulses (shocks) is clearly distinguishable from the effect of single stimulus pulses, then whenever the second stimulus of a pair falls within the refractory period left by the first stimulus, the behavior of the preparation will change from the behavior which is produced by pairs of stimuli to the behavior which is produced by single stimulus pulses. Normally, the behavioral change used as the index is a simple change in the intensity of the behavioral effect (e.g., the evoked twitch).

When this technique was being developed, it was essential to show that the results always reflected the refractory period of the stimulated nerve and not refractoriness in the muscle or at the synapse. Bramwell and Lucas (1911) were able to show this, as was Bazett (1908). The latter showed that the nerve-muscle preparation would yield the refractory period of the nerve, even when the refractory period of the muscle (to direct electrical stimulation) was twice as long as the refractory period of the nerve. Why this is so is now well understood. A synapse, even a one-to-one "synapse" like the neuro-muscular junction, integrates spikes over the range of temporal variation within which the neuronal refractory period manifests itself. In other words, if two neuronal impulses (spikes) arrive at a synapse so closely spaced that the neurons (or muscles) on the other side cannot fire in time-locked sequence, then the synapse accumulates (sums together) the effect of the two impulses. This sum persists for a longer time than the spikes which created it. And the firing of the postsynaptic neurons is proportional to the magnitude of this sum. Hence, variations in the temporal spacing of spikes, within the range of variation needed for the refractory period to become manifest (a few tenths of a millisecond), are lost at the synapse. Any sharp changes in the behavioral output of the preparation which occur as a result of a change of a few tenths of a millisecond in the spacing of paired stimulus pulses can be attributed to the properties of the presynaptic tissue, that is, the tissue directly excited by the electrical stimulation.

This principle is important to the work described below. It means that one can determine, from a given behavioral index, the characteristic refractory period of any neuronal population whose direct excitation by electrical pulses elicits some behavior, provided only that the behavior varies systematically with some twofold change in the number of stimulating pulses. It should not matter how many synapses intervene between the directly excited tissue and the recorded behavior, since any sharp change that occurs in the intensity of the effect created by the stimulation must occur by the first synapse after the point of excitation. From there on, it will be relayed to the effector system as a simple difference in intensity.

Deutsch (1964) was the first to apply the paired-pulses technique to the study of central nervous system physiology. He used it to determine the characteristic refractory periods of the neuronal populations underlying self-stimulation. In our own lab we have replicated Deutsch's basic results, using a different behavioral technique (Gallistel *et al.*, 1969). Our technique was designed to simplify the operational distinction between the aftereffect and the rewarding effect in self-stimulation. If it can be shown that these two effects derive from the excitation of neuronal populations with different characteristic refractory periods, then it will be necessary to postulate models for the self-stimulation system which assume that the system is directly stimulated at two functionally distinct points. In other words, experiments using the paired-pulses technique can have important implications for the structure of the self-stimulation system.

In order to operationally distinguish the aftereffect from the reward effect in behavior sustained by BSR, we used the same runway and priming box set-up employed in our experiments on reward magnitude and the duration of the aftereffect. The rat ran a 6-foot runway and rewarded itself with BSR by pressing a lever at the goal end of the runway. The rat was then placed in a waiting box. After an interval, the rat was automatically primed, removed from the waiting box, and placed at the start of the runway. The reward effect in self-stimulation was operationally defined as the effect on running speed produced by holding the amount of priming stimulation constant and varying the amount of reward stimulation (see Section II, D, 3 and Fig. 7-11). The aftereffect in self-stimulation was operationally defined as the effect on running speed produced by holding the amount of reward stimulation constant and varying the amount of priming stimulation (see Section II, D, 4 and Fig. 7-12).

The stimulating pulses the rat received for pressing the goal lever and the pulses it received as priming in the waiting box were identical—same electrode, same current intensity, same pulse width. Only the number of stimulating pulses was varied, either by varying pulse frequency (100–200 pulses per second) or by varying train duration (0.08–0.16 second). Within the indicated ranges, twofold variations in pulse-frequency and train duration are interchangeable. That is, 0.08 second × 200 pulses per second produces the same effect as 0.16 second × 100 pulses per second.

The first step in our experimental procedure was to determine a critical train duration. That is, we determined a train duration such that halving the pulse frequency from 200 pulses per second to 100 pulses per second produced a maximal change in running speed. For example, in determining the refractory period for the reward effect, we initially settled on a train duration of 0.12 second, because changing the reward from: 0.12 second × 200 pulses per second = 24 pulses to 0.12 second × 100 pulses per second = 12 pulses appeared to produce a maximal change in running speed. However, it later appeared that we would get an even greater change using a train duration of 0.08 second, so we made a second determination of the reward refractory period, using this train duration.

Having determined the critical train duration, we switched to a stimulation train in which the pulses, instead of being evenly spaced, came in pairs. The pulses were paired so that we could vary the interval between the first and second pulse in each pair until the second pulse fell within the refractory period left by the first, and thereby became ineffective. The interval between pairs of pulses (the interpair interval) was fixed at 10 msec. The interval within pairs of pulses (the intrapair interval, IPI) was varied from 0.1–1.5 msec. As one decreased the IPI, there came a point at which the running speed decreased from the fast speed characteristic of a 16 pulse reward to the slow speed characteristic of an 8 pulse reward. The decrease in running speed presumably occurred when the second pulse in each pair fell within the refractory period and failed to excite the neurons. Thus, the point at which the running speed decreased was, presumably, the refractory period of the neuronal population mediating the reward effect.

In other words, in order to measure the refractory period of the neurons mediating the reward effect of BSR, we gave the rat a large, fixed amount of priming before each trial, set the train duration of the stimulation produced by the goal lever at 0.08 second (or 0.12 second), and plotted the rat's running speed while varying the IPI of the stimulation produced by the goal lever.

The rat was run in blocks of 20 trials. During each block the IPI had a fixed value. The data from the first 10 trials in each block were discarded, in order to allow the rat's running speed for each new IPI to stabilize. There were 4 blocks per day, plus an initial series of control blocks with unpaired stimulation at 100 pulses per second and 200 pulses per second—the two baseline conditions. In the course of several weeks, the rat was given 4 blocks of trials at each IPI from 0.1 msec to 1.5 msec. The sequence of IPI's was randomized.

The plots of running speed obtained in this part of the experiment are shown as solid lines (or the dotted line with squares) in Fig. 7-16. The running speed between the exit from the start box and the entry to the goal (left hand graph in Fig. 7-16) and the speed of total performance from the dropping of the start door until entry into the goal (right hand graph in Fig. 7-16) both showed a sharp decrease when the IPI of the reward stimulation decreased from 0.64 to 0.54 msec, indicating that the neuronal population mediating the reward effect of BSR had a characteristic refractory period of approximately 0.6 msec.

The speeds increased again when the IPI was in the range 0.1–0.3 msec. This probably resulted from latent temporal addition in neurons sufficiently distant from the electrode to receive only subthreshold excitation from the first pulse in each pair. Such neurons would be fired by the second pulse in a pair, provided the second pulse arrived while there was still some depolarization remaining from the first pulse. Thus, the effect of two very closely spaced pulses would be greater than the effect of a single pulse (cf. Helmholtz' experiment, Fig. 7-15E; also, Lucas, 1917).

In order to measure the refractory period of the neurons mediating the aftereffect ("priming effect," "drive effect"), we set the reward at a fixed, nearly maximal value (16 pulses), set the duration of the priming stimulation at 0.16 second, and plotted the rat's running speed while varying the IPI in the priming stimulation. In this part of the experiment the interval between trials was lengthened from 30 seconds to 2 minutes in order to prevent the build up of an aftereffect over successive trials. The rat was run in blocks of 10 trials, with the IPI fixed within blocks. Between each of these blocks there was a block of 5 trials at the 100 pulses per second baseline condition. Each day's session began with a block of 10 trials at the other baseline condition (200 pulses per second).

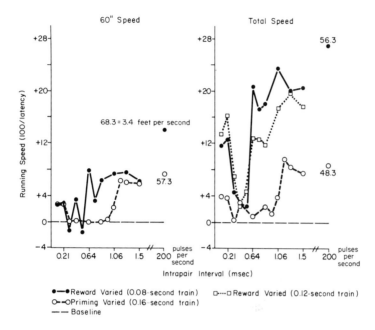

Fig. 7-16. The running spead of a rat as a function of the intrapair interval in the reward stimulation (solid lines, or dotted line with squares), and as a function of the intrapair interval in the priming stimulation (broken lines with circles). The functions are plotted as deviations from the 100 pulses per second baseline performance (0 on the ordinate), that is, the performance when the second pulse in each pair was omitted altogether. In order to give an idea of the absolute speeds involved, the points representing the other baseline condition (stimulation at frequency 200 pulses per second) have their absolute values written above or below them.[6] The left hand graph is for the true *running* speed, that is, the reciprocal of the time elapsed in running between the photocell just beyond the start box and the photocell at the entrance to the goal. The right hand graph is for the speed of overall performance, that is, the reciprocal of the running latency plus the start latency. The reward curve was determined twice, with two different train durations. During the first determination (dotted line with squares on right hand graph) only the overall latency was recorded. Each point on the graphs is the mean of 40 observations. The electrode was in the MFB above the mammillary bodies.

[6] The failure of performance at IPI's greater than the refractory period to equal the performance in the 200 pulses per second baseline condition may have been due in part to relative refractoriness. However, in part this failure was ascribable simply to fatigue. The 200 pulses per second performance was always determined at the start of a session, whereas the performance at various IPI's were determined after at least 40 trials. The extremely rapid performance characteristic of the 200 pulses per second reward condition was more vulnerable to fatigue than was the slower performance characteristic of all other conditions.

Four IPI's were tested each day in a randomized sequence until the rat had run four blocks at each IPI. There was no need to discard the data from the initial trials in each block because the adjustment in running speed following a change in the priming stimulation occurred immediately (cf., final paragraph, Section II, C, 4).

The resulting plots are shown as broken lines with open circles in Fig. 7-16. The running speed and the overall speed of performance (left and right hand graphs, respectively) both showed a decrease when the IPI decreased from 1.1 msec to 0.9 msec, indicating that the neuronal population mediating the aftereffect of BSR had a characteristic refractory period of 1.0 msec. As was the case with the reward effect, the speeds increased again when the IPI was in the range 0.1 to 0.3 msec. Again, this can reasonably be interpreted as the effect of latent temporal addition in neurons on the periphery of the excited area around the electrode tip.

Our results from this extensive experiment on a single rat (it ran more than 3000 trials), agree in considerable detail with the results obtained by Deutsch (1964). In order to obtain a refractory period estimate for the drive effect (the "aftereffect"), Deutsch determined the rate of responding (numbers of responses in a 1-minute period) for paired-pulses stimulation at various IPI's. He assumed that the drive effect would be more important than the reward effect in sustaining a high rate of lever pressing. In order to determine the refractory period of the reward effect, Deutsch used repeated extinction to train rats to stop pressing as soon as they were no longer being rewarded. He then gave the rats a minute's intense priming, followed by short periods of paired-pulses stimulation at various IPI's. At each IPI, he determined the voltage necessary to sustain pressing during these periods, reasoning that the well primed rats would persist in responding only if the reward was adequate.

The resulting plots are shown in Fig. 7-17. The refractory period estimates from Deutsch's data agree very closely with the estimates from our data. His estimates for the refractory period of the drive neurons ranged from 0.8 to 1.0 msec. His estimates of the refractory period of the reinforcement neurons ranged from 0.5 to 0.7 msec, and the effect of latent temporal summation is evident in all but one of his plots.

The results from behavioral measurements of the refractory periods of the neuronal populations underlying the reward effect and aftereffect (or drive effect) of BSR indicate that these populations have different characteristic refractory periods. The refractory period of drive neurons is always greater than 0.8 msec; the refractory period of reinforcement neurons is always 0.7 msec or less. Since similar estimates of the refractory periods were obtained from experiments employing different behavioral measures and different values for the other parameters of stimulation, the refractory period estimates are unlikely to be artifactual. We therefore assume that self-stimulation behavior arises when

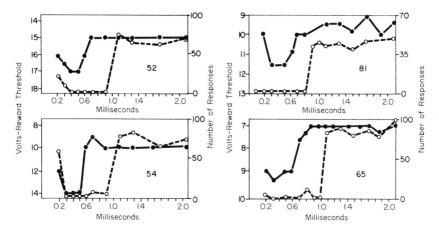

Fig. 7-17. The refractory period curves for the reward effect (solid lines, right hand ordinates) and the drive effect (broken lines, left hand ordinates) in four different rats The measured behavior on which the curves are based was bar pressing in a Skinner box. The refractory period for the reward effect (0.5 to 0.7 msec), as indicated by the sharp rises in the solid lines, agrees with another estimate which Deutsch obtained by using choice behavior in a T maze. Redrawn from Deutsch (1964); reproduced by permission of the American Psychological Association.

an electrode excites two functionally distinct components of an underlying system. Excitation at one of these points underlies the reward effect of BSR; excitation at the other point underlies the drive effect of BSR. The problem now is to determine, on the one hand, the neurophysiology of these components, and, on the other hand, the natural or normal behavioral function of these components.

B. Neurophysiology of the Self-Stimulation System

1. Indirect Evidence

a. Inferences from Refractory Period Data. One advantage of determining the characteristic refractory periods of the neuronal populations mediating self-stimulation effects is that variations in refractory period correlate with variations in other parameters of the neuron. Approximate values for these other parameters may therefore be inferred from the value for the refractory period.

Before proceeding to other inferences, it should be noted that the data just presented (Section IV, A) yield estimates of two neuronal parameters—the refractory period and the period of latent temporal addition. Are these mutually consistent, that is, is it reasonable to assume that neurons with refractory periods in the range 0.6 to 1.0 msec could show latent temporal addition at up to 0.3 msec? Grundfest (1940, p. 214) tabulated the variation in the other neuronal parameters as a function of variation in neuron size. The refractory period values we obtained—1.0 msec and 0.6 msec—are characteristic of, respectively, the smallest and next to the smallest mammalian A fibers. These fibers have diameters of 1–2 micra and 3–4 micra, respectively. The period of latent temporal addition in fibers of this type is 0.2 msec—exactly the range of IPI's within which one observes the speed-up attributed to latent temporal addition (Figs. 7-16 and 7-17). Thus, our estimates for the refractory periods and our estimates for the period of latent temporal addition are consistent with one another.

As emerged above, the values obtained for the refractory periods permit inferences as to the values for the diameters of the neurons involved in self-stimulation. These values (1–2 and 3–4 micra) permit another type of comparison: Stein has recently suggested, on the basis of pharmacological evidence, that at least part of the self-stimulation substrate utilizes a noradrenergic transmitter substance (Stein & Wise, 1969; see, however, Roll, 1970). Fuxe (1965, p. 47) has shown that the noradrenergic fibers ascending from the midbrain in the MFB have diameters of 1–4 micra. Thus, the three lines of evidence—anatomical, pharmacological, and behavioral-physiological—all converge. They are all consistent with the inference that the neuronal fibers mediating self-stimulation are the $1–4\mu$ noradrenergic fibers which ascend in the MFB from the midbrain.

b. Synaptic Properties. Indirect behavioral measures of the physiological characteristics of the self-stimulation system have also revealed something about the temporal parameters of synaptic processes. Coons and his co-workers have recently applied the paired-pulses technique to the study of the rate of decay of synaptic processes in the self-stimulation system (Smith & Coons, 1970; Ungerleider & Coons, 1970).

The use of the paired-pulses technique to study synaptic properties has an even more elaborate history than does the use of this same technique to study the refractory period (e.g., Eccles, 1965, Chapter 6; Haarevelt & Wiersma, 1936; Helmholtz, 1854; Lloyd, 1946; Lorente de Nó, 1939; Lucas, 1917; Richet, 1877). A brief review of this history will help clarify the work from Coons' laboratory.

Helmholtz' experiments in 1854 not only revealed the refractory period of neurons and latent temporal addition in neurons, they also revealed the process of temporal summation at synapses. Figure 7-15C (Section IV, A) shows an instance of such summation in Helmholtz' experiment. Two shocks were delivered to the nerve at an interval of 10 msec. Somehow, despite the fact that the shocks occurred at separate times, the effects of the two shocks were able to sum together to produce a single twitch. The magnitude of this twitch was greater than the magnitude of the twitch produced by either shock acting alone.

On first appearance, this temporal summation appears similar to the phenomenon already discussed under the heading of latent temporal addition. However, Adrian and Lucas (1912) showed that temporal summation could be distinguished from latent addition by the fact that its time course was longer by at least an order of magnitude. Furthermore, they showed that temporal summation occurred at the junction between the nerve and the muscle, that is, at a point remote from the electrodes that delivered the shocks; whereas, as already explained, latent addition occurs in the nerve immediately under the electrode.

The temporal summation of neural impulses is possible because the arrival of a neural impulse at a synapse triggers processes which rapidly rise to a maximum and then decay relatively slowly. The processes continue long after the electrical impulse that triggered them has vanished. Thus, if a second electrical impulse arrives shortly after the first, the processes it triggers add to the residual processes from the first pulse.

Electrical impulses arriving at synapses trigger at least two processes that rise rapidly and then decline slowly. One is the actual release of transmitter substance from the presynaptic tissue onto the postsynaptic tissue. The transmitter substance builds up very rapidly on the postsynaptic tissue and then is slowly destroyed by antitransmitter substance. Thus, the arrival of a second impulse can add new transmitter substance to the residual transmitter substance from the first impulse. The depolarization in the postsynaptic tissue is, of course, proportional to the amount of transmitter substance.

A second process which can show temporal summation is the mobilization of transmitter substance in the presynaptic tissue. The arrival of an electrical impulse not only triggers the release of transmitter substance onto the postsynaptic tissue, it also triggers processes which mobilize transmitter substance in the presynaptic neurons. This mobilization may be thought of as the moving up of transmitter substance into a position where it can be released. Again, the process of mobilization outlasts the electrical impulse which triggers it. Hence, if a second electrical impulse arrives while the mobilization triggered by the first persists, the second impulse will release more transmitter substance than was released by the first. In other words, some synaptic temporal summation actually occurs as a result of the summation of presynaptic mobilization processes.

The concept of temporal facilitation has been closely and somewhat confusingly tied to the concept of temporal summation throughout its history. Generally, the concept of temporal facilitation is invoked whenever the effects of two or more successive stimuli appear to sum nonlinearly. Figure 7-18A shows an instance of such an effect, as observed in the nerve-muscle preparation by Richet (1877). The first shock to the nerve elicits no twitch at all in the muscle, the second shock elicits a just perceptible twitch, the third shock elicits a large twitch, and so on. Clearly, the effect of the third shock has summed with some residual effects of the first and second shocks. However, the recorded effect of the first shock was zero and the recorded effect of the second shock was minimal. The recorded effect of the third shock is more than twice as large as the recorded effect of the second stimulus. And, of course, the recorded effect of the third shock is infinitely more than three times the apparently nonexistent effect of the first shock. Thus, it would appear that the only effect of the first shock was somehow to augment the size of the effect produced by succeeding shocks. This nonlinear summation was termed temporal facilitation by Sherrington. In most cases, it probably results from the linear summation of underlying, unrecorded processes which must pass some threshold in order to produce the effect being recorded, as was first suggested by Richet in 1877 (see Fig. 7-18B).

At present, the term facilitation is sometimes reserved for use only in cases where the summation occurs in presynaptic processes, following the suggestion of Dudel and Kuffler (1961). This presynaptic summation of mobilization processes produces nonlinear postsynaptic effects, that is, initial impulses augment the depolarizations produced by succeeding impulses.

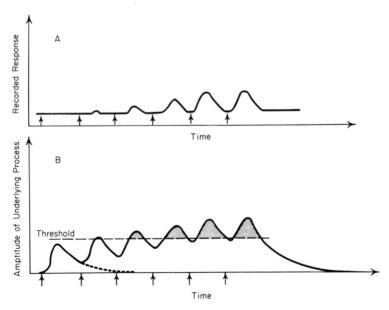

Fig. 7-18. A. A kymographic record showing temporal facilitation. The regularly repeating shocks to the nerve are indicated by the vertical arrows. B. A graphic presentation of a possible explanation. It is assumed that the processes set in motion by each shock to the nerve sum linearly. However, the sum must pass some threshold in order to produce the recorded effect. Modified from Richet, 1895, p. 150.

In order for the effects of two temporally disparate stimuli to sum together at a synapse it is not necessary for the stimuli to arrive at the synaptic area via the same neuronal pathway. When they do arrive by the same pathway, it is called homosynaptic summation. When the impulses arrive via different neurons, it is called heterosynaptic summation. The mechanism underlying heterosynaptic summation is very similar to one of the mechanisms underlying homosynaptic summation. When an initial impulse arrives at a synapse, it liberates transmitter substance onto the postsynaptic membrane, thereby producing a slowly decaying depolarization of the postsynaptic neuron. A second impulse arriving at a nearby synapse (i.e., another synapse on the same postsynaptic neuron) will give rise to a similar depolarization. This depolarization will sum with the residual depolarization from the first impulse.

The other mechanism of homosynaptic summation—facilitation, or, the summation of presynaptic mobilization processes—cannot occur in true heterosynaptic summation, because, by definition, the summating impulses arrive via different presynaptic pathways; hence, the second impulse cannot interact with the presynaptic processes set in motion by the first impulse.

Since temporal summation depends in all cases upon some residual process whose intensity decays with time, the magnitude of the sum of the effects of two stimuli must be smaller the longer the interval between stimuli. The later the second stimulus arrives, the smaller the residual effect from the first stimulus; hence, the smaller the sum of the effects of the two stimuli. Thus, by plotting the decline in the magnitude of the summated effect seen after the second stimulus, one can determine the time course of the decay of the effect of a single stimulus. When the summated effect—the effect recorded immediately after a second stimulus—no longer rises to a greater height than the height of the effect produced by a single stimulus, the residual effect of the first stimulus must have decayed completely.

In accord with the above rationale, neurophysiologists have repeatedly used paired pulses to study the time course of the decay of synaptic processes. In the course of this work a standard terminology has evolved. The first pulse in a pair is referred to as the conditioning pulse (or C pulse); the second is designated the test pulse (or T pulse). The interval between the pulses in a pair is the C-T interval. If, as is sometimes necessary, the pairs of pulses are presented in a train of pairs, the interval between pairs is the C-C interval.

It is necessary to use trains of pairs whenever one is dealing with an effect in which the sum of two pulses at even the shortest C-T intervals does not rise above threshold. In such cases, one must rely upon the summated effect of successive pairs to raise the effect above threshold so that the time course of further summation can be studied by varying the C-T interval (see Fig. 7-19). Fortunately, for exponentially decaying effects, the percentage decrease in peak amplitude produced by varying the C-T interval in a train of summating pairs is

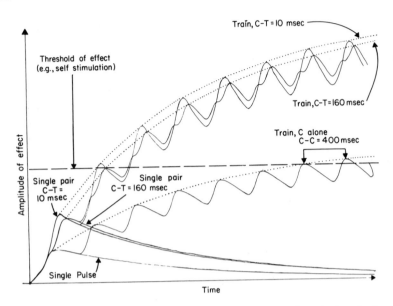

Fig. 7-19. Illustration of the use of a train of summating pulse pairs in order to study the effect of varying the within-pair interval (C-T interval). Notice that a single pair cannot be used, because, even at a minimal C-T interval (10 msec), the summated effect of two pulses is not above the threshold for a recordable effect (e.g., lever pressing in self-stimulation). To overcome this, one can use a train of pairs with the C-C interval and the train duration chosen such that the summation between C pulses (i.e., the summation when T pulses are omitted) is just sufficient to exceed the threshold. These graphs were generated by feeding pulses into an RC circuit and recording the voltage across the capacitor on an x-y plotter.

the same as the percentage decrease in peak amplitude produced by varying the C-T interval in a single pair (see Fig. 7-19).

Smith and Coons (1970) have used trains of pairs to study the time course of synaptic processes in the self-stimulation system. They set the C-C interval in their stimulation at 400 msec and the train duration at 5 seconds. They then varied the C-T interval in their stimulation. At each C-T interval they adjusted the amperage of their stimulation until it was just sufficient to induce the rat to self-stimulate. Thus, as the C-T interval increased, the synaptic summation between the effects of the C and T pulses decreased. This decreased temporal summation was compensated for by increasing the current so as to excite more neurons. Since at each change of the C-T interval the stimulation was changed so as to exactly cancel the effect of changing the C-T interval, a plot of amperage as a function of C-T interval should reveal the time course of the decay of the synaptic processes initiated by the C pulses.

The obtained plots are shown in Fig. 7-20. Notice that when the C-T interval was very short (< 1.2 msec) the T pulse had no effect. That is, the

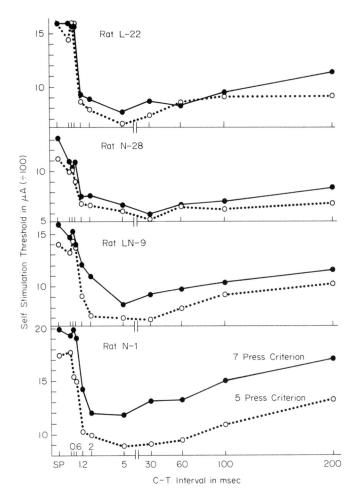

Fig. 7-20. Intensity of stimulating current required to reach the self-stimulation threshold—as a function of the C-T interval in a train of paired pulses. Reproduced from Smith & Coons, 1970; reproduced by permission of the American Association for the Advancement of Science.

threshold current for self-stimulation was just as high (1.5–2.0 mA) as when the T pulse was omitted altogether from each pair of pulses (SP on abscissa). At these short intervals the T pulse falls during the refractory period of the neurons, and fails to excite them. Since, under these circumstances, the T pulse has no effect, there is nothing to summate with the effect of the C pulse. This part of the curves is simply a replication of the refractory period findings of Deutsch (1964) and Gallistel *et al.* (1969).

At a C-T interval of 5 msec, the summation between the effects of the C and T pulses is at a maximum, as indicated by the fact that a minimal current (0.6–1.0 mA) was required to reach the self-stimulation threshold.[7] As the C-T interval increases, the current required to reach the self-stimulation threshold also increases, indicating a gradually decreasing summation. It is clear that the synaptic events in the self-stimulation system decay with a long time constant. Indeed, simply from the fact that the summated effect of a 5-second train of C pulses was greater than the maximal summated effect of a single pair of pulses, one can conclude that the time constant of decay was at least three times as long as the C-C interval (i.e., at least 3×0.4 second = 1.2 seconds).

In the experiment of Smith and Coons the C and T pulses were both delivered via the same electrode. Therefore, both pulses in each pair must have excited the same population of neurons. Thus, the experiment traced the time course of homosynaptic temporal summation. A subsequent experiment by Ungerleider and Coons (1970) traced the time course of heterosynaptic summation. Ungerleider and Coons implanted a pair of self-stimulation electrodes bilaterally in the MFB and delivered the C pulses via one electrode, the T pulses via the other.

The Ungerleider and Coons results were interesting in three regards. First, there was summation of the effects of stimulus pulses delivered to the medial forebrain bundles on opposite sides of the hypothalamus. This tells us something further about the structure of the self-stimulation circuits, viz., that the neural substrates of self-stimulation in each MFB converge and pool their excitation.

Second, from 5 msec onward, the time course of the decay in heterosynaptic summation was identical to the time course of decay in homosynaptic summation. Since this presumably heterosynaptic summation is not likely to be a presynaptic phenomenon, the similarity in the time courses of homosynaptic and heterosynaptic summation suggests that the later stages of homosynaptic summation reflect synaptic summation rather than presynaptic summation (i.e., facilitation).

Third, the decrease in homosynaptic summation at very short C-T intervals (see Fig. 7-20) does not occur in heterosynaptic summation. This strengthens the previous conclusion that the decrease in homosynaptic summation at short C-T intervals was the result of the neural refractory period and other presynaptic processes.

The experiments in the Coons laboratory have not as yet attempted to distinguish between the reinforcement component and the drive-like component in the self-stimulation system. That is, one doesn't know in which component

---

[7] The failure of summation to be maximal immediately after the end of the refractory period may be the result of relative refractoriness or it may reflect the type of presynaptic summation demonstrated by Lucas (1917).

the summation mapped by their experiments occurred. However, the extremely long time constant of decay, which their experiments reveal, makes it likely that their experiments measured summation in the drive-like component. The decay-of-priming experiments by Deutsch *et al.* (1964) and Gallistel (1969a) showed that the time constant of decay in the drive component was several seconds or more (see Section II, D, 3 and 4). Interestingly, Ungerleider and Coons found that the time constant of decay for C-T intervals of less than 5 msec was significantly shorter than the time constant of decay for longer intervals. Perhaps, the results at C-T intervals shorter than 5 msec reflected summation in the reinforcement component as well, whereas the results at longer intervals reflected only summation in the drive-like component. If the time constant in the reinforcement component is substantially shorter than the time constant in the drive component, no summation would have occurred in the reinforcement component at the longer C-T intervals.

2. Direct Evidence

The experiments reported so far have used self-stimulation behavior under special conditions of stimulation to draw inferences about the physiology of the self-stimulation system. From these experiments it has been inferred that the neurons subserving the drive effect in self-stimulation have refractory periods of approximately 1.0 msec, whereas the neurons subserving the reinforcement effect have refractory periods of approximately 0.6 msec. It has also been inferred that the synaptic processes in at least one component of the self-stimulation system show a very slow rate of decay. Finally, it has been suggested that these slowly decaying synaptic processes are characteristic of the drive component of the system rather than the reinforcement component.

These inferences have motivated two types of electrophysiological research—research designed to obtain more direct evidence for the existence of neural systems that are excited by stimulation from self-stimulation electrodes and, in addition, possess the characteristics inferred by means of the paired-pulses behavioral technique.

The indirect evidence for the various physiological characteristics (refractory period, etc.) is useful in guiding attempts to directly record activity in the neural substrate of self-stimulation. Without the guidance of this indirect evidence one does not know what to look for in the recordings obtained directly from the CNS. The inferences drawn from the use of behavioral techniques guide the interpretation of and give significance to what would otherwise be an undigestible mass of data about electrophysiological events occurring during self-stimulation. The data obtained from direct recordings, on the other hand, help substantiate the inferred entities and processes and permit further probing of their underlying structure and mechanisms. Thus, the two types of evidence complement and reinforce one another.

The first confirmatory evidence obtained by direct recording was obtained by Deutsch (Deutsch & Deutsch, 1966), who used macroelectrodes to record the evoked response in the MFB. His preparations were rats with stimulating electrodes implanted in the posterior or lateral hypothalamus. After it had been confirmed that the stimulating electrodes would sustain self-stimulation, the rats were anaesthetized with nembutal and a recording electrode was inserted into the MFB approximately 5 mm anterior to the stimulating electrode. The MFB was stimulated with single pulses or pairs of pulses and the evoked responses recorded.

On the basis of the behavioral measurements of the neural refractory periods, it was expected that a single pulse from the self-stimulation electrode would set up a volley of neural impulses in each of two distinct populations of neurons. Since the neurons in one population (the reinforcement population) were assumed to have a larger diameter than the neurons in the other population (the drive population), it was expected that the impulses in the reinforcement population would travel faster (conduction velocity is approximately linearly proportional to fiber diameter) and reach the recording electrode first. Only later would the volley of impulses traveling in the slower conducting drive populations reach the recording electrode. Thus, electrical responses evoked at the recording electrode should show two peaks. Figure 7-21A shows the evoked responses as recorded in seven different rats. In each case, two peaks are clearly evident. The latencies of the two peaks indicate that the conduction velocities in the drive population were 2–3 meters per second and the conduction velocities in the reinforcement population were 5–15 meters per second. These values for the conduction velocities are in approximate agreement with the values for the refractory periods inferred from the behavioral work (cf., Grundfest, 1940, pp. 214–215).

In this same experiment, it was shown by direct recording that the refractory periods of the fibers that produced the second (i.e., longer latency) peak were in the range 0.8–1.1 msec. When the preparation was stimulated with a pair of pulses (Fig. 7-21B) with an intrapair interval of less than 0.85 msec, the second pulse failed to produce a second evoked response. That is, the pair of pulses produced only a single evoked response (P_1 in Fig. 7-21B), which was identical in size and shape to the response evoked by a single pulse, indicating that the second pulse in each pair was failing to excite the neurons. When the IPI increased to 0.85 msec, the second pulse elicited a just perceptible response (P_2 in Fig. 7-21B). When the IPI reached 1.1 msec, the response evoked by the second pulse was well defined. Evidently, the refractory periods of the fibers mediating the longer latency evoked response were greater than 0.8 msec. Thus, the data on evoked responses confirm the inferences drawn from behavioral data.

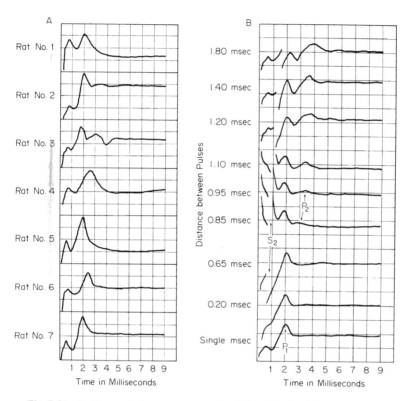

Fig. 7-21. A. The evoked responses produced by self-stimulation electrodes in the MFB. B. The evoked responses produced by a pair of pulses at varying intrapair intervals. The short latency evoked response—evident in the single pulse record—is obliterated by the artifact from the second stimulus pulse (indicated by S_2) in the middle records. Reproduced (with additions) by permission of the Dorsey Press from Deutsch and Deutsch (1966).

Whereas Deutsch used macroelectrodes to record the activity of whole populations of neurons, Gallistel *et al.* (1969) used microelectrodes to record the activity of single neurons during and after stimulation from self-stimulation electrodes.

Our preparations were rats with stimulating electrodes in the MFB. After it had been confirmed that the electrodes would sustain self-stimulation, the rats were anaesthetized with urethane. Paired microelectrodes were then lowered into their brains to enable us to record the responses of individual neurons to stimulation from the self-stimulation electrode.

Many neurons did not show any response following stimulation. The neurons that did show a response could be divided into two classes on the basis of the type of response shown. In the first type of response, there was a neuronal impulse at a short (0.2–2.0 msec) and unvarying interval after every stimulus pulse. This type of response led us to conclude that we were probably recording activity in a neuron whose anatomical path brought it close enough to our stimulating electrode to be directly excited ("fired") by our stimulus pulses. We termed neurons that showed this type of response *directly driven* neurons.

In the second type of response, there was not a neuronal impulse after every stimulus pulse; rather, at some comparatively long interval (5–100 msec) after the onset of a train of stimulus pulses, the ongoing rate of firing in the neuron we were recording from would suddenly increase (excitation) or decrease (inhibition). The increases or decreases outlasted the stimulation by as much as several seconds. This type of response led us to conclude that we were recording from a neuron that was not being directly fired by our stimulus pulses. Rather, we assumed that our stimulus pulses were exciting neurons which in turn relayed the effect of this stimulation "downstream" through an unknown number of synapses to the neuron we were recording from. The intervening synapses would be carrying out temporal summation of inputs, which would explain the absence of a 1–1 correspondence between stimulus pulses and recorded impulses. The intervening synapses could also have converted the excitatory effect of the electrical stimulation to an inhibitory effect on the neuron we were recording from. We termed the temporary increases (or decreases) in firing rate excitatory (or inhibitory) bursts and classified the neurons showing this type of response as *synaptically driven* neurons.

The results of behavioral measurements of neuronal refractory periods led us to stimulate with paired pulses and look for refractory period effects in the neurons excited by self-stimulation electrodes. It was hoped that neurons would fall into two groups exhibiting refractory period effects at different intrapair intervals.

We measured the refractory periods of the directly driven neurons by stimulating with paired pulses and reducing the IPI until the neuron ceased to produce a spike after the second stimulus in each pair. Figure 7-22 shows records from a directly driven neuron with a refractory period of 0.6 msec. When the interval within a pair of pulses was less than 0.6 msec, no spike followed the second pulse in each pair. When the interval was exactly 0.6 msec, a spike followed the second pulse on only one of the five superimposed sweeps of the oscilloscope trace. At intervals greater than 0.6 msec a spike always followed the second pulse.

The records in Fig. 7-22 reveal another characteristic phenomenon. Notice that when the IPI is 0.7 msec—just longer than the refractory period—the latency at which the spike follows the second stimulus is longer than usual. This indicates that the neuron was in a state of relative refractoriness. A period of relative refractoriness always follows the (absolute) refractory period. During the relative refractory period the neuron can be fired. However, a more intense

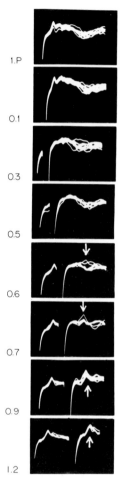

Fig. 7-22. Stimulating a directly driven neuron at various IPI's (given, in milliseconds, to the left of each frame). In the topmost frame there was only one stimulus pulse. In the second frame from the top there were two stimulus pulses, but since they were contiguous, only one stimulus artifact can be seen. In the lower frames an arrow indicates the action potential following the second stimulus. Each photograph shows at least five superimposed sweeps.

stimulus pulse is required. When the neuron does fire, the spike is of lower amplitude and is conducted more slowly. This is the effect one sees at an IPI of 0.7 msec.

We also looked for refractory period effects in the neurons we classified as synaptically driven. In the case of synaptically driven neurons it was not possible to measure the refractory periods of the neurons we were actually recording from because the neurons we were recording from were being driven via synapses whose temporal summation characteristics prevented our delivering precisely separated stimulus pulses. However, the magnitude of the bursts (i.e., increases or decreases in firing rate) evoked in synaptically driven neurons was, of course, a function of the number of firings which the stimulation produced in the "upstream," directly driven neurons. When we used trains of paired pulses and varied the IPI, the number of firings in the upstream, directly stimulated neurons was halved whenever the IPI was so short that the second pulse in each pair fell within the refractory period. This halving of the number of firings in the upstream neurons resulted in a diminished burst response in the synaptically driven neuron we were recording from. Thus, we could use the size of the evoked bursts of firing (or, in the case of inhibitory responses, nonfiring) to infer the refractory periods of the neurons whose stimulation produced the bursts. The rationale of this burst-size technique parallels the rationale of the behavioral technique for inferring refractory periods.

In order to measure burst-size, we estimated the average duration of the increase or decrease in firing rate. We then set a counter to count the number of spikes occurring during this interval after each stimulation. The poststimulation interval during which the counter counted spikes was called the count interval.

We adjusted the frequency and duration of the stimulating train to the range which maximized the change in burst size produced by halving the number of stimulus pulses. Then we stimulated with paired pulses and plotted burst size (i.e., the number of spikes in the count interval) as a function of the IPI.

Figure 7-23A shows three plots in which the burst size increases when the IPI exceeds 1.0 msec. Figures 7-23B and 7-23C together show three plots in which the burst size changed (increased or decreased) when the IPI exceeded 0.6 msec. From these plots we inferred that the neurons represented in Fig. 7-23A were being driven by way of directly excited neurons that had refractory periods of 1.0 msec. And we inferred that the neurons represented in Figs. 7-23B and C were being driven by way of directly excited neurons that had refractory periods of 0.6 msec.

The use of the burst-size technique to infer neuronal refractory periods substantially enhances the value of refractory period measurements for suggesting the behavioral function of single neurons. If a directly driven neuron has a refractory period of 1.0 msec, this suggests that this neuron is likely to subserve drive-like effects in self-stimulation rather than reinforcement effects. Similarly, if a synaptically driven neuron is being driven by a population of neurons with refractory periods of 1.0 msec, then it is likely to be a part of the drive component rather than the reinforcement component of the self-stimulation system. Thus, one can infer the possible behavioral functions of neurons that are only indirectly activated by self-stimulation electrodes. That is, one can trace a component of the self-stimulation system beyond its directly stimulated elements.

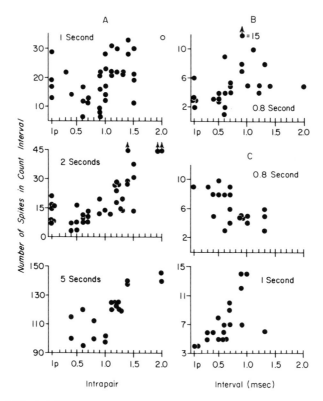

Fig. 7-23. A. Three plots of burst size as a function of the intrapair interval in the stimulation. The interval indicated on each plot (e.g., 1 second on the uppermost plot) is the duration of the count-interval. The lp (1 pulse) "interval" on the abscissas was the condition in which the second pulse in each pair was omitted. B. The burst-size plot from an indirectly driven neuron in the immediate vicinity of the directly driven neuron of Fig. 7-22. The increase in burst size at IPI's greater than 0.6 msec was verified by χ^2 tests. C. Two more burst size plots showing refractory period effects in the 0.6–0.7 msec range. The upper plot was made on a unit showing inhibitory "bursts" in response to the stimulation. The burst size decreased when the intrapair interval exceeded the refractory period of the "upstream" neurons.

In view of the potential value of the burst-size technique, we looked for evidence which would help establish the validity of the inferences based on this technique. The burst-size plot in Fig. 7-23B is from a synaptically driven neuron that was in the immediate vicinity of the directly driven neuron of Fig. 7-22. The value for the refractory period of the presynaptic neurons, as inferred from the increase in burst size, was 0.6 msec. This is the same value obtained by direct means from the nearby neuron (Fig. 7-22). The proximity of the neurons represented in Figs. 7-22 and 7-23B makes it likely that the directly driven neuron of Fig. 7-22 was one of the population of presynaptic neurons driving the neuron of Fig. 7-23B. Thus, the data in Fig. 7-22 may constitute verification of the inferences drawn from the burst-size data. This verification helps confirm the validity of using burst size to infer the refractory period of the directly driven neurons in the presynaptic chain of neurons. As explained in the introductory discussion of the paired-pulse technique, the refractory periods inferred from changes in the intensity of downstream effects (e.g., muscle twitches and bursts) probably reflect the refractory periods of the directly stimulated neurons and not the refractory periods of intervening neurons, nor the refractory period of the element being recorded from.

The purpose of getting refractory period estimates while recording with microelectrodes was to see if we could find two groups of neurons yielding refractory periods corresponding to the refractory periods inferred from behavioral measurements. We soon discovered that units picked up on lateral penetrations into the thalamus yielded refractory period values of 0.6–0.7 msec, whereas units picked up on more medial penetrations yielded refractory periods of 1.0 msec or longer. In many synaptically driven units, the variability in spontaneous firing rate was too great to permit refractory period estimations. The refractory period values obtained from the fifteen synaptically driven units we were able to analyze and the values from four directly driven neurons are presented as a frequency of occurrence histogram in Fig. 7-24. In order to facilitate comparison with the behavioral measurements of refractory periods, the running speed plots from Fig. 7-16 are superimposed on this histogram. Although, there was some tendency for the electrophysiologically determined refractory periods to be longer than the behaviorally estimated refractory periods,[8] it was clear that the self-stimulation electrode was firing at least two populations of neurons with distinctly different characteristic refractory periods, and these characteristic refractory periods were approximately the same as the behaviorally inferred refractory periods.

In our initial report (Gallistel et al., 1969) we suggested that the two brain stem units (see histogram, Fig. 7-24) were not related to self-stimulation behavior. However, subsequent work by Rolls (1971) suggests that such brain stem units may help mediate drive effects.

The anatomical loci of the units from which the data in Fig. 7-24 derive is of interest on two counts. First, as illustrated in Figs. 7-24 and 7-25, the units

---

[8] Subsequent work by Rolls (1971) indicates that this was an artifact of the relative refractory period, that is, these estimates would have been shortened had we increased the intensity of our stimulus pulses. This, however, leads one to ask why the effect of the relative refractory period did not appear in our behavioral measurements. One likely explanation is that at the longer C-T intervals, where the T pulses fires more neurons because refractoriness has declined, the increase in the number of fired neurons is offset by a decrease in the amount of synaptic summation between the volley produced by the C pulse and the volley produced by the T pulse.

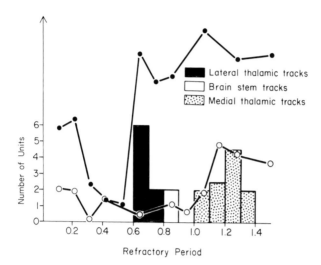

Fig. 7-24. Histogram showing the number of units yielding each refractory period value. To facilitate comparison, reward and priming curves from Fig. 7-16 are superimposed on the histogram.

yielding the shorter refractory period estimates were found more laterally (3.2–3.7 mm), whereas the units yielding longer refractory period estimates were found more medially (1.3–2.0 mm). The ultimate goal of measuring refractory periods is to help establish behavioral function. The fact that units yielding different refractory period values were anatomically segregated suggests that differences in refractory period do correlate with differences in function and are not a fortuitously varying characteristic. The difference in function is suggested by the fact that neurons having different refractory periods apparently project their excitatory and inhibitory effects to different areas of the thalamus.

Second, the photomicrograph in Fig. 7-25A shows the lesion marking the site from which the data in Figs. 7-22 and 7-23B were obtained. The microelectrode was in an area where fibers give way to cells. Thus, the anatomical locus of the electrode tip was consistent with our suggestion that the data in Figs. 7-22 and 7-23B represent pre- and postsynaptic recordings, respectively.

If differences in refractory period effects do indicate differences in behavioral function, then one should expect to find that units in different refractory period classes differ in their response to stimulation. To test this expectation we studied the response to repeated trains of stimulation. On the basis of our behavioral studies of the priming effect in self-stimulation (Section II, D, 4) and the growth of reinforcement magnitude (Section II, D, 3), we expected that the response of synaptically driven neurons yielding priming effect refractory periods (1.0 msec) would show summation during repeated trains of stimulation,

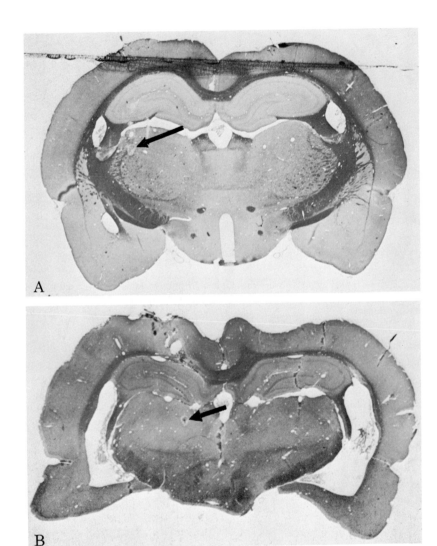

Fig. 7-25. Photomicrograph showing the lesion that marks the tip of the recording electrode from which the data in Fig. 7-22 and 7-23B were obtained. All of the units yielding refractory period values in the 0.6–0.7 msec range were in this dorsolateral area of the thalamus (or, perhaps, in a few cases, in the ventral portion of the dorsolateral hippocampus). B. Photomicrograph showing the lesion that marks the tip of the recording electrode from which the data in the uppermost plot of Fig. 7-23A were obtained. All of the units yielding refractory period values in the 1.0–1.4 msec range were in this area of the thalamus (or, perhaps, in a few cases, in the ventral part of the dorsomedial hippocampus).

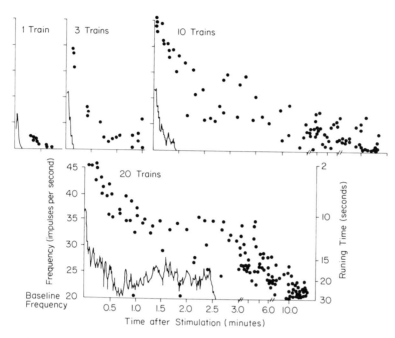

Fig. 7-26. Summation in the response of a synaptically driven unit classified, on the basis of the refractory period effect, as belonging to the priming or "drive" class. The jagged lines are the poststimulation firing frequency, as indicated by an RC averaging circuit with a time constant of less than ½ second. To facilitate comparison with behavioral data, the point plots of postpriming running speed from Fig. 7-12 are superimposed.

whereas the response of synaptically driven neurons yielding reinforcement effect refractory periods (0.6 msec) should not show much summation.

As illustrated in Fig. 7-26, units yielding refractory periods in the range 1.0–1.4 msec did indeed show a summated response to repeated trains of stimulation. Increasing the number of trains (0.3 second long) increased both the peak firing frequency in the resulting burst and the duration of the burst, that is, the time required for firing frequency to subside to the prestimulation baseline. In Fig. 7-26, in order to show the qualitative similarity between these data and the behavioral data, the point plots of running speed from Fig. 7-12 are superimposed on the same time axis as the graph of spike frequency.

The response of units yielding refractory periods in the range 0.6–0.7 msec was variable, but it never resembled the responses of the "priming effect neurons" which were always similar to the example in Fig. 7-26. Generally, the units in the "reinforcement class" showed little or no summation. That is, the burst of firing after 20 trains was no more intense and lasted no longer than the burst produced by a single train. In one case, repeated stimulating trains elicited large increases in firing rate that persisted for 12–15 minutes without decline.

The fact that neurons yielding different values for the refractory period responded differently to repeated trains of stimulation further encourages the assumption that the refractory period measurements isolated two populations of neurons having distinct functions. However, we are far from being able to conclude with assurance that the neurons identified electrophysiologically correspond to the neurons identified behaviorally. We believe that we have, nonetheless, taken a step in that direction.

Furthermore, the electrophysiological data have helped substantiate and extend our previous conclusions about the physiology of the self-stimulation substrate. Behavioral evidence indicates that the self-stimulation substrate consists of neurons whose refractory periods are in the ranges 0.5–0.6 msec and 0.8–1.1 msec (Deutsch, 1964; Gallistel et al., 1969). Microelectrode recording confirms that neurons with these refractory periods are in fact excited by self-stimulation electrodes. From the refractory period values it is inferred that the diameters of these neurons are in the ranges 1–2 and 2–4 μ. Macroelectrode recording reveals a bimodal evoked response in the MFB at latencies consistent with the inferred values for the diameters of the neurons (Deutsch & Deutsch, 1966). Anatomical evidence confirms the presence in the MFB of neurons with diameters ranging 1-4 micra and shows that at least some of these neurons are adrenergic (Fuxe, 1965). Pharmacological evidence implicates noradrenergic transmitter in self-stimulation (Stein & Wise, 1969). Behavioral evidence suggests that the synaptic processes in the drive component have a long time constant of decay and can therefore show temporal summation over considerable intervals (Gallistel, 1969a; Smith & Coons, 1970). Microelectrode recordings show that synaptically driven units yielding refractory periods characteristic of the drive component show a summated response to repeated trains of stimulation. The summated response decays slowly.

C. One System, Or Several?

The preceding experiments established that the system excited by a self-stimulation electrode has two components, each component mediated by a different neuronal population. One component manifests itself in the ability of BSR to act as a reinforcement. The other component manifests itself in the drive-like aftereffect of BSR. This aftereffect produces not only more rapid performance but also a momentarily heightened tendency to choose BSR in preference to other rewards (Deutsch et al., 1964) and other activities (Ball & Adams, 1965). That is, the aftereffect does not potentiate behavior indiscriminately, but rather selectively potentiates some behavior patterns. As such, the aftereffect behaves like a drive. This leads one to ask whether all self-stimulation electrodes are exciting the same drive-reinforcement system or whether some electrodes are exciting one system, while other electrodes excite others.

Deutsch and Howarth (1962) blocked rats' access to a lever after the rats had learned to press the lever for BSR. When the block was removed, the rats did not return to the lever—another instance of drive-decay. However, when the rats were frightened with a loud buzzer or footshock, those with rostro-ventral tegmental electrodes returned immediately to the lever and pressed it; those with placements elsewhere in the MFB did not. Deutsch and Howarth suggested that this demonstrated that tegmental electrodes excited a drive-reward system concerned with fear (drive) and escape from danger (reward). The induction of fear by noise or footshock reactivated the drive that had dissipated while the rats were blocked from the lever, thereby reactivating the behavior. The failure of fear to reactivate responding in rats with more anterior placements suggested to Deutsch and Howarth that the anterior placements excited other drive-reward systems, systems not concerned with fear and escape.

Several other theorists, who do not share Deutsch's conviction as to the importance of the drive component in self-stimulation, have also suggested that electrodes at different sites stimulate different reward systems. Olds (1958d) found that hunger increased the rate of self-stimulation, provided that the electrodes were located about 1.25 mm or more lateral to the midline, whereas hunger either had no effect or slightly decreased self-stimulation rates when electrodes were located more medially (about 0.75 mm lateral to the midline). Manipulation of the testosterone level had reverse effects. High levels of testosterone potentiated responding on the more medial placements and did not affect, or slightly inhibited, responding on the more lateral placements. Olds (1960) was naturally led to suggest that the reward produced by medial (hypothalamic and septal) placements was sexual in nature, whereas the reward produced by more lateral stimulation was akin to food.

Hoebel (1968) and his coworkers (Balagura, 1968; Balagura & Hoebel, 1967; Hoebel, 1965; Mount & Hoebel, 1967) have carried out an extensive investigation of the relation between lateral hypothalamic self-stimulation and hunger. They have shown that nearly all of the manipulations (lesions, stomach loads, insulin and glucagon injections, deprivation) which increase or decrease eating have parallel effects on lateral hypothalamic self-stimulation. These manipulations usually do not affect the rate of self-stimulation when the electrode is in the subcommissural septum (Hoebel, 1968). Hoebel has concluded that lateral hypothalamic BSR is more intimately related to food reward than is septal BSR.

These data are consonant with another assumption of the Deutsch model, viz., that the hypothalamus contains several homeostats, each homeostat having its own drive and reinforcement components. Each two-component system is assumed to be localized in a different area of the baso-lateral diencephalon (Deutsch & Howarth, 1963). Figure 7-27 depicts the Deutsch (1963) interpretation of the Olds (1958d) data and related data. If the hungry rat self-stimulates on the lateral electrode (bottom electrode in Fig. 7-27), then its lever pressing

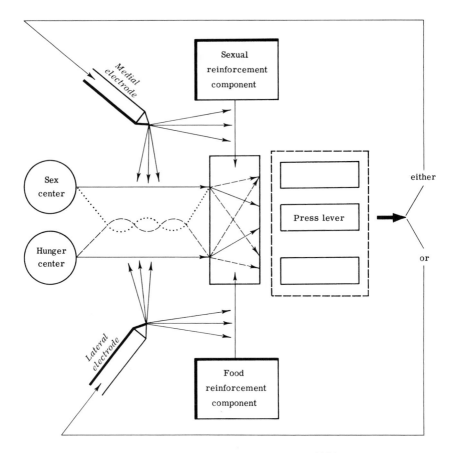

Fig. 7-27. Schematization of Deutsch's interpretation of Olds' data on the effects of hunger and sex hormone on rats self-stimulating at different electrode sites. The upper electrode stimulates the drive and reinforcement signals for the sex center, while the lower electrode stimulates drive and reinforcement signals for the hunger center. The entwining broken and dotted lines indicate an anatomical alternative.

will be potentiated by the naturally arising hunger as well as by the electrically excited hunger. If, however, the hungry rat self-stimulates on the medial electrode (upper electrode in Fig. 7-27), then the artificial, sexual reinforcement will be inappropriate to the rat's naturally arising hunger.[9] The hunger drive will not add to the sex drive signal artificially excited by the medial electrode. In fact,

---

[9] Extinction is implicitly assumed, that is, it is assumed that the failure of lever pressing to excite the food reinforcement component will produce an alteration in the drive transfer parameters such that hunger potentiation is no longer transferred to the lever pressing behavior pattern.

insofar as the hunger drive potentiates competing behaviors, it will hamper the behavior potentiated by the sex drive signals, that is, self-stimulation. The same considerations apply, *mutatis mutandis*, when the rat's sexual drive is strong and its hunger drive weak.

Many other data lend themselves to interpretation in a similar fashion. Wilkinson and Peele (1962) found effects in the cat similar to those reported by Hoebel for the rat. Hunger increased, and satiety decreased self-stimulation, when electrodes were located midway along the rostro-caudal extent of the lateral hypothalamus. Hunger and satiety did not have such effects when electrodes were located more caudally or more rostrally. Other experiments have shown that hunger or thirst can increase rates of self-stimulation (Brady, Boren, Conrad, & Sidman, 1957), or increase a rat's tolerance for poor partial reinforcement schedules (Elder *et al.*, 1965), or increase the number of responses emitted in extinction (Deutsch & DiCara, 1967). All of these data can be explained by assuming that natural drives supplement or substitute for the rapidly decaying drive signals produced during self-stimulation.

Brady and Conrad (1960) reported that, with some placements, fear did not produce any conditioned suppression in some rats. These same rats had demonstrated such suppression while responding for a water reward. One can apply to these data the interpretation which Deutsch and Howarth (1962) applied to their data. If some of Brady and Conrad's electrodes tapped the fear-escape system, then more fear would potentiate more responding. There was, however, a very poor correspondence between the location of Deutsch and Howarth's electrodes and the location of Brady and Conrad's electrodes. Many of the latter electrodes were in the more rostral areas that Deutsch and Howarth suggested were not related to fear.

Falk (1961) showed that rats with septal placements would, when the current was high, continue self-stimulation to the exclusion of drinking until the rats were nearly dead of thirst. Somewhat similar findings have been reported by Valenstein and Beer (1962), Endroczi and Lissak (1966, in cats), Routtenberg and Lindy (1965), and Spies (1965). The last two studies are particularly interesting from the standpoint of the Deutsch model since they again showed that the effect of a given drive (hunger) depended on the electrode locus. Spies found that rats with lateral hypothalamic placements continued to prefer BSR over food in a T maze, even when the rats had been severely food deprived. Rats with placements outside the MFB switched their preference from BSR to food as deprivation increased. Similarly, Routtenberg and Lindy found that rats with placements in the MFB took BSR, to the exclusion of food, until they starved to death. Rats with placements in the septum or in the hypothalamus outside the MFB did not ignore food in this fashion and did not starve. One might conclude that electrodes in the LH-MFB area excited the reinforcement component of the nutrient homeostat more effectively than food itself. Thus, the potentiation from hunger was channeled toward the artificially rewarded behavior rather than toward behavior rewarded with food. In order to explain the effect of varying electrode locus, one can assume that electrodes outside the LH-MFB area tapped different homeostatic systems.

A final line of evidence consistent with the multiple-homeostat assumption comes from the numerous studies showing different stimulation-bound consummatory effects produced by prolonged stimulation from self-stimulation electrodes in different loci. Hoebel and Teitelbaum (1962) showed that self-stimulation electrodes in the lateral hypothalamic area would sometimes elicit eating that started and stopped with the stimulation (see also, Coons & Cruce, 1968; Margules & Olds, 1962). Self-stimulation electrodes in this same area can also elicit stimulation-bound drinking (Mendelson, 1967; Mogenson & Stevenson, 1966). Self-stimulation electrodes in the posterior hypothalamus can elicit copulation (Caggiula & Hoebel, 1966) and seminal ejaculation (Herberg, 1963). Caggiula and Hoebel suggested that the posterior hypothalamus relates to sexual motivation, while more rostral areas relate to food or water motivation. However, the specificity and anatomical differentiation of the stimulation bound consummatory effects have recently come into doubt (Valenstein, Cox, & Kakolewski, 1970, see below for fuller discussion).

With the multiple-homeostat model and the supporting evidence in mind we undertook to test some further implications. If one studies Fig. 7-27, labelling one electrode A and the other electrode B, it can be seen that if a rat is run in an alley with priming administered on electrode A and reward received on electrode B, then performance should not be as fast as when both stimulations come from the same electrode. If the rat is primed on one electrode and rewarded on the other, then the induced drive will be inappropriate to the reinforcement, whereas if a single electrode is used for both priming and reinforcement, then the induced drive will be appropriate to the reinforcement. Thus, the permutations AA (primed on A, rewarded on A) and BB should produce better performance than the permutations AB and BA.

We ran the experiment just outlined (Gallistel, 1969b) and obtained the results presented in Table 7-1. In conditions OA and OB there was no priming. Thus, these results again demonstrate the large effect priming has on runway performance, even in thoroughly trained rats. However, in other respects, the results ran contrary to expectations. In comparing the permutations AA and BB to the permutations AB and BA one finds that in no case did both AA and BB produce significantly better performance than BA and AB. Indeed, in five instances, priming on the other electrode was significantly more effective than priming on the electrode being used for reward.

These data were consistent with the assumption that, in all cases, both electrodes were exciting a single two-component system. This can be seen by rank ordering the means, AA, BB, AB, and BA, for each pair of electrodes. In

TABLE 7-1
Runway Speed under Permutations of Priming and Reward Electrodes

Subject	Electrode locus	Condition[a]					
		OA	AA	BA	OB	BB	AB
No. 35	A-DBB B-LH	78.6	80.3	96.0*†	35.8	97.5	84.0*
	A-LH B-VT	35.8	93.6	87.1*	55.8	85.3	82.5*
	A-DBB B-VT	85.2	85.1	103.4*†	62.8	90.2	80.6*
No. 40	A-DBB B-PH	37.0	87.0	89.2*	39.6	90.4	93.2*
No. 45	A-LH B-PH	23.2	43.5	98.8*†	73.4	104.0	87.9*
No. 48	A-LH B-DBB	24.8	56.9	83.6*†	10.0	75.7	43.6*
No. 54	A-PH B-DBB	42.6	109.6	97.6*	0.0	86.2	101.3*†
No. 55	A-PH B-DBB	13.8	96.2	94.4*	8.6	96.9	89.3*

[a]Performance after priming with the electrode not used for reward is compared to unprimed performance and to performance after priming with the reward electrode: *faster than unprimed performance ($p < .01$); †faster than performance primed with reward electrode ($p < .01$). Results are given in speed scores: $S = 145\,e^{-6.5/t}$, where t = running time Abbreviations: DBB, diagonal band of Broca; LH, lateral hypothalamus; PH, posterior hypothalamus; VT, ventral tegmental area of Tsai.

five of the eight pairs, this rank ordering is immediately comprehensible in terms of the assumption that only one two-component system is involved. For example, rank ordering these four conditions for Number 48, one gets AB > BB > AA > BA. From the fact that AA > BA, one concludes that the drive effect of A is better than the drive effect of B. From the further fact that BB > AA, one concludes that the reward effect of B must be greater than the reward effect of A. From these two conclusions it must follow that AB is the best combination of all, which proves to be the case. In three of the eight pairs, rank ordering the conditions does not yield a pattern that is comprehensible in this fashion.

However, in all three cases, interchanging the ranks of two means that are not significantly different yields a comprehensible ordering.

The loci of the placements in this study were such that one or more pairs straddled every suggested functional partition of the ventrolateral diencephalon.

Although these data were not consistent with our expectations concerning multiple systems, they did provide more evidence that the system (or systems) underlying self-stimulation has two independent components. There was no pronounced correlation between the efficacy of any given electrode when the electrode was being used to reward the completion of a run and the efficacy of that electrode when it was being used to prime the rat before a run. There were two pairs (No. 35 DBB-VT and No. 48) in which one of the mixed permutations, AB or BA, was significantly ($p < .01$) better than any other permutation, indicating that one electrode was best for priming and the other best for reward. If the priming effect (i.e., aftereffect) of BSR were a secondary consequence of its rewarding effect, then the two effects ought to be closely correlated. If an electrode were best for reward, then it ought also to be best for priming.

As a check on the conclusions drawn from running speed, we conducted T-maze experiments that looked for selective priming effects in the rats' choice behavior (Gallistel, 1969b).

We trained four rats from the preceding experiment in a T maze. One electrode always rewarded the choice of one arm, the other electrode the choice of the other arm. During the initial 50-trial training period there was a 15-minute intertrial interval to insure that the rats' choices were only minimally influenced by the aftereffect of preceding BSR. After training, the rats were given a series of trials with each trial preceded by priming on one or the other electrode. We found that this priming, although it produced a very marked increase in the rapidity of performance, did not differentially affect the rats' choices. Priming a rat with electrode A just before a choice trial did not induce it to choose the arm rewarded by electrode A.

Unfortunately, with this training procedure, the rats showed pronounced side preferences, that is, there appeared to be an unexplained bias toward one side or the other. This bias may have prevented rats' alternating their choices in accordance with the priming.

Using five new rats, we ran another T-maze experiment in which the rats were consistently primed with only one electrode during the training phase. During the training phase, the magnitude of the BSR that a rat received in each arm was adjusted until the rat was choosing both arms (i.e., both electrodes) equally often. Then priming was switched to the other electrode. Again, the shift in the locus of priming did not influence the rats' choice of rewarding electrode. And, again, the loci of electrodes were such that at least one pair straddled every suggested functional partition of the ventrolateral diencephalon.

In this experiment we also tested some rats for stimulation-bound motivation effects. In one rat we found that stimulation on the lateral hypothalamic electrode initially yielded only drinking, whereas stimulation on the posterior hypothalamic electrode elicited only copulation. However, as testing progressed, stimulation on the lateral hypothalamic electrode began to elicit copulation. When we followed up the suggestions of Valenstein, Cox, and Kakolewski (1968) by removing the female from the environment and stimulating on the posterior hypothalamic electrode, we began to see some eating and drinking in response to stimulation on the copulation electrode. Another rat in this study showed eating and drinking in response to stimulation on the more caudal electrode and no stimulation-bound consummatory effect in response to stimulation on the more rostral electrode. Thus, in two cases, the electrodes A and B were not only in different areas, they produced somewhat different stimulation-bound motivation effects. Valenstein's work suggests that it would be difficult to find a pair of electrodes showing more clearcut differentiation of stimulation-bound motivation effects.

The results from the T-maze experiments confirmed our conclusions from the runway experiments. Priming on an electrode did not selectively potentiate responses rewarded by that electrode over responses rewarded by another electrode, even when the two electrodes were at different loci and produced somewhat different stimulation-bound consummatory effects.

These findings have led us to take another look at the evidence for the assumption that electrodes at different loci tap different systems.

Some of the evidence that most impressed us was the finding by Spies (1965) and Routtenberg and Lindy (1965) that rats with electrodes in the medial forebrain bundle at the rostrocaudal midway point in the lateral hypothalamus preferred BSR to food no matter how hungry they became, whereas rats with placements elsewhere switched their preference to food as they became hungrier. We took this as evidence that the former electrodes mimicked food reward, whereas the latter did not. However, in retrospect we are struck by Routtenberg and Lindy's emphasis that the closer an electrode was to the MFB, the more likely a rat was to ignore food in preference for BSR. The same statement can be made about the Spies data. The MFB is known to be the primary locus of self-stimulation and the area that produces the highest rates of responding. It may be that electrodes in this area produced a food-like reward that was more potent than Noyes pellets; whereas placements elsewhere also produced a food-like reward, but one that was less potent than Noyes pellets.

However, one need not assume that any of the electrodes produced a reward similar to food. In the Routtenberg and Lindy experiment, the rats were lever pressing on a continuous reinforcement schedule. Each new response came immediately after the BSR produced by the preceding response. Similarly, the

Spies T-maze experiment used massed trials; therefore each choice was made shortly after the BSR received on the preceding trial. As we have pointed out, BSR has a drive-like aftereffect. This effect potentiates further responding, and it does so selectively. Deutsch *et al.* (1964) showed that the decaying aftereffect of BSR could selectively potentiate BSR directed responses, whereas water deprivation selectively potentiated water-directed responses. If MFB electrodes have a more intense aftereffect than electrodes outside the MFB, then this aftereffect could have produced the preference for BSR seen by Routtenberg and Lindy and Spies, even if the reward produced by the brain stimulation were not food-like in character. In other words, the drive for BSR may have over-ridden the drive for food instead of summating with it.

The evidence for separate systems that derives from specific stimulation-bound consummatory effects occurring in association with self-stimulation is also open to question. Extensive experiments by Valenstein *et al.* (1970) have shown that there is no clear anatomical division of sites yielding stimulation-bound eating, drinking, and gnawing. They have repeatedly obtained all three effects from electrode sites ranging along the MFB from the anterior hypothalamus to the ventral tegmental area of Tsai. It should be recalled that we also obtained sexual behavior from the lateral hypothalamic "eating" area and eating and drinking (albeit weakly) from the posterior hypothalamic "sex" area. Valenstein *et al.* (1970) have further suggested that the stimulation-bound consummatory effect produced at any one locus can be redirected by depriving a rat of the originally preferred goal-object while stimulation continues, and by other manipulations. They argue that artificially elicited motivation in these areas has no goal-specificity. Although this contention has yet to be established beyond dispute (Wise, 1968), it is clear from their work that there is little segregation by function at the level of gross anatomy—contrary to what had previously been thought.

There remains the evidence from the Deutsch and Howarth (1962), the Olds (1958d), and the Hoebel (1968) studies. The Olds study showed that hunger affected rate of responding with some placements but not others, whereas testosterone affected rate of responding with the latter placements and not with the former. The Hoebel study showed hunger and satiety having large effects on the rate of lateral hypothalamic self-stimulation while leaving the rate of septal self-stimulation unaffected. The Deutsch and Howarth study showed fear-eliciting BSR directed behavior when rats had ventral tegmental electrodes, but not when the rats had electrodes elsewhere. These three studies all suggest that different electrodes produce rewards that relate to different natural drive states. We have not been able to find a ready alternative explanation for these data.

There is one hypothesis that could reconcile these data with the results of our own double electrode studies. The previous hypothesis assumed that both the drive and reinforcement components of a given homeostatic system were anatomically segregated from similar components in other systems. It was assumed, for example, that it was possible to stimulate the drive and reinforcement components of the hunger system without stimulating either the drive or the reinforcement component of the sexual system (see Fig. 7-27). The revised hypothesis assumes that the drive pathways from the various homeostats are thoroughly intertwined and run together throughout the ventrolateral diencephalic self-stimulation system. This minimal modification is indicated by the intertwining broken and dotted lines in Fig. 7-27. This intertwining makes it impossible to stimulate the drive component of one system without also stimulating the drive components of the other systems. The reinforcement pathways, on the other hand, are assumed to be less intertwined. Thus, electrodes in the ventral tegmental area of Tsai could excite the reinforcement component of only the fear-escape system, but the drive component of every system; electrodes in the lateral hypothalamic area could excite the reinforcement component of only the food homeostat, but the drive component of every system; and so on. From this it follows that naturally induced hunger will only potentiate responses reinforced by lateral hypothalamic electrodes. On the other hand, priming on any electrode will activate the drive component of the hunger homeostat and thereby potentiate responses reinforced by a lateral hypothalamic electrode. In other words, natural drives can selectively favor one electrode over another, but priming induced drive cannot, because the priming always induces a multifarious drive state.

D. Stimulation-bound Motivation and the Aftereffect of BSR

One issue, touched on but not discussed in the last section, is the relation between the drive-like aftereffect of brain stimulation reward and the drive-like effect of this same stimulation that is manifested in the frequently found stimulation-bound motivation effects. It is tempting to regard these two effects as different manifestations of the same underlying process. If BSR activates the drive component of various homeostats as well as their reinforcement component, then, during prolonged stimulation, animals may attempt to maximize rewarding input by consuming natural rewards (cf., Coons & Cruce, 1968). The parallel between our data on the lack of electrode specificity in the aftereffect and Valenstein et al. data on the lack of specificity in stimulation elicited consummatory effects encourages this assumption.

There are, however, reasons for doubting that the two effects are manifestations of the same process. First, the drive-like aftereffect is a nearly invariable accompaniment of rewarding brain stimulation, whereas many self-stimulation electrodes do not elicit any discernible consummatory behavior (Valenstein et al., 1970). Second, and more important, termination of prolonged stimulation leads to immediate termination of the induced consummatory behavior. In fact, there appears to be some poststimulation inhibition of the induced consummatory behavior (Cox, Kakolewski, & Valenstein, 1969). The drive-like effect of BSR in self-stimulation, on the other hand, outlasts the stimulation by several seconds to a few minutes. There is no evidence of an inhibitory aftereffect, only an excitatory aftereffect.

In sum, the relation of the drive effect of BSR to naturally arising drives and to the drive or drives induced by prolonged stimulation of the lateral areas of the hypothalamus is, at the moment, obscure. We have, nonetheless, learned a good deal about the general structure of the system or systems underlying self-stimulation and about its neurophysiological properties.

V. SUMMARY

The system, or systems, underlying self-stimulation has at least two major components. Activation of one of these components—the reinforcement component—has behavioral effects similar to the effects of natural gratifications such as food, water, and copulation. As with natural reinforcement, the fact that this component has previously been activated by a given behavior does not, by itself, produce any strong or persistent behavior. In order for the behavior to show strength relative to competing behaviors and persistence in the face of obstruction, there must also be a drive state appropriate to the reinforcement. In self-stimulation such a drive state remains as a decaying residue from previous BSR.

Evidence has been adduced that the decaying aftereffect of BSR is not a secondary consequence of exciting a reinforcement component. Rather, it appears to be the result of direct excitation by BSR of a second component. The realization of the role played by this second component of the self-stimulation system resolves several apparent paradoxes in self-stimulation behavior. It explains, for example, why an artificial reward which rats prefer over food to the point of starvation is nonetheless worse than food for sustaining performance on partial reinforcement schedules. More generally, the decay of drive explains why the time elapsed since the last reward is an important determinant of performance for BSR.

The two functionally distinct components are mediated by neuronal populations with different characteristic fiber diameters. Data from behavioral measurements of the neuronal refractory periods indicate a characteristic diameter of 2–4 micra for the neurons in the reward component and a characteristic diameter of 1–2 micra for the neurons in the drive component. This range of diameters matches closely the known diameters of the noradrenergic fibers in the MFB. There is pharmacological evidence that also implicates noradrenergic fibers in the mediation of self-stimulation.

Both components of the self-stimulation system apparently employ a surprisingly primitive code. The total amount of excitation in the relevant population of neurons is the important variable, with the spatio-temporal distribution of excitation having little importance. The time interval over which the spatio-temporal integration of excitation is performed is apparently short (1 second or less) in the case of the reward component and long (10 seconds or more) in the case of the drive component. Limited amounts of stimulation (8–64 pulses, depending on current intensity) suffice to drive the integrator in the reward component to maximum output. At least an order of magnitude more stimulation is required to drive the integrator in the drive component to its maximum output. The output of the integrator in the reward component probably subsides rapidly (in less than 1 second) when stimulation ceases, whereas the output of the integrator in the drive component can take several minutes to subside completely when it has been driven to its maximum.

Preliminary evidence from single unit recordings indicates that the drive component may project in part from the MFB to the medial thalamus, while the reward component may project in part to the dorsolateral thalamus. (There may also be hippocampal and brain stem involvement in both these projections.)

It is not clear whether there is one two-component system or several two-component systems underlying self-stimulation. If there are several such systems, then their drive components must be thoroughly intertwined throughout the MFB.

Self-stimulation is a promising phenomenon to investigate, provided one is interested in the neurophysiological basis of complex processes such as motivation and reinforcement in instrumental behavior. The self-stimulation phenomenon offers one of the few opportunities outside the sensory domain for the close integration of behavioral and electrophysiological data. Experiments on parallel behavioral and electrophysiological effects produced by varying the temporal parameters of stimulation have begun to exploit this opportunity.

REFERENCES

Adrian, E. D., & Lucas, K. On the summation of a propagated disturbance in nerve and muscle. *Journal of Physiology*, 1912, Vol. 44, 68-124.

Albino, A. C., & Lucas, J. W. Mutual facilitation of self-rewarding regions within the limbic system. *Journal of Comparative & Physiological Psychology*, 1962, Vol. 55, 182-185.

Asdourian, D., Stutz, R. M., & Rocklin, K. W. Effects of thalamic and limbic system lesions on self-stimulation. *Journal of Comparative & Physiological Psychology*, 1966, Vol. 61, 468-472.

Balagura, S. Influence of osmotic and caloric loads upon lateral hypothalamic self-stimulation. *Journal of Comparative & Physiological Psychology*, 1968, Vol. 66, 325-328.

Balagura, S., & Hoebel, B. G. Self-stimulation of the lateral hypothalamus modified by insulin and glucagon. *Physiology & Behavior*, 1967, Vol. 2, 337-340.

Ball, G. G. Electrical self-stimulation of the brain and sensory inhibition. *Psychonomic Science*, 1967, Vol. 8, 489-490.

Ball, G. G., & Adams, D. W. Intracranial stimulation as an avoidance or escape response. *Psychonomic Science*, 1965, Vol. 3, 39-40.

Bazett, H. C. Observations on the refractory period of the sartorius of the frog. *Journal of Physiology*, 1908, Vol. 36, 414-430.

Beer, B., Hodos, W. H., & Matthews, T. J. Rate of intracranial self-stimulation as a function of reinforcement magnitude and density. *Psychonomic Science*, 1964, Vol. 1, 321-322.

Bindra, D. Neuropsychological interpretation of the effects of drive and incentive-motivation on general activity and instrumental behavior. *Psychological Review*, 1968, Vol. 75, 1-22.

Bishop, M. P., Elder, S. T., & Heath, R. G. Intracranial self-stimulation in man. *Science*, 1963, Vol. 140, 394-395.

Bogacz, J., St. Laurent, J., & Olds, J. Dissociation of self-stimulation and epileptiform activity. *Electroencephalography & Clinical Neurophysiology*, 1965, Vol. 19, 75-87.

Boycott, A. E. Note on the muscular response to two stimuli of the sciatic nerve (frog). *Journal of Physiology*, 1899, Vol. 24, 144-145.

Boyd, E. S., & Gardner, L. C. Effects of some brain lesions on intracranial self-stimulation in the rat. *American Journal of Physiology*, 1967, Vol. 213, 1044-1052.

Brady, J. V. Temporal and emotional factors related to electrical self-stimulation of the limbic system. In H. H. Jasper, L. D. Proctor, R. S. Knighton, W. C. Noshay, & R. T. Costello (Eds.), *The reticular formation of the brain*. Boston, Massachusetts: Little-Brown, 1958.

Brady, J. V. Temporal and emotional effects related to intracranial electrical self-stimulation. In E. R. Ramey & D. S. O'Doherty (Eds.), *Electrical studies on the unanesthetized brain*. New York: Hoeber, 1960.

Brady, J. V., Boren, J. J., Conrad, D. G., & Sidman, M. The effect of food and water deprivation upon intracranial self-stimulation. *Journal of Comparative & Physiological Psychology*, 1957, Vol. 50, 134-137.

Brady, J. V., & Conrad, D. G. Some effects of limbic system self-stimulation upon conditioned emotional behavior. *Journal of Comparative & Physiological Psychology*, 1960, Vol. 53, 128-137.

Bramwell, J. C., & Lucas, K. On the relation of the refractory period to the propagated disturbance in nerve. *Journal of Physiology*, 1911, Vol. 42, 495-518.

Brodie, D. A., Moreno, O. M., Malis, J. L., & Boren, J. J. Rewarding properties of intracranial stimulation. *Science*, 1960, Vol. 131, 929-930.

Bruce, R. H. An experimental investigation of the thirst drive in rats with especial reference to the goal gradient hypothesis. *Journal of General Psychology*, 1937, Vol. 17, 49-62.

Bruce, R. H. The effect of lessening the drive upon performance by white rats in a maze. *Journal of Comparative & Physiological Psychology*, 1938, Vol. 25, 225-248.

Caggiula, A. R., & Hoebel, B. G. "Copulation-Reward Site" in the posterior hypothalamus. *Science*, 1966, Vol. 153, 1284-1285.

Coons, E. E., & Cruce, J. A. F. Lateral hypothalamus: Food, current intensity in maintaining self-stimulation of hunger. *Science*, 1968, Vol. 159, 1117-1119.

Cooper, R. M., & Taylor, L. H. Thalamic reticular system and central grey: self-stimulation. *Science*, 1967, Vol. 156, 102-103.

Cox, V. C., Kakolewski, J. W., & Valenstein, E. S. Inhibition of eating and drinking following hypothalamic stimulation in the rat. *Journal of Comparative & Physiological Psychology*, 1969, Vol. 68, 530-535.

Crespi, L. P. Quantitative variation of incentive and performance in the white rat. *American Journal of Psychology*, 1942, Vol. 55, 467-517.

Culbertson, J. L., Kling, J. W., & Berkley, M. A. Extinction responding following ICS and food reinforcement. *Psychonomic Science*, 1966, Vol. 5, 127-128.

Deutsch, J. A. *The structural basis of behavior*. Chicago, Illinois: Chicago University Press, 1960.

Deutsch, J. A. Learning and self-stimulation of the brain. *Journal of Theoretical Biology*, 1963, Vol. 4, 193-214. (a)

Deutsch, J. A. Drive decay and differential training. *Science*, 1963, Vol. 142, 1125-1126. (b)

Deutsch, J. A. Behavioral measurement of the neural refractory period and its application to intracranial self-stimulation. *Journal of Comparative & Physiological Psychology*, 1964, Vol. 58, 1-9.

Deutsch, J. A., Adams, D. W., & Metzner, R. J. Choice of intracranial stimulation as a function of delay between stimulations and strength of competing drive. *Journal of Comparative and Physiological Psychology*, 1964, Vol. 57, 241-243.

Deutsch, J. A., & Deutsch, D. *Physiological psychology*. Homewood, Illinois: Dorsey Press, 1966.

Deutsch, J. A., & DiCara, L. Hunger and extinction in intracranial self-stimulation. *Journal of Comparative & Physiological Psychology*, 1967, Vol. 63, 344-347.

Deutsch, J. A., & Howarth, C. I. Evocation by fear of a habit learned for electrical stimulation of the brain. *Science*, 1962, Vol. 136, 1057-1058.

Deutsch, J. A., & Howarth, C. I. Some tests of a theory of intracranial self-stimulation. *Psychological Review*, 1963, Vol. 70, 444-460.

Dudel, J., & Kuffler, S. W. Mechanism of facilitation at the crayfish neuromuscular junction. *Journal of Physiology*, 1961, Vol. 155, 530-542.

Eccles, J. C. *The physiology of synapses.* Berlin: Springer, 1965.

Elder, S. T., Montgomery, N. P., & Rye, M. M. Effects of food deprivation and methamphetamine on fixed-ratio schedules of intracranial stimulation. *Psychological Reports*, 1965, Vol. 16, 1225-1237.

Endroczi, E., & Lissak, K. Behavioral reactions evoked by electrical stimulation in the medial forebrain bundle region. *Physiology & Behavior*, 1966, Vol. 1, 223-229.

Falk, J. L. Septal stimulation as a reinforcer of and alternative to consummatory behavior. *Journal of the Experimental Analysis of Behavior*, 1961, Vol. 4, 213-217.

Ferster, C. B., & Skinner, B. F. *Schedules of reinforcement.* New York: Appleton-Century-Crofts, 1957.

Furshpan, E. J. Neuromuscular transmission in invertebrates. In J. Field & V. E. Hall (Eds.), *Handbook of physiology.* Section 1, H. W. Magoun (Ed.), *Neurophysiology.* Vol. 1. Washington, D.C.: American Physiological Society, 1959.

Fuxe, K. Evidence for the existence of monoamine neurons in the central nervous system, IV. Distribution of monoamine nerve terminals in the central nervous system. *Acta Physiologica Scandinavica* (Supplement 247), 1965, Vol. 64, 37-84.

Gallistel, C. R. Electrical self-stimulation and its theoretical implications. *Psychological Bulletin*, 1964, Vol. 61, 23-34.

Gallistel, C. R. Motivating effects in self-stimulation. *Journal of Comparative & Physiological Psychology*, 1966, Vol. 62, 95-101.

Gallistel, C. R. Intracranial stimulation and natural rewards: Differential effects of trial spacing. *Psychonomic Science*, 1967, Vol. 9, 167-168.

Gallistel, C. R. The incentive of brain stimulation reward. *Journal of Comparative & Physiological Psychology*, 1969, Vol. 69, 713-721. (a)

Gallistel, C. R. Failure of pretrial stimulation to affect reward electrode preference. *Journal of Comparative & Physiological Psychology*, 1969, Vol. 69, 722-729. (b)

Gallistel, C. R., Rolls, E. T., & Greene, D. Neuron function inferred from behavioral and electrophysiological estimates of refractory period. *Science*, 1969, Vol. 166, 1028-1030.

Gandelman, R., & Trowill, J. A. The effects of chlordiazepoxide on acquisition and extinction responding for brain stimulation. *Journal of Comparative & Physiological Psychology*, 1968, Vol. 66, 753-755.

Gibson, W. E., Reid, L. D., Sakai, M., & Porter, P. B. Intracranial reinforcement compared with sugar water reinforcement. *Science*, 1965, Vol. 148, 1357-1359.

Gotch, F., & Burch, G. J. The electrical response of nerve to two stimuli. *Journal of Physiology*, 1899, Vol. 24, 410-426.

Grossman, S. P. *A textbook of physiological psychology*. New York: Wiley, 1966.

Grundfest, H. Bioelectric potentials. *Annual Review of Physiology*, 1940, Vol. 2, 213-242.

Haareveld, A., & Wiersma, C. A. G. The double motor innervation of the adductor muscle of the claw of the crayfish. *Journal of Physiology*, 1936, Vol. 88, 78-99.

Hawkins, T. D., & Pliskoff, S. S. Brain stimulation intensity, rate of self-stimulation, and reinforcement strength: An analysis through chaining. *Journal of the Experimental Analysis of Behavior*, 1964, Vol. 7, 285-288.

Helmholtz, H. Über die Geschwindigkeit einiger Vorgänge in Muskeln und Nerven. *Bericht über die zur Bekanntmachung geeigneten Verhandlungen der König. Preuss. Akademie der Wissenshaften zu Berlin*, 1854, 328-332. (Forerunner of *Berichte der Berlinische Akademie*).

Herberg, L. J. Seminal ejaculation following positively reinforcing electrical stimulation of the rat hypothalamus. *Journal of Comparative & Physiological Psychology*, 1963, Vol. 56, 679-685.

Hill, A. V. Excitation and Accommodation in nerve. *Proceedings of the Royal Society of London, Series B*, 1936, Vol. 119, 305-355.

Hodos, W. H. Motivational properties of long durations of rewarding brain stimulation. *Journal of Comparative & Physiological Psychology*, 1965, Vol. 59, 219-224.

Hodos, W., & Kalman, G. Effects of increment size and reinforcement volume on progressive ratio performance. *Journal of the Experimental Analysis of Behavior*, 1963, Vol. 6, 387-392.

Hodos, W., & Valenstein, E. S. An evaluation of response rate as a measure of rewarding intracranial stimulation. *Journal of Comparative & Physiological Psychology*, 1962, Vol. 55, 80-84.

Hoebel, B. G. Hypothalamic lesions by electrocauterization: disinhibition of feeding and self-stimulation. *Science*, 1965, Vol. 149, 452-453.

Hoebel, B. G. Inhibition and disinhibition of self-stimulation and feeding: Hypothalamic control and post-ingestional factors. *Journal of Comparative & Physiological Psychology*, 1968, Vol. 66, 89-100.

Hoebel, B. G., & Teitelbaum, P. Hypothalamic control of feeding and self-stimulation. *Science*, 1962, Vol. 135, 375-377.

Holz, W. C., & Azrin, N. H. A comparison of several procedures for eliminating behavior. *Journal of the Experimental Analysis of Behavior*, 1963, Vol. 6, 399-406.

Howarth, C. I., & Deutsch, J. A. Drive decay: The cause of fast "extinction" of habits learned for brain stimulation. *Science*, 1962, Vol. 137, 35-36.

Hull, C. L. *Principles of behavior*. New York: Appleton-Century-Crofts, 1943.

Hull, C. L. *A behavior system*. New Haven, Connecticut: Yale University Press, 1952.

Johnson, R. N. Effects of intracranial reinforcement intensity and distributional variables on brightness reversal learning in rats. *Journal of Comparative & Physiological Psychology*, 1968, Vol. 66, 422-426.

Justesen, D. R., Sharp, J. C., & Porter, P. B. Self-stimulation of the caudate nucleus by instrumentally naive cats. *Journal of Comparative & Physiological Psychology*, 1963, Vol. 56, 371-374.

Kavanau, J. L. Behavior of captive white-footed mice. In E. R. Willems & H. L. Raush (Eds.), *Naturalistic viewpoints in psychology*. New York: Holt, Rinehart, Winston, 1969.

Keesey, R. E. The relation between pulse frequency, intensity, and duration and the rate of responding for intracranial stimulation. *Journal of Comparative & Physiological Psychology*, 1962, Vol. 55, 671-678.

Keesey, R. E. Duration of stimulation and the reward properties of hypothalamic stimulation. *Journal of Comparative & Physiological Psychology*, 1964, Vol. 58, 201-207.

Keesey, R. E. Hypothalamic stimulation as a reinforcer of discrimination learning. *Journal of Comparative & Physiological Psychology*, 1966, Vol. 62, 231-236.

Keesey, R. E., & Goldstein, M. D. Use of progressive fixed-ratio procedures in the assessment of intracranial reinforcement. *Journal of the Experimental Analysis of Behavior*, 1968, Vol. 11, 293-301.

Kendler, H. H. The influence of simultaneous hunger and thirst drives upon the learning of two opposed spatial responses of the white rat. *Journal of Experimental Psychology*, 1946, Vol. 36, 212-220.

Kent, E., & Grossman, S. P. Evidence for a conflict interpretation of anomalous effects of rewarding brain stimulation. *Journal of Comparative & Physiological Psychology*, 1969, Vol. 69, 381-390.

Kimble, G. A. Behavior strength as a function of the intensity of the hunger drive. *Journal of Experimental Psychology*, 1951, Vol. 41, 341-348.

Kimble, G. A. *Hilgard and Marquis' conditioning and learning.* (2nd ed.) New York: Appleton-Century-Crofts, 1961.

Kling, J. W., & Matsumiya, Y. Relative reinforcement values of food and intracranial stimulation. *Science*, 1962, Vol. 135, 668-670.

Knott, P. D., & Clayton, K. N. Durable secondary reinforcement using brain stimulation as the primary reinforcer. *Journal of Comparative & Physiological Psychology*, 1966, Vol. 61, 151-153.

König, J. F. R., & Klippel, R. A. *The rat brain: A stereotaxic atlas.* Baltimore, Maryland: Williams & Wilkins, 1963.

Konorski, J. *Integrative activity of the brain.* Chicago, Illinois: University of Chicago Press, 1967.

Kornblith, C., & Olds, J. T-maze learning with one trial per day using brain stimulation reinforcement. *Journal of Comparative & Physiological Psychology*, 1968, Vol. 66, 488-492.

Lashley, K. S. A simple maze; with data on the relation of distribution of practice to the rate of learning. *Psychobiology*, 1918, Vol. 1, 353-367.

Lashley, K. S. Experimental analysis of instinctive behavior. *Psychological Review*, 1938, Vol. 45, 445-471.

LeMagnen, J., & Tallon, S. La periodicité spontanée de la prise d'aliments ad libitum du rat blanc. *Journal de Physiologie,* 1966, Vol. 58, 323-349.

Lilly, J. C. Learning motivated by subcortical stimulation: the start and stop patterns of behavior. In H. H. Jasper, L. D. Proctor, R. S. Knighton, W. C. Noshay, & R. T. Costello (Eds.), *The reticular formation of the brain.* Boston, Massachusetts: Little-Brown, 1958.

Lilly, J. C. Learning motivated by subcortical stimulation. In E. R. Ramey, & D. S. O'Doherty (Eds.), *Electrical studies on the unanesthetized brain.* New York: Hoeber, 1960.

Lilly, J. C. Operant conditioning of the bottlenose Dolphin with electrical stimulation of the brain. *Journal of Comparative & Physiological Psychology*, 1962, Vol. 55, 73-79.

Lloyd, D. P. C. Facilitation and inhibition of spinal motoneurons. *Journal of Neurophysiology*, 1946, Vol. 9, 421-438.

Logan, F. A. *Incentive.* New Haven, Connecticut: Yale University Press, 1960.

Lorens, S. A. Effect of lesions in the central nervous system on lateral hypothalamic self-stimulation in the rat. *Journal of Comparative & Physiological Psychology*, 1966, Vol. 62, 256-262.

Lorente de Nó, R. Transmission of impulses through cranial motor nuclei. *Journal of Neurophysiology*, 1939, Vol. 2, 402-464.

Lorenz, K. Über die Bildung des Instinktbegriffs. *Die Naturwissenschaften*, 1937, Vol. 25, 289-300, 307-318, 324-331.

Lucas, K. The analysis of complex excitable tissues by their response to electric currents of short duration. *Journal of Physiology*, 1906, Vol. 35, 310-331.

Lucas, K. On summation of propagated disturbances in the claw of *Astacus*, and on the double neuro-muscular system of the adductor. *Journal of Physiology*, 1917, Vol. 51, 1-35.

Malmo, R. B. Slowing of heart rate following septal self-stimulation in rats. *Science*, 1961, Vol. 133, 1128-1130.

Mandler, G. M. The interruption of behavior. *Nebraska Symposium on Motivation*, 1964, Vol. 12, 163-219.

Margules, D. L., & Olds, J. Identical "feeding" and "rewarding" systems in the lateral hypothalamus of rats. *Science*, 1962, Vol. 135, 374-375.

Mayer, B. A., & Stone, C. P. The relative efficiency of distributed and massed practice in maze learning by young and adult albino rats. *Journal of Genetic Psychology*, 1931, Vol. 39, 28-38.

McIntire, R. W., & Wright, J. E. Parameters related to response rate for septal and medial forebrain bundle stimulation. *Journal of Comparative & Physiological Psychology*, 1965, Vol. 59, 131-134.

Mendelson, J. Lateral hypothalamic stimulation in satiated rats: The rewarding effects of self-induced drinking. *Science*, 1967, Vol. 157, 1077-1079.

Meyers, W. J., Valenstein, E. S., & Lacey, J. I. Heart rate changes after reinforcing brain stimulation in rats. *Science*, 1963, Vol. 40, 1233-1235.

Miller, N. E. Implications for theories of reinforcement. In D. E. Sheer (Ed.), *Electrical stimulation of the brain.* Austin, Texas: Texas University Press, 1961.

Milner, P. *Physiological Psychology.* New York: Holt, Rinehart, Winston, 1970.

Mogenson, G. J. An attempt to establish secondary reinforcement with rewarding brain stimulation. *Psychological Reports*, 1965, Vol. 16, 163-167.

Mogenson, G. J., & Stevenson, J. A. F. Drinking and self-stimulation with electrical stimulation of the lateral hypothalamus. *Physiology & Behavior*, 1966, Vol. 1, 251-254.

Morgan, C. T. Physiological mechanisms of motivation. *Nebraska Symposium on Motivation*, 1957, Vol. 5, 1-43.

Morgan, C. T., & Fields, P. E. The effect of variable preliminary feeding upon the rat's speed of locomotion. *Journal of Comparative & Physiological Psychology*, 1938, Vol. 26, 331-348.

Morgane, P. J. Medial forebrain bundle and "feeding centers" of the hypothalamus. *Journal of Comparative Neurology*, 1961, Vol. 117, 1-26.

Mount, G. B., & Hoebel, B. G. Lateral hypothalamic reward decreased by intragastric feeding: self-determined "threshold" technique. *Psychonomic Science*, 1967, Vol. 9, 265-266.

Nauta, W. J. H. Some neural pathways related to the limbic system. In E. R. Ramey & D. S. O'Doherty (Eds.), *Electrical studies on the unanesthetized brain.* New York: Hoeber, 1960.

Newman, B. L. Behavioral effects of electrical self-stimulation of the septal area and related structures in the rat. *Journal of Comparative & Physiological Psychology*, 1961, Vol. 54, 340-346.

Newman, B. L., & Feldman, S. M. Electrophysiological activity accompanying intracranial self-stimulation. *Journal of Comparative & Physiological Psychology*, 1964, Vol. 57, 244-247.

Olds, J. Physiological mechanisms of reward. In M. R. Jones (Ed.), *Nebraska Symposium on Motivation*. Lincoln, Nebraska: University of Nebraska Press, 1955.

Olds, J. Runway and maze behavior controlled by basomedial forebrain stimulation in the rat. *Journal of Comparative & Physiological Psychology*, 1956, Vol. 49, 507-512.

Olds, J. Adaptive functions of paleocortical and related structures. In H. F. Harlow & C. N. Woolsey (Eds.), *Biological and biochemical bases of behavior*. Madison, Wisconsin: University of Wisconsin Press, 1958. (a)

Olds, J. Self-stimulation of the brain. *Science*, 1958, Vol. 127, 315-324. (b)

Olds, J. Satiation effects in self-stimulation of the brain. *Journal of Comparative & Physiological Psychology*, 1958, Vol. 51, 675-678. (c)

Olds, J. Effects of hunger and male sex hormones on self-stimulation of the brain. *Journal of Comparative & Physiological Psychology*, 1958, Vol. 51, 320-324. (d)

Olds, J. Differentiation of reward systems in the brain by self-stimulation techniques. In E. R. Ramey & D. S. O'Doherty (Eds.), *Electrical studies on the unanesthetized brain*. New York: Hoeber, 1960.

Olds, J., & Milner, P. Positive reinforcement produced by electrical stimulation of septal area and other regions of the rat brain. *Journal of Comparative & Physiological Psychology*, 1954, Vol. 47, 419-427.

Olds, J., & Olds, M. E. Drives, rewards, and the brain. In T. M. Newcombe (Ed.), *New directions in psychology II*. New York: Holt, Rinehart, Winston, 1965.

Olds, M. E., & Olds, J. Effects of lesions in medial forebrain bundle on self-stimulation behavior. *American Journal of Physiology*, 1969, Vol. 217, 1253-1264.

Panksepp, J., Gandelman, R., & Trowill, J. A. The effect of intertrial interval on running performance for ESB. *Psychonomic Science*, 1968, Vol. 13, 135-136.

Panksepp, J., & Trowill, J. A. Intraoral self-injection: I. Effects of delay of reinforcement on resistance to extinction and implications for self-stimulation. *Psychonomic Science*, 1967, Vol. 9, 405-406. (a)

Panksepp, J., & Trowill, J. A. Intraoral self-injection: II. The simulation of self-stimulation phenomena with a conventional reward. *Psychonomic Science*, 1967, Vol. 9, 407-408. (b)

Papez, J. W. A proposed mechanism of emotion. *Archives of Neurology & Psychiatry*, 1937, Vol. 38, 725-743.

Perez-Cruet, J., Black, W. C., & Brady, J. V. Heart rate: Differential effects of hypothalamic and septal self-stimulation. *Science*, 1963, Vol. 140, 1235-1236.

Perez-Cruet, J., McIntire, R. W., & Pliskoff, S. S. Blood pressure and heart rate changes in dogs during hypothalamic self-stimulation. *Journal of Comparative & Physiological Psychology*, 1965, Vol. 60, 373-381.

Phillips, A. G., & Mogenson, G. J. Self-stimulation of the olfactory bulb. *Physiology & Behavior*, 1969, Vol. 4, 195-197.

Pliskoff, S. S., & Hawkins, T. D. Test of Deutsch's drive-decay theory of rewarding self-stimulation of the brain. *Science*, 1963, Vol. 141, 823-824.

Pliskoff, S. S., & Hawkins, T. D. A method for increasing the reinforcement magnitude of intracranial stimulation. *Journal of the Experimental Analysis of Behavior*, 1967, Vol. 10, 281-289.

Pliskoff, S. S., Wright, J. E., & Hawkins, T. D. Brain stimulation as a reinforcer: intermittent schedules. *Journal of the Experimental Analysis of Behavior*, 1965, Vol. 8, 75-88.

Porter, R. W., Conrad, D. G., & Brady, J. V. Some neural and behavioral correlates of electrical self-stimulation of the limbic system. *Journal of the Experimental Analysis of Behavior*, 1959, Vol. 2, 43-55.

Prescott, R. G. W. Diurnal activity cycles and intracranial self-stimulation in the rat. *Journal of Comparative & Physiological Psychology*, 1967, Vol. 64, 346-349.

Pribram, K. H., & Kruger, L. Functions of the olfactory brain. *Annals of the New York Academy of Science*, 1954, Vol. 58 (2), 109-138.

Quartermain, D., & Webster, D. Extinction following intracranial reward: The effect of delay between acquisition and extinction. *Science*, 1968, Vol. 159, 1259-1260.

Ray, O. S., Hine, B., & Bivens, L. W. Stability of self-stimulation responding during long test sessions. *Physiology & Behavior*, 1968, Vol. 3, 161-165.

Reid, L. D., & Porter, P. B. Reinforcement from direct electrical stimulation of the brain. *Rocky Mountain Psychologist*, 1965, Vol. 1, 3-22.

Reid, L. D., Gibson, W. E., Gledhill, S. M., & Porter, P. B. Anticonvulsant drugs and self-stimulation behavior. *Journal of Comparative & Physiological Psychology*, 1964, Vol. 57, 353-356.

Reynolds, R. W. The relationship between stimulation voltage and hypothalamic self-stimulation in the rat. *Journal of Comparative and Physiological Psychology*, 1958, Vol. 51, 193-198.

Reynolds, W. F., & Pavlik, W. B. Running speed as a function of deprivation period and reward magnitude. *Journal of Comparative & Physiological Psychology*, 1960, Vol. 53, 615-618.

Richet, C. Addition latente des excitations électriques dans les nerfs et dans les muscles. *Travaux du laboratoire de M. Marey*, 1877, Vol. 3, 97-105.

Richet, C. *Dictionaire de Physiologie*. Vol. 1, Paris: Ballière, 1895.

Roberts, W. W. Both rewarding and punishing effects from stimulation of posterior hypothalamus of cat with same electrode at same intensity. *Journal of Comparative & Physiological Psychology*, 1958, Vol. 51, 400-407.

Roll, S. K. Intracranial self-stimulation and wakefulness: Effect of manipulating ambient brain catecholamines. *Science*, 1970, Vol. 168, 1370-1372.

Rolls, E. T. Involvement of brainstem units in medial forebrain bundle self-stimulation. *Physiology & Behavior*, 1971, Vol. 7, 297-310.

Routtenberg, A., & Huang, Y. H. Reticular formation and brainstem unitary activity: Effects of posterior hypothalamic and septal-limbic stimulation at reward loci. *Physiology & Behavior*, 1968, Vol. 3, 611-617.

Routtenberg, A., & Lindy, J. Effects of the availability of rewarding septal and hypothalamic stimulation on bar pressing for food under conditions of deprivation. *Journal of Comparative & Physiological Psychology*, 1965, Vol. 60, 158-161.

Scott, J. W. Brain stimulation reinforcement with distributed practice: Effects of electrode locus, previous experience and stimulus intensity. *Journal of Comparative & Physiological Psychology*, 1967, Vol. 63, 175-183.

Segal, E. F. Prolonged extinction following one session of food reinforced conditioning: A methodological note. *Journal of Comparative & Physiological Psychology*, 1962, Vol. 55, 40-43.

Sem-Jacobson, C. W., & Torkildsen, A. In E. R. Ramey & D. S. O'Doherty (Eds.), *Electrical studies on the unanesthetized brain*. New York: Hoeber, 1960.

Seward, J. P., Uyeda, A. A., & Olds, J. Resistance to extinction following cranial self-stimulation. *Journal of Comparative & Physiological Psychology,* 1959, Vol. 52, 294-299.

Seward, J. P., Uyeda, A. A., & Olds, J. Reinforcing effect of brain stimulation on runway
performance as a function of interval between trials. *Journal of Comparative & Physiological Psychology,* 1960, Vol. 53, 224-227.

Sidman, M., Brady, J. V., Conrad, D. G., & Schulman, A. Reward schedules and behavior
maintained by intracranial self-stimulation. *Science,* 1955, Vol. 122, 830-831.

Sidman, M., & Stebbens, W. C. Satiation effects under fixed ratio schedules of reinforcement. *Journal of Comparative & Physiological Psychology,* 1954, Vol. 47, 114-116.

Skinner, B. F. Are theories of learning necessary? *Psychological Review,* 1950, Vol. 57,
193-216.

Smith, N. S., & Coons, E. E. Temporal summation and refractoriness in hypothalamic
reward neurons as measured by self-stimulation behavior. *Science,* 1970, Vol. 169,
782-784.

Spear, N. E. Comparison of the reinforcing effect of brain stimulation on Skinner box,
runway, and maze performance. *Journal of Comparative & Physiological Psychology,*
1962, Vol. 55, 679-684.

Spence, K. W. *Behavior theory and conditioning.* New Haven, Connecticut: Yale University
Press, 1956.

Spies, G. Food versus intracranial self-stimulation reinforcement in food deprived rats.
Journal of Comparative & Physiological Psychology, 1965, Vol. 60, 153-157.

Stark, P., & Boyd, E. S. Effects of cholinergic drugs on hypothalamic self-stimulation rates
in dogs. *American Journal of Physiology,* 1963, Vol. 205, 745-748.

Stein, L. Secondary reinforcement established with subcortical stimulation. *Science,* 1958,
Vol. 127, 466-467.

Stein, L. An analysis of stimulus-duration preference in self-stimulation of the brain. *Journal
of Comparative & Physiological Psychology,* 1962, Vol. 55, 405-414.

Stein, L. Reciprocal action of reward and punishment. In R. G. Heath (Ed.), *The role of
pleasure in behavior.* New York: Hoeber, 1964.

Stein, L., & Ray, O. S. Self-regulation of brain stimulation current intensity in the rat.
Science, 1959, Vol. 130, 570-572.

Stein, L., & Wise, D. C. Release of norepinepherine from hypothalamus and amygdala by
rewarding medial forebrain bundle stimulation and amphetamine. *Journal of Comparative & Physiological Psychology,* 1969, Vol. 67, 189-198.

Stellar, E. Drive and motivation. In J. Field & V. E. Hall (Eds.), *Handbook of physiology.*
Section 1, H. W. Magoun (Ed.), *Neurophysiology.* Vol. 3. Washington, D.C., American
Physiological Society, 1960.

Stutz, R. M., Lewin, I., & Rocklin, R. W. Generality of drive decay as an explanatory
concept. *Psychonomic Science,* 1965, Vol. 2, 127-128.

Tasaki, I. Conduction of the nerve impulse. In J. Field & V. E. Hall (Eds.), *Handbook of
physiology.* Section 1, H. W. Magoun (Ed.), *Neurophysiology.* Vol. 1. Washington, D.C.:
American Physiological Society, 1959.

Terman, M., & Terman, J. S. Circadian rhythm of brain self-stimulation behavior. *Science,*
1970, Vol. 168, 1242-1244.

Timberlake, W. Straight alley acquisition drive and ad lib test performance. *Psychonomic
Science,* 1967, Vol. 9, 585-586.

Tolman, E. C. Demands and conflicts. *Psychological Review,* 1937, Vol. 44, 158-169.

Trowill, J. A., Panksepp, J., Gandelman, R. An incentive model of rewarding brain stimulation. *Psychological Review,* 1969, Vol. 76, 264-281.

Ulrich, J. L. The distribution of effort in learning in the white rat. *Behavioral Monographs*, 1915, Vol. 10, (No. 2).

Ungerleider, L. G., & Coons, E. E. A behavioral measure of homosynaptic and heterosynaptic temporal summation in the self-stimulation system of the rat. *Science,* 1970, Vol. 169, 785-787.

Ursin, R., Ursin, H., & Olds, J. Self-stimulation of hippocampus in rats. *Journal of Comparative & Physiological Psychology*, 1966, Vol. 61, 353-359.

Valenstein, E. S. Problems of measurement and interpretation with reinforcing brain stimulation. *Psychological Review*, 1964, Vol. 71,415-437.

Valenstein, E. S. The anatomical locus of reinforcement. In E. Stellar & J. M. Sprague (Eds.), *Progress in physiological psychology*. New York: Academic Press, 1966.

Valenstein, E. S., & Beer, B. Unipolar and bipolar electrodes in self-stimulation experiments. *Americal Journal of Physiology*, 1961, Vol. 201, 1181-1186.

Valenstein, E. S., & Beer B. Reinforcing brain stimulation in competition with water reward and shock avoidance. *Science*, 1962, Vol. 137, 1052-1054.

Valenstein, E. S., & Beer B. Continuous opportunities for reinforcing brain stimulation. *Journal of the Experimental Analysis of Behavior*,1964, Vol. 7, 183-184.

Valenstein, E. S., Cox, V. C., & Kakolewski, J. W. Polydipsia elicited by the synergistic action of a saccharin and glucose solution. *Science*, 1967, Vol. 157, 552-554.

Valenstein, E. S., Cox, V. C., & Kakolewski, J. W. Modification of motivated behavior elicited by electrical stimulation of the hypothalamus. *Science*, 1968, Vol. 159, 1119-1121.

Valenstein, E. S., Cox, V. C., & Kakolewski, J. W. Reexamination of the role of the hypothalamus in motivation. *Psychological Review*, 1970, Vol. 77, 16-31.

Valenstein, E. S., & Valenstein, T. On the interaction of positive and negative reinforcing neural systems. *Science*, 1964, Vol. 145, 1456-1458.

Ward, H. P. Basal tegmental self-stimulation after septal ablation in rats. *Archives of Neurology*, 1960, Vol. 3, 158-162.

Ward, H. P. Tegmental self-stimulation after amygdaloid ablation. *Archives of Neurology*, 1961, Vol. 4, 657-659.

Ward, J. W., & Hester, R. W. Intracranial self-stimulation in cats surgically deprived of autonomic outflows. *Journal of Comparative & Physiological Psychology*, 1969, Vol. 67, 336-343.

Wasden, R. E., Reid, L. D., & Porter, P. B. Overnight performance decrement with intracranial reinforcement. *Psychological Reports*, 1965, Vol. 16, 653-658.

Webb, W. B. Response in absence of the acquisition drive. *Psychological Review,* 1952, Vol. 59, 54-61.

Wetzel, M. C. Self-stimulation aftereffects and runway performance in the rat. *Journal of Comparative & Physiological Psychology*, 1963, Vol. 56, 673-678.

Wetzel, M. C. Self-stimulation anatomy: Data needs. *Brain Research*, 1968, Vol. 10, 287-296.

Wetzel, M. C., Howell, L. G., & Bearie, K. J. Experimental performance of steel and platinum electrodes with chronic monophasic stimulation of the brain. *Journal of Neurosurgery*, 1969, Vol. 31, 658-669.

Wilkinson, H. A., & Peele, T. L. Modification of intracranial self-stimulation by hunger satiety. *American Journal of Physiology*, 1962, Vol. 203, 537-540.

Wise, D. C., & Stein, L. Facilitation of brain self-stimulation by central administration of norepinephrine. *Science*, 1969, Vol. 163, 299-301.

Wise, R. A. Hypothalamic motivational systems: Fixed or plastic neural circuits? *Science*, 1968, Vol. 162, 377-379.

Wurtz, R. H., & Olds, J. Amygdaloid stimulation and operant reinforcement in the rat. *Journal of Comparative & Physiological Psychology*, 1963, Vol. 56, 941-949.

Zeaman, D., & House, B. J. Response latency at zero drive after varying numbers of reinforcements. *Journal of Experimental Psychology*, 1950, Vol. 40, 570-583.

Zeigler, H. P. Electrical stimulation of the brain and the psychophysiology of learning and motivation. *Psychological Bulletin*, 1957, Vol. 54, 363-382.

CHAPTER

8

SPREADING DEPRESSION:
A BEHAVIORAL ANALYSIS[1]

ALLEN M. SCHNEIDER

Potassium chloride (KC1) applied topically to a cerebral hemisphere produces a temporary depression of electrocortical activity which spreads over

[1]Research from our laboratory reported in this chapter was supported by NSF grants GB7278 and GB19642 to New York University. The secretarial skills of Mrs. Geraldine Hansen added immeasurably to the preparation of this chapter.

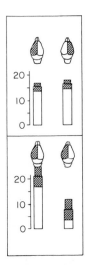

Fig. 8-1. Comparison of number of trials to learn for animals trained and tested under opposite states of unilateral depression (top panel) with animals trained and tested under the same state of unilateral depression (lower panel). Savings occurred if the same hemisphere was depressed during training and testing, but no savings occurred if opposite hemispheres were depressed. Shading in hemispheres represents depression (after Bures, 1959).

the stimulated hemisphere but does not spread interhemispherically (Bures and Buresova, 1960). Although this phenomenon, commonly referred to as spreading cortical depression, has been known for a number of years (Leao, 1944), it remained for Bures (1959) to recognize its importance for behavioral research. Bures reasoned that since memory is apparently stored normally in the form of a dual trace, one trace in each cerebral hemisphere (Sperry, 1964), it should be possible to eliminate a trace in one of the hemispheres by depressing that hemisphere during training. Based on this reasoning, Bures tested the following prediction: if depression of a single hemisphere during training prevents storage in that hemisphere and thereby confines storage to the functional hemisphere, then allowing the depressed hemisphere to recover normal activity should not be sufficient to sustain retention given that the recovery coincides with depression of the initially functional hemisphere. As shown in Fig. 8.1, consistent with this prediction, Bures found that animals trained to avoid shock with one hemisphere depressed retained the avoidance with the same hemisphere again depressed (lower panel) but did not retain the avoidance with depression shifted to the initially functional hemisphere (upper panel).

The problem with a memory confinement interpretation of these data is the assumption that absence of retention accompanying the shift in depression necessarily reflects interference with memory storage, or, equivalently, with associative processes. While the evidence is clear that the shift in depression interfered with performance during the test, it certainly does not demand an explanation solely in terms of neural-associative processes. Rather, when we speak of retention from a neurobehavioral point of view, we mean the physiological state of events that detects the stimuli, associates the stimuli with an earlier conditioned response, and executes the response. The purpose of this chapter is to delineate the degree to which interference with each of these processes contributes to the total behavioral effect of spreading depression.

The chapter is divided into four sections. The first section describes the neural aspects of depression that provide the impetus for using the technique in behavioral research. The second section considers some of the important methodological requirements for using spreading depression in behavioral research. The third section is divided into two parts: the first part deals with the effects of cortical depression on nonassociative processes; the second part deals with the effects of cortical depression on associative processes. It should be emphasized that although the behavioral effects of depression are divided into nonassociative and associative categories, they are not treated as mutually exclusive; rather, the nonassociative effects define the control measures that must be taken to study the associative effects. The fourth section is a direct outgrowth of the research described in Section III and is concerned with the application of spreading depression to the problems of interhemispheric memory transfer and subcortically-controlled associative and recovery-of-function processes.

I. THE NEURAL PROPERTIES OF SPREADING DEPRESSION RELEVANT TO BEHAVIORAL RESEARCH

When we study the behavioral effects of removing portions of the nervous system by means of surgery we are limited by the fact that once central nervous system damage is produced it cannot be reversed. What is needed is a technique by which neural activity can be arrested and then recovered, and the reversible properties of spreading depression seem to meet these needs.

Two bioelectric measures indicate that neural activity is arrested during spreading depression. First, Leao (1944) recorded EEG activity from a number of points on rabbit cortex and found that electrical stimulation of the cortex induced depressed EEG activity that spread at the rate of 2 to 6 mm per minute over the surface of the stimulated hemisphere. Second, depressed EEG activity is accompanied by both a negative shift in the steady potential (Leao, 1947) and an increase in the electrical impedance of the cortex (van Harreveld and Ochs, 1957). Furthermore, although depression can be triggered by vigorous perturbation of the cortex in the form of electrical, mechanical, or chemical stimulation, the most reliable triggering agent is 25 percent KCl solution (Marshall, 1959) which, when applied via filter paper topically to the cortex, abolishes EEG activity for as much as 3 hours and induces repeated negative shifts in the steady potential for at least 90 minutes (Bures, 1959). In addition to the electrophysiological effects that accompany spreading depression, recent histochemical analyses indicate that protein synthesis is temporarily inhibited during spreading depression in anesthetized (Ruscak, 1964) and free-moving rats (Bennett & Edelman, 1969).

The boundaries that define the sphere of spread are under continual revision. Initially it was thought that depression of cortical activity in one hemisphere neither spreads interhemispherically (Bures, 1959) nor beneath the upper layers of the stimulated cortex (Ochs & Hunt, 1960). More recently Gollender and Ochs (1963) and Cofoid (1965) have found that KCl applied to one hemisphere not only induced depressed EEG activity in the cortex of the stimulated hemisphere, but also induced depressed activity, although to a lesser degree and for a shorter time, in the cortex of the nonstimulated hemisphere (i.e., secondary spread). The significance of the secondary spread for behavioral research on free-moving animals is questionable since Gollender and Ochs (1963) report that the secondary spread is clearly evident in anesthetized but not in normal animals.

Because of the elaborate structural and functional connections between the cortex and subcortex, it is not surprising that cortical depression has extensive effects on subcortical activity. Specifically, cortical depression is accompanied by depressed activity in the hypothalamus (Weiss & Fifkova, 1961), caudate nucleus (Bures & Buresova, 1962), amygdala (Fifkova & Syka, 1964), and increased activity in the bulbopontine reticular formation (Bures, Buresova, Fifkova, Olds, Olds, & Travis, 1961); tegmental activity also increases but returns to normal between shifts in the steady potential (Weiss, 1961). Needless to say, these subcortical side effects of cortical depression introduce a critical and perplexing problem in specifying the neural site of action related to the behavioral effects of cortical depression.

That spreading cortical depression can be temporarily blocked only by cuts in the upper cortical layers (i.e., apical dendrites) has been taken as evidence that the propagating mechanism is largely confined to the upper layers (Ochs, 1962). Moreover, the increase in electrical impedance of the cortex that accompanies spreading depression (van Harreveld & Ochs, 1957) has been taken to reflect a decrease in conducting properties of the intercellular space or, more specifically, an increase in membrane permeability to intercellular ions and water (van Harreveld & Schade, 1959). Furthermore, the uptake of intercellular material is thought to trigger the release of intracellular material, either potassium (Grafstein, 1956) and/or glutamic acid (van Harreveld, 1959), which in turn acts upon neighboring cells to excite depolarization in a chain-like reaction.

Although depression is a self-propagating phenomenon, the natural boundaries that define the extent of spread are subject to modification: (1) Weiss and Fifkova (1960) have elicited depression via cannulae directly in the hippocampus, the activity of which is not otherwise affected during cortical depression; (2) Bures and Buresova (1960) have found that cortical areas within the depressed hemisphere can be protected from spread if treated with magnesium or calcium chloride.

II. METHODOLOGICAL REQUIREMENTS FOR USING SPREADING DEPRESSION IN BEHAVIORAL RESEARCH

Utilization of the unique functional and reversible properties of spreading depression requires the following experimental conditions. First, to undergo KCl-induced depression reliably, experimental animals must have a smooth rather than convoluted cortex (Marshall, 1959). Fortunately, the rat and the rabbit, two of the most frequently used animals in behavioral research, meet this requirement. Second, behavioral studies demand that the animals be free to respond while under the influence of depression. To resolve this problem, several chronic preparations have been developed, all of which share the common feature of exposing the dura of the cortex through trephined openings located usually in the parietal-occipital area of the skull. Caution has been taken to hold the focus of stimulation constant in spite of the fact that Bures and Buresova (1960) found that conditioned responses were inhibited to the same degree, irrespective of whether depression was induced in cortical areas related or unrelated to either the conditioned stimulus or the conditioned response.

The major distinction among the preparations is the treatment of the incised scalp. In one case, the incision is closed with loose sutures (Bures, 1959); the disadvantage of this technique is the irritation that ensues upon reopening the wound. To avoid excessive irritation, subsequent preparations were designed to minimize contact with the wound. One procedure (Schneider & Behar, 1964) has employed a rubber grommet centered over the trephined openings and secured with sutures to the scalp; a second procedure has used either small plastic cups (Russell & Ochs, 1963) or polyethelene tubing (Tapp, 1962), holed at the base, fitted into the trephined openings and secured with dental cement to anchoring screws. In both preparations the exposed dura is kept moist between KCl treatments with either saline or Ringer solution. Although the two preparations were designed for long-term studies, their effectiveness is limited by bone regrowth and infection, both of which appear within 3 or 4 days after surgery (Ochs, 1966; Schneider & Ebbesen, 1967). Furthermore, recent histological work (Hamburg, Best, & Cholewiak, 1968) has shown that two or more applications of KCl to a single hemisphere induces lesions in the focal area exposed to

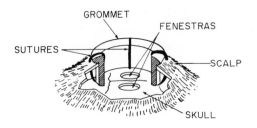

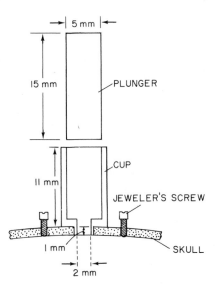

Fig. 8-2. The upper panel depicits the grommet preparation used by Schneider and Behar (1964); the lower panel depicts the cup preparation employed by Russell and Ochs (1963).

KCl. In light of these side effects, future studies using KCl-induced depression must incorporate histological verification of the degree of neural damage, limit the time between surgery and termination of the experiment to 3 or 4 days, and either limit the number of KCl exposures to one treatment per hemisphere, or equate the number of KCl exposures between groups.

III. THE BEHAVIORAL EFFECTS OF
SPREADING DEPRESSION

That depressed activity proliferates indiscriminately across the cortex of the stimulated hemisphere(s) introduces two behavioral spheres of influence, that of nonassociative and of associative processes. Within the behavioral framework, nonassociative factors constitute processes involved in detecting stimuli and executing responses; associative factors consist of processes, other than stimulus detection and response execution, that are involved in forming, storing, and subsequently triggering new relations between the stimulus and the response. We will first consider the effects of depression on nonassociative processes and then, to the extent that the behavioral analysis will permit, we will turn our attention to the effects of depression on associative processes. Finally, where possible, we will consider studies that cut across both analyses in an attempt to specify the degree to which the subcortex contributes to the behavioral effects of cortical depression.

A. Designs and Procedures

The framework within which we will evaluate the studies is based on the following working assumption: all behavior, whether conditioned or unconditioned, consists of both stimulus and response components. Therefore, differences in responding between depressed and normal animals can be a function of impairment in any one or combination of three factors: stimulus detection, response execution, and, in the case of conditioned responses, associative processes. To assess the degree to which these variables independently contribute to the total effect of depression on behavior, two experimental designs have been used: factorial analysis of nonassociative processes, and what we will term matched-group analysis of associative processes. Furthermore, since these designs have not been utilized to nearly the degree that is demanded by the complexity of subject matter, we will risk belaboring what may be obvious for some and consider the designs in detail; the factorial will be considered here and the matched group later, in connection with the associative analysis.

In a factorial-type analysis of the behavioral effects of cortical depression, one factor must be the state of the cortex, either depressed or normal. The other factor depends on the focus of interest: analysis of response execution, stimulus detection, or associative processes demands independent manipulation of response criteria (e.g., latency, amplitude), stimulus input (e.g., intensity), or conditioning criteria (e.g., number of correct responses), respectively. The scope of the design can range from two to four factors, and, even in the case of a complex four-way design, the factorial analysis (Edwards, 1968) permits assessment of the behavioral effects of depression relative to normal (cortical factor) as an independent as well as a joint function of variations in any one or combination of the three remaining factors.

The research that has taken the factorial approach to nonassociative problems has largely employed two-factor designs. Therefore, to illustrate the power of the design, we will consider a hypothetical two-way analysis of one of the pioneering behavioral observations made by Bures, Buresova, and Zahorova (1958): rats under bilateral depression have more difficulty than normals in learning to run from an electrified to a safe compartment (i.e., active avoidance). Let us suppose that we want to determine the degree to which inferior learning under bilateral depression is due to impaired stimulus detection or, more specifically, decreased shock sensitivity. To examine this problem we must go beyond the single-factor analysis of comparing behavior under depressed and normal states and introduce a second factor of shock intensity. If, for example, with increases in shock intensity the difference in avoidance between depressed and normal animals was (1) eliminated, then the disparity can be attributed to differential sensitivity, (2) decreased or increased, then the disparity is partially a function of differential sensitivity, (3) the same, then the disparity is not a function of shock sensitivity unless there is complete insensitivity under depression.

The factorial design, however, is not a panacea. The success of the design depends on the extent to which the factors are isolated, and since this problem is both crucial and perplexing, let us consider one of its more serious complications. In accord with the two-factor design, to analyze the effects of depression on response execution, responding under depressed and normal cortical conditions must be compared as a function of variations in response difficulty. However, variations in response difficulty are most assuredly accompanied by variations in response-produced stimuli such as kinesthetic feedback. Therefore, until more refined analyses are developed to separate the two factors, both response-execution and its accompanying stimuli must be treated as one.

In assessing the effects of depression on either associative or nonassociative processes there are two response systems, overt (i.e., skeletal and smooth muscle) or neural, that can be monitored as a function of depressed or normal cortex. We will consider only those studies that have used, at the very least, an overt measure. The reason for emphasis on overt behavior is twofold: First, comprehensive reviews of the neural effects of depression can be found elsewhere (Marshall, 1959; Ochs, 1962). Second, the validity of inferring behavioral states from neural activity is tenuous. For example, injection of atropine induces high voltage slow activity which characterizes electrophysiologically defined sleep, but does not impair overt responsiveness (Bradley & Elkes, 1953).

B. The Effects of Spreading Depression on Stimulus
Detection and Response Execution

Two behavioral procedures have been used to study the effects of depression on stimulus detection and response execution: an unconditioned response procedure in which the stimulus inherently controls the response; a conditioned response procedure in which the stimulus, through repeated associations with the response, acquires control of the response. The advantage of the unconditioned response procedure is that it can be used to study stimulus detection or response execution without the complications of associative factors; the disadvantage of the procedure is that it is limited to stimulus and response systems that are characterized by eliciting properties. The conditioned response procedure, on the other hand, is not limited to analysis of elicited-related systems but, conversely, is limited to analysis of conditioning-related systems. Specifically, since the conditioned-response analysis of nonassociative processes uses associative processes or, equivalently, the conditioned response as its dependent variable, the analysis hinges on the feasibility of conditioning animals under depression.

Unfortunately, research on the stimulus and response properties of depression is still in such a formative and fragmentary state that we have divided the nonassociative studies into two categories: (1) single-factor experiments that have compared responding of depressed and normal animals, have in some cases, because of their unconditioned response measures, observed nonassociative effects, but have not attempted to manipulate stimulus or response parameters independently; (2) two-factor experiments that have compared responding of depressed and normal animals as a function of variations in either stimulus or response parameters.

1. Single-Factor Experiments

There is a group of single-factor experiments that are probably as decisive as any two-factor experiments in analyzing nonassociative properties. Their effectiveness is in part due to the use of unconditioned response measures, ruling out associative contaminants, and in part a function of their response-oriented analysis, the type of data that is virtually impossible to refine into stimulus-response components with any experimental design.

Bures (1959) reported that bilateral depression impairs both the righting and placing reflex of rats, and Buresova, Bures, and Beran (1958) observed that unilateral depression impairs reaching for food with the paw contralateral to the depressed hemisphere. Furthermore, in accord with Bures' findings that bilateral depression interferes with postural reflexes, Tapp (1962) observed that bilaterally depressed rats were impaired in both their ability to avoid shock and to balance on a rotating stick as a direct function of the percentage of KCl. The data are clear: depression does indeed produce impairment of what generally can be considered coordination and posture-related processes. The interpretations are not clear: the depression-induced impairment may reflect interference with either the musculature and/or the sensory apparatus (e.g., visual, kinesthetic) for balance and coordination.

To further complicate these seemingly simple postural effects, the possibility of subcortical involvement has been intimated by recent observations of Koppman and O'Kelly (1966). Studying the effects of unilateral depression on choice responding in a T-maze, they found that unilaterally depressed rats turned toward the side of the maze that corresponded to the unimpaired limbs, irrespective of the location of the reward. According to Koppman and O'Kelly, this type of ipsilateral effect is difficult to explain in light of the more commonly observed contralateral turning that occurs with lesion-induced paresis. They further note a striking parallel between the ipsilateral effect obtained with depression and that obtained with caudate lesions (Jung & Hassler, 1960). This similarity, taken together with the fact that cortical depression is accompanied by depressed activity in the caudate (Bures & Buresova, 1962), suggests a possible connecting link between the concurrent effects of cortical depression on turning behavior and caudate activity. Unfortunately, as noted by Koppman and O'Kelly, this relationship is at best only suggestive, since Weiss and Fifkova (1963) have found no evidence of ipsilateral turning with direct depression of the caudate but, on the contrary, found contralateral turning. However, one possibility in need of further investigation is that the effects of cortical depression on caudate activity reproduce the neural as well as the behavioral effects of caudate lesions more closely than do the effects of direct depression of the caudate.

Using a modified unconditioned response-type analysis, Schneider and Ebbesen (1967) observed that unilateral depression reduced motor activity as measured by a decrease in pretraining lever pressing, and Freedman, Pote, Butcher, and Suboski (1968) observed that activity covaried with the shift in the steady potential during depression. Again, however, the interpretation is equivocal: reduced activity could be taken to reflect motor impairment and/or, for example, something as subtle as depression-induced fluctuations in body temperature (Buresova, 1957a).

Turning from the single-factor unconditioned to the single-factor conditioned response approach, two experiments that fall into this latter category share the common feature of monitoring unconditioned as well as conditioned responses. Although it is tempting in these experiments to equate interference of conditioned and unconditioned responses with associative and nonassociative effects, respectively, the equivalences simply do not hold.

Using a classical conditioning procedure in rabbits, Papsdorf, Longman, and Gormezano (1965) found that bilateral depression abolished an eyeblink previously conditioned to noise under normal cortical conditions but did not interfere with the unconditioned eyeblink to infra-orbital shock. That the unconditioned response remained intact clearly indicates that depression neither affects the stimulus nor the response properties of a shock-elicited eyeblink. On the other hand, that the conditioned response was interrupted can be taken to reflect interference with associative processes and/or with nonassociative processes such as auditory detection of the conditioned stimulus.

Employing a similar single-factor approach to the effects of depression on heart rate conditioning, Hendrickson and Pinto-Hamuy (1967) obtained virtually the same results as that of Papsdorf *et al.*, (1965). They found that bilateral depression abolished a decelerative heart-rate response previously conditioned to a light under normal cortical conditions but did not affect the unconditioned decelerative response to shock. On the basis of this single-factor approach, where neither an anatomical nor a nonassociative (e.g., visual detection of the conditioned stimulus) parameter is independently assessed, they arrived at the only possible conclusion: the cortex and/or the subcortex play(s) a role in the effects of depression on heart rate conditioning. On the basis of the unconditioned response data, however, it may be concluded that depression neither affected the stimulus nor the response properties of the unconditioned shock-elicited heart deceleration.

2. Two-Factor Unconditioned Response Experiments

Although the single-factor experiments, in particular those using an unconditioned response analysis, have served the important function of implicating nonassociative processes in the effects of depression on behavior, the two-factor experiment must be employed for an independent analysis of the effects of depression on stimulus detection and response execution. To recapitulate, the major distinction between what we have termed single and two-factor nonassociative experiments is that in the two-factor case a stimulus or response parameter is manipulated in addition to the cortical factor (i.e., state of depression).

Schneider (1965) attempted to determine the degree to which impairment in response execution contributed to the debilitating effects of cortical depression on water-intake. He used what may be considered a crude approximation of an unconditioned response two-factor analysis: one factor was the cortical state, depression or normal; the other factor was response difficulty defined in terms of the time allowed to drink. He found that water-deprived rats under unilateral depression consume water at a slower rate than normals but, given enough time, they consume the same amount as normals. That the difference between normal and depressed animals in water consumption was virtually eliminated as the time allowed for drinking increased or, equivalently, as response difficulty decreased, was taken as evidence that unilateral depression affects execution of the consummatory response. It should be emphasized, however, that the data offer no evidence for whether the response effect is cortically or hypothalamically induced.

Thompson and Enter (1967) used an unconditioned response two-factor procedure to assess shock sensitivity in depressed and normal rats. They employed a repeated measure design in which each rat was tested for shock sensitivity under bilateral depression, unilateral depression, and normal cortical conditions. The test consisted of subjecting the rats to shock intensities that varied randomly from 0 to 0.9 mA and observing the frequency of both a flinch and locomotor response at each intensity. Since the depression-shock relation with the flinch response was virtually the same as that with the locomotor response, we will consider only the locomotor data.

Under the three cortical conditions, the frequency of locomotor responses increased as shock intensity increased. Relative to normals, unilateral depression suppressed the locomotor response at shock intensities less than but not at or above 0.8 mA, and bilateral depression suppressed the locomotor response at intensities less than 0.9 mA, at which point frequency of responding approached the normal level. Thus, unilaterally depressed and normal animals have equivalent shock sensitivity at 0.8 mA, but not at lesser intensities, whereas the disparity in sensitivity between bilaterally depressed and normal animals begins to diminish at 0.9 mA.

These data have important implications for at least two types of depression-related research. First, with regard to analysis of associative processes, if shock values of less than 0.8 mA or 0.9 mA are employed in conditioning experiments and if animals under unilateral depression or bilateral depression are inferior to normals in avoidance, the disparity in responding may in part be due to the effects of depression on shock sensitivity. Fortunately, to this writer's knowledge, conditioning experiments comparing depressed and normal animals have not used shock intensities less than 0.8 mA. Second, this type of shock-sensitivity data provides a basis for assessing the response execution effects of depression independent of stimulus artifacts: responding under depressed and normal cortical conditions could be compared as a function of variations in the response criteria (e.g., degree of locomotion) to escape shock fixed at 0.9 mA.

3. Two-factor Conditioned Response Experiments

Although the unconditioned response two-factor procedure is ideally suited for independent analysis of the effects of depression on stimulus and response systems, as previously noted, the procedure is severely limited by the fact that it can only be used with stimuli that elicit discrete overt responses. Therefore, to broaden the spectrum of analysis, particularly with respect to stimulus detection, investigators have turned to the conditioned response procedure.

To assess the effects of depression on stimulus detection, three conditioned response-type procedures have been employed: generalization decrement, discrimination, and additivity-of-cues. Each procedure utilizes a different aspect of the conditioned stimulus-response relation to determine if, under spreading depression, the stimulus is detected or, equivalently, if it has gained control of the conditioned response. Two experiments, one using a generalization decrement and the other a discrimination approach, employed what may be termed a counter-type analysis. Each of these experiments arranged reinforcement contingencies such that if depression has stimulus-control properties, then greater responding was expected under depressed than under normal cortical conditions; this result is counter to the debilitating effects that would be expected if depression acted on associative and/or response processes. A third experiment used an additivity-of-cue approach in combination with the more conventional two-factor design.

Generalization decrement is characterized by the fact that if an animal learns to respond in the presence of a given set of stimuli, then, given that the stimuli are changed during testing, the strength of the conditioned response decreases with increases between the training and testing stimuli. With this as a working framework, Schneider (1966) reasoned that if depression has stimulus properties then, like any other stimulus, a change in the state of depression from training to testing should result in a decrement in the conditioned response, and the degree of decrement should be directly related to the degree of depression-induced stimulus change.

In his initial attempt to test the hypothesis, Schneider (1966) found that rats trained to actively avoid shock under unilateral depression showed significantly greater retention when tested under bilateral depression than animals trained normally and tested under bilateral depression. Unfortunately, it later (Schneider, 1967) became apparent that there were at least two explanations for these data: (1) depression is accompanied by stimuli and, as expected on the basis of stimulus control, these stimuli were more similar and thereby occasioned greater retention in the group trained under unilateral depression and tested under bilateral depression than in the group trained normally and tested under bilateral depression, and/or (2) during training the subcortex takes over storage for the depressed animals but not for the normals, thereby giving the animals trained under depression the advantage of subcortical storage when tested for retention under bilateral depression. Consistent with this second possibility, Carlson (1967) not only replicated the findings of Schneider (1966) but, with an additional control group, found that animals trained and tested under the same state of unilateral depression retained as well as those trained under unilateral depression and tested under bilateral depression. These results have serious implications for stimulus-control notions: they may be taken to indicate that unilateral and bilateral depression either have no stimulus-control properties or have stimulus properties that are virtually the same.

Accordingly, Schneider (1967) conducted a second experiment designed to examine stimulus relations other than unilateral and bilateral that may exist between cortical states during training and testing. Taking a lead from his earlier experiment, he held subcortical factors constant during training and varied only the stimulus conditions between training and testing by training animals under identical states of depression and testing them under different cortical states. Although this experiment consisted of five groups, consideration of three of these groups will suffice in clarifying the basic rationale and results. The three groups were trained under unilateral depression; one group was tested for retention with depression shifted to the opposite hemisphere, one group was tested with the cortex normal, and one group was tested with depression in the same hemisphere that was depressed during training. Since the three groups were trained under unilateral depression, cortical and subcortical conditioning should contribute equally to retention and, therefore, any difference among the groups in retention must be due to depression-induced stimulus change. In accord with stimulus-control expectations, animals trained and tested under the same state of unilateral depression retained more than animals trained under unilateral depression and tested normally, which in turn retained more than animals trained under one state of unilateral depression and tested under the opposite state. These data were taken to indicate not only that unilateral depression has stimulus-control properties different from those with the cortex normal, but that the difference in these properties was greater between opposite states of unilateral depression than between unilateral depression and normal cortical conditions.

To cross validate the generalization–decrement data, Schneider and Kay (1968) conducted a discrimination experiment. They reasoned that if stimuli available during unilateral depression are indeed different from those available during normal cortical conditions, then it should be possible to train rats to discriminate between normal and depressed conditions. Specifically, they gave rats discrimination training in which lever presses during unilateral depression were reinforced and lever presses during normal cortical conditions were not reinforced. To assess the degree to which responding was under the control of depression-produced cues independent of reinforcement, they gave each rat extinction sessions with the cortex first normal and then unilaterally depressed. Consistent with the stimulus-control prediction, responding showed the expected decrease with nondepression and increase with one hemisphere depressed.

These stimulus-detection experiments not only demonstrate that depression has stimulus-control properties but also resolve some of the perplexities of earlier findings. For example, Travis and Sparks (1963) found that animals trained under bilateral depression and tested normally were impaired more during the test than animals trained under unilateral depression and tested normally, which in turn were impaired more than those trained and tested under normal cortical conditions. Conversely, Bures (1959) and later Russell, Ross, and Strongman (1964) found that animals trained normally and tested under unilateral depression were impaired during the test relative to animals trained and tested normally. Impaired performance following the depression-to-normal transition in the Travis & Sparks experiment was taken to indicate that a reciprocal inhibitory process operated between the subcortex, which presumably mediated conditioning during bilateral depression, and the cortex, which was functional during testing. On the other hand, impaired performance following the normal-to-depression transition in the Bures and later in the Russell *et al.*, experiment was taken to indicate that spreading depression affects the cortical determinants of memory. However, reconsidering these interpretations in light of the stimulus-control data, one explanation may be appropriate for both types of training-test transitions: if the conditioned response is under the control of stimuli available during spreading depression, the impaired performance during the test noted in each of the three studies can simply be interpreted as due to generalization decrement.

There is an obvious gap in the stimulus detection data: given that depression does affect stimulus detection, the question remains, what detection systems are affected? There is an interesting but ad hoc interpretation (Schneider, 1967) of data reported by Ray and Emley (1964) that may bear on at least one of the stimulus-detection systems affected by depression. In this study, rats were trained in a T-maze, with the right hemisphere depressed, to respond right with light-on and left with light-off. Curiously, it was found that during a subsequent retention test with depression shifted to the left hemisphere, choice responding reversed: with light-on the animals responded left, and with light-off they responded right. To account for these data Schneider (1967) reasoned that if depression in the right hemisphere is accompanied by unique stimuli, such as kinesthetic feedback from paralysis in the left limbs, then the animals may be learning to respond away from the paralysis with light-on and toward the paralysis with light-off. Therefore, when depression is shifted to the left hemisphere and paralysis is shifted to the right limbs, the animals reverse their choice: with light-on they respond away from the paralysis which now corresponds to a left choice, and with light-off they respond toward the paralysis which now corresponds to a right choice.

What is needed to resolve the detection problem, however, are not ad hoc explanations but, rather, experiments which incorporate controllable stimuli (e.g., light, tone) into the stimulus-control procedures, arrange the reinforcement contingencies such that these stimuli gain control of the conditioned response under normal cortical conditions, and then compare the degree to which this control is maintained under normal and depressed conditions.

To achieve this type of detection analysis, Thompson and Hjelle (1965) employed an additivity-of-cue procedure, which is based on the premise that if cues are added to the warning stimulus in avoidance conditioning and if the cues are detected, then, within limits, avoidance behavior should improve. Specifically, Thompson and Hjelle observed avoidance behavior in bilaterally depressed and normal rats as a function of the number and type of avoidance cues that signalled the ensuing shock. They found in normal rats that avoidance behavior improved significantly if a buzzer was added to the raising of a guillotine door, but did not improve further if a light was added as a third cue. Relative to this avoidance behavior under normal cortical conditions, avoidance behavior under bilateral depression was uniformly inferior but changed to the same degree with variations in the preshock cues. Thus, that the addition of the buzzer to the guillotine-door cue had comparable facilitory effects on avoidance behavior under both bilateral depression and normal cortical conditions indicates that auditory sensitivity, at least at the intensity and pitch tested, was equivalent under both cortical states. On the other hand, since the addition of the light cue had no effect on either normal or depressed behavior, no conclusions could be drawn with regard to visual sensitivity. Furthermore, that depressed animals never reached the avoidance level of the normals indicates that some factor other than stimulus detection is contributing to the disparity.

Thompson and Hjelle (1965) conducted a second two-factor conditioned-response experiment to examine the effects of depression on response execution. In this experiment they held the warning signal (which consisted of raising the guillotine door) constant and observed avoidance behavior in bilaterally depressed and normal rats as a function of variations in response difficulty. Just as stimulus detection was defined in terms of changes in rate of conditioning in normal animals as a function of adding cues, response difficulty was defined in terms of changes in rate of conditioning in normal animals as a function of adding response demands. The response that was the least difficult to learn was a one-way avoidance in which, following either an escape or avoidance response, the animals were returned to the original shock compartment for the next trial; the response that was moderately difficult to learn consisted of a two-way avoidance in which, following either an escape or avoidance response, the animals were picked up and were returned to the compartment that was safe on that trial but that was electrified on the next trial; the response that was most difficult to learn was a shuttle avoidance which was identical to the two-way avoidance except that the animals were not picked up between trials.

Relative to the avoidance behavior under normal cortical conditions, avoidance under bilateral depression was uniformly inferior at each response level. Similar to the normal animals, the bilaterally depressed animals had the most difficulty in learning the shuttle response; however, in contrast to the normals, the bilaterally depressed animals were equally facile in learning the one-way and two-way responses. This is a rather striking finding: apparently the transition from a one-way to a two-way response created less difficulty for bilaterally depressed than normal animals. Thompson and Hjelle raise an interesting explanation for this disparity that not only bears on their specific data but has significant implications for response analysis in general. They note that because normal animals are more active, they are more subject to competing responses than depressed animals, thereby putting them at a disadvantage in procedures, such as the two-way response, where competing responses may be a source of interference. However, if normal animals are at a disadvantage where inactivity is required, then depressed animals may be at a similar disadvantage where activity is required; this possibility may account for the impaired learning under bilaterai depression that Thompson and Hjelle (1965) observed in even the simplest one-way avoidance. Consistent with this hypothesis, Schneider (1966) found that unilaterally depressed animals relative to normals were impaired in a one-way active avoidance task but were not impaired in a passive-avoidance task (Schneider, 1967) where activity is not an advantage. Thus, that the difference in avoidance behavior between normal and unilaterally depressed rats is eliminated as response demands are decreased provides compelling evidence that the disparity in avoidance behavior is a function of the effects of depression on response execution. This conclusion, however, must be considered tentative since it is based on data from two independent studies that may have varied on parameters other than response difficulty.

Just as the generalization-decrement data resolved disparities in the extant retention data, the stimulus and response analyses of Thompson and Hjelle have a similar impact on the disparities in the extant conditioning data. Specifically, it is clear from their analyses that learning an active–avoidance response under bilateral depression improves with decreases in response difficulty and with increases in saliency (e.g., auditory cues) of the warning stimulus. As Thompson and Hjelle note, these observations may account for the fact that avoidance conditioning under bilateral depression was poor in studies (Bures, 1959; Travis & Sparks, 1963) that used the simple one-way response without salient auditory cues, and in studies (Bures et al., 1958; Tapp, 1962) that used salient auditory cues without the simple one-way response, but was not poor in the two studies (Thompson, 1964; Thompson & Hjelle, 1965) that combined the simple one-way response with the salient auditory cues.

C. The Effects of Spreading Depression on Associative Processes

Although the nonassociative analysis is still in a formative stage, it provides the guidelines for analysis of the associative effects of depression. The nonassociative data suggest that the disparity in avoidance behavior between depressed and normal animals during training and during testing may be a joint function of the effects of depression on stimulus detection and response execution. These nonassociative effects, however, may be confounded by a subtle associative variable. Specifically, the debilitating effects of depression on conditioning are more apparent with difficult than easy conditioning tasks; if easy tasks are associatively processed in the subcortex (i.e., areas not affected by cortical depression) and if difficult tasks are associatively processed in the cortex (i.e., areas affected by cortical depression), then, on the basis of this differential associative involvement, cortical depression may indeed interfere more with associative processing of difficult than easy tasks. Two groups of experimental findings tend to rule out this possibility. First, passive-avoidance conditioning, a procedure characterized by a simple response and rapid conditioning, has been shown to be associatively mediated by areas subject to cortical depression; Bures and Buresova (1963) and more recently Pearlman (1966) and Schneider (1967) have independently shown that bilateral cortical depression administered after normal passive-avoidance training produces retrograde amnesia. Second, the difficult, and thereby presumably the cortically-mediated, active avoidance is associatively processed under cortical depression. Bilaterally depressed rats can learn an active avoidance (Thompson, 1964; Thompson and Hjelle, 1965) and, in cases where the active avoidance was too difficult to perform under bilateral depression, Kukleta (1966) has shown that associative processes must have operated, since in a later relearning test under unilateral depression the animals that received training under bilateral depression showed savings relative to nontrained controls.

1. Design and Procedure

It is premature to pass judgment on the associative effects of depression solely on the basis of these conditioning data. Associative processes operate after as well as during conditioning and, therefore, may be affected differentially as a function of when depression is introduced into the conditioning-retention complex. Accordingly, in the following section we will systematically examine the associative effects of depression during training, after training but before testing (posttraining effects), and during testing.

The nonassociative effects of depression dictate that associatively directed experiments use two types of control measures to match depressed and normal animals on stimulus detection and response execution: first, to eliminate stimulus-control contaminants, each animal should be trained and tested under the same cortical state or, if the nature of the problem calls for a shift in cortical state from training to testing, control groups must be employed to independently assess the effects of stimulus change. Second, to eliminate response-execution bias when comparing normal and depressed animals during training or testing, the conditioning task should have minimal motor requirements, such as the passive-avoidance response which requires that animals refrain from responding to avoid shock.

2. Associative Effects of Posttraining Depression

We will consider the posttraining effects of depression first, since they provide the basis for experimental designs used to determine the associative effects of depression during training and testing.

As noted earlier, animals trained and tested normally in a passive-avoidance task show retrograde amnesia if bilateral depression is administered after training. That posttraining depression induces amnesia in animals that are trained and tested under normal cortical conditions rules out the possibility of nonassociative performance effects and provides an unambiguous way of using depression to study such associative processes as memory consolidation.

Similar to other agents that have posttraining amnesic effects (e.g., electroconvulsive shock), the degree of depression-induced amnesia varies inversely with the training-treatment interval. The data are, however, discrepant regarding the length of the training-treatment interval in which depression must be administered to produce amnesia. According to Bures and Buresova (1963) a two-hour interval is sufficient; according to Pearlman (1966) ten minutes is the limit. Curiously, both claims are probably accurate; the duration of depression in the Pearlman and the Bures and Buresova studies was approximately ten minutes and several hours, respectively, and on the basis of recent data (Avis & Carlton, 1968) indicating that the degree of retrograde amnesia varies directly with duration of depression, it is not surprising that Pearlman's amnesia gradient was steeper than that of Bures and Buresova.

Turning from bilateral to unilateral posttraining effects, Schneider, Advokat, Kapp, and Sherman (1969) found that animals trained and tested normally in a passive-avoidance task showed partial amnesia (i.e., greater retention than nontrained controls but less retention than trained nondepressed controls) if a single hemisphere was depressed one or three minutes after training but showed no amnesia if the single hemisphere was depressed fifteen minutes or two hours after training. These data were taken to indicate that unilateral depression not only has associative effects but, since the retrograde amnesic effect was partial, that the associative effects were limited to a single hemisphere.

Although at the behavioral level the retrograde amnesic effects of cortical depression may be taken as an indication of associative interference, at the anatomical level the locus of interference is an open question. Specifically, as noted earlier, with more refined analyses of electrophysiological effects, it has become apparent that cortical depression is accompanied by depressed activity in a number of subcortical areas. Because of the extensive anatomical effects of cortical depression together with the dearth of research on the behavioral-anatomical relations, caution must be taken to attribute the retrograde amnesic effects, until otherwise disproven, to all areas subject to cortical depression. This nonspecific approach, however, can be partially qualified on the basis of recent data reported by Kupfermann (1966). Specifically, among its subcortical effects, cortical depression is accompanied by depressed activity in the amygdala (Fifkova & Syka, 1964). This taken together with the fact that the amygdala is involved in associative processes during aversive conditioning (Goddard, 1964; Kesner & Doty, 1968), raises the possibility that the retrograde amnesic effects obtained with cortical depression reflect interference with amygdala rather than cortical activity. In an attempt to resolve this problem, Kupfermann (1966) surgically separated the amygdala from the cortex and found that although the sectioning procedure was successful in preventing depression of the amygdala, it was not sufficient to prevent retrograde amnesia. Thus, the amnesic effects of posttraining cortical depression do not reflect the effects of depression on amygdaloid structures.

3. Associative Effects of Depression during Training

Two types of data indicate that associative processes operate during conditioning under depression. First, rats can learn to avoid shock actively under bilateral depression (Thompson, 1964; Thompson & Hjelle, 1965; Kukleta, 1966). Second, rats trained with one hemisphere depressed to avoid shock passively (Bures, Buresova, & Fifkova, 1964) or to lever press for water (Schneider & Ebbesen, 1967) show retention with the opposite hemisphere depressed; furthermore, retention in the passive-avoidance case occurred irrespective of whether or not the corpus callosum was intact, thereby ruling out the possibility of interhemispheric transfer.

These data, however, do not preclude the possibility that associative processes operate differently under depressed than under normal conditions. For example, as a working hypothesis suppose that cortical depression does indeed impair associative processes in the cortex but, in doing so, it forces other neural areas that normally do not participate in the associative process to assume the associative burden from the inactivated structures. To examine this hypothesis, Schneider (1967) first determined the locus of association of a passive-avoidance response under normal cortical conditions. He trained animals normally, bilaterally depressed them immediately after training, and tested them normally 24 hours later. Consistent with earlier reports (Bures & Buresova, 1963; Pearlman, 1966) he found total amnesia and, on this basis, concluded that during training under normal cortical conditions the cortex of both hemispheres or, more specifically, neural structures that can subsequently be affected by posttraining cortical depression, participate in the associative process. Schneider then proceeded to examine the retrograde amnesic effect of bilateral depression following training under unilateral depression. Moreover, because he trained the animals with one hemisphere depressed, he tested the animals with the same hemisphere depressed to avoid the contaminating effects of generalization decrement. In contrast to the total loss in retention observed when bilateral depression was administered to animals trained normally, partial retention was obtained when bilateral depression was administered to animals trained under unilateral depression. In accord with the relocalization-of-function hypothesis, Schneider took the partial retention to indicate that (1) during training under unilateral depression the cortex of the normal hemisphere (i.e., neural areas susceptible to the effects of posttraining cortical depression) and the subcortex of the depressed hemisphere (i.e., neural areas resistant to the effects of posttraining cortical depression) participate in the associative process, and (2) during posttraining bilateral depression the associative process in the subcortex (i.e., resistant areas) remains operative.

Although these data taken together with those considered earlier of Schneider (1966) and Carlson (1967) provide cogent evidence that associative processes under depression occur in areas different from those involved with the cortex normal, the data reveal nothing about the locus of the compensatory mechanism. The first step in determining the locus should be directed toward neural areas that are free from disruption during cortical depression (Carlson, 1967). Using this approach, Freedman *et al.* (1968) found that conditioning was significantly facilitated under bilateral cortical depression if training trials were delivered between rather than during the steady potential shift that accompanies cortical depression. These data are crucial in at least two respects: first, they demonstrate that electrical shifts in the cortex are reliable indices of neural susceptibility to associations; second, they identify the compensatory mechanism as either the cortex and/or structures, for example, the tegmentum (Weiss, 1961), that undergo electrical shifts concomitant with those in the cortex.

4. Associative Effects of Depression during Testing

If, during training under unilateral depression, associative processes operate in the subcortex of the depressed hemisphere and the cortex of the normal hemisphere, then during testing with depression shifted to the hemisphere that was functional during training, the memory stored in the subcortex of the originally depressed hemisphere should maintain retention. Retention has been observed in some cases (Bures, Buresova, & Fifkova, 1964; Schneider, 1967; Schneider & Ebbesen, 1967) but not in others (Bures, 1959), and the degree to which it occurs is inversely related to the response demands of the training task. To account for the covariation between retention and response demands, Schneider (1967) employed a generalization-decrement explanation. First, the shift in depression from training to testing induces a stimulus change which, during subsequent testing, demands that the animal emit the conditioned response in the presence of new stimuli to which the response was not conditioned. Second, the depression-related stimuli are, at least in part, kinesthetic in nature, an assumption based on depression-induced paresis; therefore, as the response demands of the task decrease, stimulus control by kinesthetic feedback and the resultant generalization decrement also decrease.

Given that depression-induced stimulus change can interfere with retention, the question remains: What effect does depression during the test have on the memory that was stored in the functional hemisphere during training? It is possible that depression during testing has a twofold effect: (1) stimulus effects that induce generalization decrement and thereby nullify the effect of the subcortical storage in the hemisphere depressed during training and (2) associative effects that inactivate the memory stored in the hemisphere functional during training.

Schneider *et al.* (1969), have attempted to assess the effects of unilateral depression during testing on associative processes independent of stimulus change. Two groups of rats were trained under normal cortical conditions and were tested under unilateral depression; thus, any stimulus change induced by the shift from normal cortex to unilateral depression was held constant between the groups. Furthermore, to assure that both groups entered the final test with storage in one hemisphere, each group was also depressed in a single hemisphere three minutes after training; this posttraining manipulation was based on the earlier posttraining finding (Schneider *et al.*, 1969) that unilateral depression administered three minutes after training interferes with unilateral storage. The independent variable was introduced during the test; Group S (S-storage) was tested with depression in the storage hemisphere (i.e., the hemisphere that was functional three minutes after training); Group NS (NS-nonstorage) was tested with depression in the nonstorage hemisphere (i.e., the hemisphere that was depressed three minutes after training). If depression during testing interferes with storage independent of stimulus change, then Group S should show less retention than Group NS, and indeed this is precisely what was observed.

IV. APPLICATIONS OF THE TECHNIQUE
OF SPREADING DEPRESSION

It should be made clear that although we have attempted to follow the maxim that analysis precede application, this has not been the case in practice. Accordingly, the initial interpretations of the interhemispheric transfer data reviewed in this applied section were based on incomplete tests of the associative assumptions and, thereby, in light of the more recent analyses, come under extensive revision here.

A. The Use of Spreading Cortical Depression
to Study Interhemispheric Memory Transfer

The interest in using spreading depression to study interhemispheric relations derives from the fact that if one accepts the notion that unilateral depression abolishes associative processes in one hemisphere during training and in the other hemisphere during testing, then, because of the reversible nature of depression, one can accomplish an analysis of interhemispheric memory transfer that cannot otherwise be achieved. Specifically, to determine if memory can transfer from one hemisphere to the other, one must first confine memory to a single hemisphere. Sperry (1964) and his coworkers have accomplished this by sectioning the corpus callosum and optic chiasm and training monkeys with one eye occluded. The major disadvantage of this procedure is that sectioning the corpus callosum precludes the possibility of studying its subsequent transfer properties. Therefore, what is needed is a technique by which memory can be confined to one hemisphere without permanent damage to either the interhemispheric tracts or to the other hemisphere. At the neural level, the reversible property of spreading depression meets these demands. At the behavioral level, spreading depression can be used to confine memory to a single hemisphere, but the solution to the problem, although simple, was not apparent until complications with the prevailing procedure were revealed. In the following analysis of the interhemispheric transfer data, we will use the associative and nonassociative analyses first to reevaluate the existing data and then to guide our choice in design and procedure for future interhemispheric work.

Bures (1959) was the first to recognize the possibility of using depression to study interhemispheric memory transfer. He found that rats could learn an active avoidance with one hemisphere functional and one hemisphere depressed, could not retain the avoidance when tested with depression shifted to the hemisphere functional during training, but could retain the avoidance when tested with depression shifted back to the hemisphere depressed during training. On the basis of these data, he concluded that memory must be confined to the functional hemisphere during training since only depression of that hemisphere during testing was sufficient to abolish retention.

With these data as a basis, Bures (1959) used an active-avoidance task and later Russell and Ochs (1963) used an appetitive lever-press task to study interhemispheric transfer. The findings of both experiments were virtually the same: animals trained with one hemisphere depressed had to be given one (Russell & Ochs, 1963) or ten (Bures, 1959) training trials with neither hemisphere depressed (interdepression training) in order to show later retention with the opposite hemisphere depressed. The interpretations were also in agreement: interdepression training serves to "provoke" the memory to transfer to the nontrained hemisphere.

The source of the problem with the confinement and transfer interpretations can be traced to the basic assumption that absence of retention following the shift in depression from one hemisphere during training to the opposite hemisphere during testing indicates that: (1) depression of a single hemisphere during training prevents storage in that hemisphere and (2) depression of the opposite hemisphere during testing inactivates storage in that hemisphere.

On the basis of the more recent associative and nonassociative analyses, it is clear that these assumptions are, at best, tenuous: depression of one hemisphere during training does not prevent associative processes from operating in that hemisphere; depression of the opposite hemisphere during testing both inactivates associative processes in that hemisphere as well as induces generalization decrement. Furthermore, it is the generalization-decrement effect that may provide the clue to explaining the function of interdepression training. Specifically, if the absence of retention following a shift in unilateral depression from training to testing reflects generalization decrement, then the presence of retention following interdepression training may be due to a process that promotes rather than impedes generalization, namely stimulus generalization.

According to this stimulus-control interpretation of confinement and transfer, the degree of generalization decrement between opposite states of unilateral depression should determine the stimulus generalization role of inter-depression training. If you will recall, however, generalization decrement covaries with the response demands of the task. Therefore, we will consider the role of interdepression training in terms of the response demands of the training procedures.

In those procedures such as passive avoidance and lever pressing, in which response demands and thereby kinesthetic stimulus control is minimal, retention generalizes between opposite states of unilateral depression without interdepression training. Therefore, interdepression training should serve only to strengthen the generalized response. Consistent with this interpretation, Schneider and Ebbesen (1967) found that following lever-press training under unilateral depression (1) a single reinforcement of the first lever press emitted during testing with the opposite hemisphere depressed was sufficient to increase subsequent lever pressing under extinction, and (2) responding during test conditions increased more when the single reinforcement was delivered under the unilateral state that prevailed during subsequent testing than when it was delivered under the more conventional normal cortical state. This latter result is particularly compelling since, in accord with the stimulus-generalization hypothesis, it indicates that the strength of test responding varies as a direct function of the degree of similarity between the states of the cortex that prevail during the single reinforcement and later test conditions.

In procedures such as the active avoidance in which response demands and thereby kinesthetic stimulus control is maximal, retention does not generalize between opposite states of unilateral depression unless interdepression training is given. In this case, according to a stimulus-control interpretation, it is assumed that interdepression training under normal cortical conditions serves to mediate generalization between opposite states of unilateral depression that are otherwise too disparate in their stimulus properties to permit generalization. Implicit within this assumption is that stimulus properties under unilateral depression are more similar to those with the cortex normal than to those under the opposite state of unilateral depression. If you will recall, there is an empirical basis for this continuum of stimulus similarity: Schneider (1967) found greater generalization of retention in animals trained under unilateral depression and tested normally than in animals trained and tested under opposite states of unilateral depression. Based on these data, the interhemispheric paradigm with active-avoidance training is interpreted as follows: the response conditioned during initial unilateral training generalizes from the unilateral state during training to the normal cortical conditions during interdepression training; the conditioned response under normal cortical conditions is then reinforced and strengthened over the course of ten training trials (Bures, 1959); the conditioned response generalizes from the normal cortical conditions during interdepression training to the unilateral state during testing.

With regard to the active-avoidance procedure, although the stimulus-control theory contends that interdepression training mediates stimulus generalization and the memory-transfer theory claims that interdepression training "provokes" interhemispheric transfer, the two theories are difficult to distinguish because both posit that training with neither hemisphere depressed is necessary for subsequent transfer. This dilemma, however, is more apparent than real. The crux of the memory-transfer theory is based on the assumption that depression abolishes storage of the active-avoidance response in the treated hemisphere during initial unilateral training and, as described earlier, Thompson (1964) and Kukleta (1966) have shown that storage of the active-avoidance response does indeed occur with the cortex depressed.

Despite the explanatory, integrating, and predictive powers of the stimulus-control approach to interhemispheric transfer, there is one experiment (Albert, 1966) that some claim (Squire & Liss, 1968) defies explanation by any hypothesis other than memory transfer. Before passing judgment, however, let us first briefly consider the experiment and then compare the memory-transfer interpretation with an explanation derived from a stimulus-control analysis.

Albert trained rats to avoid shock actively with one hemisphere depressed and one hemisphere normal, returned them to their home cage or permitted them a single interdepression trial with neither hemisphere depressed, and then tested them for retention with depression shifted to the opposite hemisphere. Consistent with earlier reports, Albert found that only those animals that received interdepression training showed subsequent retention during the test under unilateral depression.

In accordance with a memory transfer position, Albert took the data to indicate that the interdepression trial "provoked" memory transfer, and with this as a working basis he proceeded to track the temporal course of transfer. To accomplish this he repeated the transfer procedure but depressed either the trained (transmitting) or nontrained (receiving) hemisphere at varied times after the single interdepression trial. Although he found that depression of the transmitting hemisphere after the single interdepression trial did not produce total amnesia during the final test, the fact that it did produce partial amnesia when administered thirty seconds or one minute but not when administered three minutes after interdepression training, led him to conclude that the memory trace must be released by the transmitting hemisphere within the first few minutes after the interdepression trial. On the other hand, he found that depression of the receiving hemisphere when administered up to but not beyond two hours after the interdepression trial produced total amnesia during the final test and interpreted these data to indicate that it took two hours for the receiving hemisphere to consolidate the transferred trace.

The problem with this interpretation can best be illustrated by considering how well the transfer theory would have survived had either of two other possible results occurred. First, suppose the time parameter was reversed and depression of the transmitting hemisphere was effective in producing amnesia up to two hours and depression of the receiving hemisphere was effective up to one minute after interdepression training; these results may have been taken to indicate that only the first one minute "bit" of information must be received to complete the transfer, given that no partial competing information was left in the transmitting hemisphere. Second, suppose there was no difference between the time interval in which the two hemispheres had to be depressed to produce amnesia; these results may have been taken to indicate that all the information must be transmitted for transfer to occur, and the rate of transmission is equal to the rate of reception. Thus, what we in fact have in the transfer interpretation of Albert's data is a theory that accounts for everything, and thereby accounts for nothing.

On the other hand, when we reduce Albert's experiment to a basic stimulus-control interpretation, the data, in large part, can be accounted for on the basis of the documented associative and nonassociative effects of depression. To evaluate Albert's results in terms of the behavioral analysis, we must assume that initial unilateral training serves only to facilitate conditioning during interdepression training, and that interdepression training consists of nothing more than a learning trial under normal cortical conditions. Taken within this framework, the critical aspects of Albert's experiment consist of (1) giving normal animals a single training trial, the learning during which is facilitated by initial unilateral training, (2) depressing one hemisphere at varied times after the single training trial, and (3) depressing either the same (analogous to Albert's transmitting condition) or opposite (analogous to Albert's receiving condition) hemisphere during testing.

On the basis of the associative and nonassociative effects of depression, given that animals are trained normally or, equivalently, receive interdepression training, we can interpret Albert's results as follows: In accord with Albert's "transmitting" condition, depression of a single hemisphere within one minute after training inactivates storage in that hemisphere, depression of the same hemisphere during testing is accompanied by generalization decrement, and generalization decrement taken together with unilateral storage accounts for Albert's partial amnesic effect. In accord with Albert's receiving condition, depression of a single hemisphere within one minute after training inactivates storage in that hemisphere, depression of the opposite hemisphere during testing inactivates storage in that hemisphere, and the total absence of storage accounts for Albert's total amnesic effect.

There is one aspect of Albert's data that as yet cannot be accounted for by the associative effects of posttraining and test depression. If you will recall, in Albert's "receiving" condition total amnesia was induced by depressing one hemisphere as much as two hours after training and depressing the opposite hemisphere during testing. According to the posttraining data (Schneider *et al.*, 1969), depression of a single hemisphere two hours after training should not interfere with associative processes. Therefore, storage in that hemisphere should be operative during the test and depression of the opposite hemisphere during the test, although inactivating storage and inducing generalization decrement, should not be sufficient to produce total amnesia. However, there are several possible empirical reasons for this disparity [e.g., Albert, (1966) used active-avoidance training and Schneider *et al.*, (1969) used passive-avoidance training] and hopefully the issue will be resolved by data not speculation.

From this analysis of the interhemispheric research, it seems clear that experiments which employ the strategy of training animals under one state of unilateral depression and testing them under the opposite state are not adequately designed to obtain memory confinement. There may, however, be an alternative design that is appropriate. This design was considered in a different context in our earlier analysis of the associative effects of depression, but we purposely postponed considering its implications for memory confinement until the reader was familiar with the shortcomings of the traditional approach.

The key to obtaining memory confinement is to introduce unilateral depression after, rather than during, training. Specifically, depression of a single hemisphere during training displaces storage to subcortical areas in that hemisphere (Schneider, 1967); depression of a single hemisphere immediately after normal training interferes with unilateral associative processes triggered in that hemisphere during normal training (Schneider *et al.*, 1969). Hopefully this posttraining depression approach, where displacement of storage accompanying training under unilateral depression is avoided and generalization decrement accompanying the shift from normal training to unilateral testing can be independently assessed, will provide a basis for future analysis of interhemispheric relations.

B. The Effects of Spreading Cortical Depression on Hypothalamic-Controlled Behavior

During bilateral cortical depression, at the neural level there is a pronounced decrease in lateral hypothalamic activity (Weiss & Fifkova, 1961), and at the behavioral level there is a cessation in lever pressing for electrical stimulation of the lateral hypothalamus (Bures *et al.*, 1961), in drinking (Buresova, 1957b; Schneider, 1965) and in water excretion (Buresova, 1957b). That cortical depression is accompanied by such extensive hypothalamic effects has provided the basis for two types of research: that concerned with partialling out the degree to which the hypothalamic effects influence behavior under cortical depression and that concerned with using the hypothalamic effects to study hypothalamic-controlled behavior.

Perplexed by the undefined anatomical effects of cortical depression, Rudiger and Fifkova (1963) attempted to determine whether suppression of intracranial self-stimulation of the lateral hypothalamus during bilateral spreading depression was due to depressed cortical activity, depressed hypothalamic activity, or both. The rationale for their design was based on the following data: conditioned avoidance responses are suppressed equally by cortical depression of either hemisphere (Buresova, Bures, & Beran, 1958), whereas unilateral cellular activity in the hypothalamus is depressed more by cortical depression elicited in the ipsilateral than in the contralateral hemisphere (Bures *et al.*, 1961). On this basis, they reasoned that if cessation of self-stimulation during cortical depression is due to depression of hypothalamic activity rather than depression of cortical activity, the lever press rate for self-stimulation under unilateral depression should depend on the relationship, ipsilateral or contralateral, between the depressed hemisphere and the electrode site. Consistent with this prediction, and thus implicating hypothalamic factors in the response suppression, Rudiger and Fifkova (1963) found that depression in the hemisphere ipsilateral to the electrode site produced a greater suppression in lever-press rate than depression in the hemisphere contralateral to the site; ipsilateral depression resulted in responding at 37.2 percent of the control rate and contralateral depression resulted in responding at 64.9 percent of the control rate. From these results, it seems clear that, at least in the case of self-stimulation, part of the response decrement produced by spreading depression is due to impairment of hypothalamic activity. However, that contralateral depression also decreased response rate suggests that impaired cortical processes may also be involved. It is encouraging to note that Rudiger and Fifkova's findings with artificial electrical stimulation of the hypothalamus have been substantiated with more natural hypothalamically-controlled eating responses. Koppman and O'Kelly (1966) found that unilateral depression impaired eating with the side of the mouth ipsilateral but not contralateral to the depressed hemisphere. The absence of independent stimulus or response manipulations in both studies, however, makes it impossible to go beyond anatomical implications.

In contrast to the Rudiger and Fifkova study, Teitelbaum and Cytawa (1965) reversed the strategy and used the subcortical effects of cortical depression to study recovery-of-function following hypothalamic lesions. Teitelbaum and Stellar (1954) have found that although bilateral lesions placed in the lateral hypothalamus produce aphagia and adipsia, if the animals are given tube-feeding, both eating and drinking gradually recover. Furthermore,

Teitelbaum and Epstein (1962) have shown that the tissue adjacent to the lesion plays a critical role in recovery since, upon its removal, aphagia and adipsia reappear. Therefore, to account for the gradual recovery, Teitelbaum and Cytawa (1965) proposed that depressed activity is surgically-induced in the tissue adjacent to the lesion and as this depression slowly dissipates its aphagic and adipsic effects diminish. If dissipation of depressed activity in the lesion site is the source of the recovery and if cortical depression is accompanied by depressed activity in lateral hypothalamus, which it indeed is (Bures *et al.*, 1963), then depression of the cortex in rats that recover from the effects of the lesion should reinstate aphagia and adipsia. Consistent with this hypothesis, Teitelbaum and Cytawa found that cortical depression administered to lateral hypothalamic rats, after they had recovered feeding and drinking, reinstated aphagia and adipsia for at least three days after depression. Furthermore, to confirm the generality of the effect, Teitelbaum and Cytawa cortically depressed septal animals after they had recovered from hyperemotionality and found that the hyperemotionality was reinstated for as long as two weeks after depression. These data are puzzling in one major respect: since cortical depression lasts for only a few hours, it is difficult to understand why the adipsia and the aphagia persisted for at least three days, and the hyperemotionality for two weeks. Teitelbaum and Cytawa raise two possible explanations for this disparity, both of which are in need of further investigation: (1) recovery from cortical spreading depression may not be as rapid as generally thought; (2) recovery of hypothalamic and septal activity may be slow, especially in animals that have neural deficits. In addition to these problems, it should be emphasized that although Teitelbaum and Cytawa's data clearly indicate that behavioral effects ordinarily produced by subcortical lesions can be reproduced by cortical depression, the data, at best, are only suggestive regarding the anatomical locus of the effect.

C. Nonassociative and Associative
Effects of Hippocampal Depression

Thus far, depending upon the focus of interest, both the cortical and subcortical neural effects of depression have been treated as surplus factors that severely limit the implications that cortical depression may have for anatomical-behavioral relations. There are, however, at least two studies that have circumvented the nonspecific anatomical effects of cortical depression by inducing depression directly in the hippocampus, an area from which depression does not proliferate (Weiss & Fifkova, 1961).

Although the anatomical analysis now shifts to a different level, the behavioral problems remain the same. The nonassociative and associative properties of hippocampal depression, similar to those of cortical depression, may vary as a function of when the hippocampus is depressed during the condition-

ing-retention complex. Fortunately, there are sufficient data to assess systematically the nonassociative and associative effects of hippocampal depression during
training, after training but before testing (posttraining), and during testing.

1. The Effects of Hippocampal Depression during Training and Testing

To distinguish between associative and nonassociative effects of hippocampal depression, Grossman and Mountford (1964) used an instrumental conditioning analogue to the Papsdorf *et al.* (1965) classical conditioning approach of
monitoring the effects of depression on conditioned and unconditioned responses. Specifically, Grossman and Mountford trained and tested rats under
bilateral hippocampal depression on a black-white discrimination in a T maze.
To distinguish between the associative and nonassociative effects, they monitored latency of responses, presumed to be a nonassociative measure, and
percent of correct choices, presumed to be an associative measure. Grossman and
Mountford found that hippocampal depression, relative to normal, impaired
nonassociative processes, as measured by increased latencies, but did not affect
associative processes, as measured by percent correct choice. Thus, there is a
striking similarity between the behavioral effects of cortical and hippocampal
depression at least during training: in both cases impaired behavior under
depression reflects interference with nonassociative rather than associative processes. However, since the Grossman and Mountford analysis consists of a
single-factor design (i.e., depressed versus normal hippocampus), it is impossible
to determine the degree to which interference with stimulus detection and
response execution contributed to the nonassociative effects of hippocampal
depression.

2. Posttraining Effects of Hippocampal Depression

Administering depression after training but before testing to the hippocampus offers the same advantage as that with cortical depression: the reversible
properties of depression assure that animals are trained and tested under normal
neural conditions and, therefore, any subsequent impairment of behavior during
the test must reflect posttraining interference with associative processes.

Avis and Carlton (1968) found that depression administered bilaterally to
the hippocampus twenty-four hours after normal passive-avoidance training,
induced amnesia four days after treatment with depression. The parallel between
cortical and hippocampal effects is again striking: in both cases posttraining
depression apparently interferes with associative processes. Furthermore, the
long-term (twenty-four-hour) effect of depression in the hippocampus when
taken together with the short-term (two-hour) effect of depression in the cortex
(Bures & Buresova, 1963), has significant implications for the conceptualization
of the neural distinction between short and long-term memory. Specifically, that
short compared with long-term memory is more sensitive to interference by such

agents as electroconvulsive shock or bilateral cortical depression has traditionally been taken as evidence that, depending on their age, memories are encoded differentially in the nervous system. Some investigators (e.g., Hebb, 1949) have speculated that the code is electro-chemical in nature: short-term memories encoded electrically and long-term memories encoded biochemically. The temporal disparity in the amnesic effects of cortical and hippocampal depression raises the possibility that short- and long-term memory may also be distinguished on the basis of anatomical locus. However, because this speculation is derived from comparing the effects of two independent studies and because Hughes (1969) has recently reported that the amnesic effects of hippocampal depression are not permanent (i.e., amnesia occurred if retention were tested four days, but not if it were tested twenty-one days after depression), further investigation of the behavioral distinction between posttraining hippocampal and cortical depression is urgently needed.

V. CONCLUSION

The conceptual and methodological issues considered in this chapter are not unique to spreading depression. That conditioned behavior is a composite of nonassociative and associative processes demands a two-dimensional analysis, no matter what the neural manipulation. Accordingly, the main thrust of the present chapter has been to partition the behavioral effects of spreading depression between nonassociative and associative processes. Hopefully this approach has served, at the very least, a twofold purpose: first, to specify the experimental design, namely posttraining depression, most appropriate for independently studying associative processes; second, to define the potentials and limitations of the technique for studying anatomical-behavioral relations in general, and interhemispheric memory transfer and recovery of function in particular.

REFERENCES

Albert, D. J. The effect of spreading depression on the consolidation of learning. *Neuropsychologia*, 1966, Vol. 4, 49-64.
Avis, H. H., & Carlton, P. L. Retrograde amnesia produced by hippocampal spreading depression. *Science*, 1968, Vol. 161, 73-75.

Bennett, G. S., & Edelman, G. M. Amino acid incorporation into rat brain proteins during spreading cortical depression. *Science*, 1969, Vol. 163, 393-395.

Bradley, P. B., & Elkes, J. The effect of atropine, hyoseyamine, physostigmine, and neostigmine on the electrical activity of the brain of the conscious cat. *Journal of Physiology (London)*, 1953, Vol. 120, 14.

Bures, J. Reversible decortication and behavior. In M. H. Brazier (Ed.), *Conference on the central nervous system and behavior*. New York: Josiah Macy, Jr. Foundation, 1959. Pp. 207-248.

Bures, J., & Buresova, O. The use of Leao's spreading cortical depression in research on conditioned reflexes. *Electroencephalography & Clinical Neurophysiology, Supplement*, 1960, Vol. 13, 359-376.

Bures, J. & Buresova, O. Excitability changes in thalamus and caudate induced by cortical spreading depression. *Proceedings of International Union of Physiological Science*, XXII International Congress in Leiden, 1962. Pp. 1061. (Abstract)

Bures, J., & Buresova, O. Cortical spreading depression as a memory disturbing factor. *Journal of Comparative & Physiological Psychology*, 1963, Vol. 56, 268-272.

Bures, J., Buresova, O., & Fifkova, E. Interhemispheric transfer of a passive avoidance reaction. *Journal of Comparative & Physiological Psychology*, 1964, Vol. 57, 326-330.

Bures, J., Buresova, O., Fifkova, E., Olds, J., Olds, M. E., & Travis, R. P. Spreading depression and subcortical drive centers. *Physiologia Bohemoslovenica*, 1961, Vol. 10, 321-331.

Bures, J., Buresova, O., Zahorova, A. Conditioned reflexes and Leao's spreading cortical depression. *Journal of Comparative and Physiological Psychology*, 1958, Vol. 51, 263-268.

Buresova, O. Disturbance in thermoregulation and metabolism as a result of prolonged EEG depression. *Physiologia Bohemoslovenica*, 1957, Vol. 6, 369. (a)

Buresova, O. Influencing water metabolism by spreading EEG depression. *Physiologia Bohemoslovenica*, 1957, Vol. 6, 12-20. (b)

Buresova, O., Bures, J., & Beran, V. A contribution to the problem of the dominant hemisphere in rats. *Physiologia Bohemoslovenica*, 1958, Vol. 7, 29-37.

Carlson, K. R. Cortical spreading depression and subcortical memory storage. *Journal of Comparative & Physiological Psychology*, 1967, Vol. 64, 422-430.

Cofoid, D. A. Interhemispheric spread and graded response in spreading cortical depression. *Psychonomic Science*, 1965, Vol. 2, 343-344.

Edwards, A. L. *Experimental design in psychological research*. (3rd ed.). New York: Holt, Rinehart and Winston, 1968.

Fifkova, E., & Syka, J. Relationships between cortical and striatal spreading depression in rats. *Experimental Neurology*, 1964, Vol. 9, 355-366.

Freedman, N., Pote, R., Butcher, R., & Suboski, M. D. Learning and motor activity under spreading depression depending on EEG amplitude. *Physiology & Behavior*, 1968, Vol. 3, 373-376.

Goddard, G. V. Amygdaloid stimulation and learning in the rat. *Journal of Comparative & Physiological Psychology*, 1964, Vol. 58, 23-30.

Gollender, M., & Ochs, S. Evaluation of EEG depression as an index of spreading depression in chronic preparations. *American Psychologist*, 1963, Vol. 17, 431.

Grafstein, B. Mechanism of spreading cortical depression. *Journal of Neurophysiology*, 1956, Vol. 19, 154-171.

Grossman, S. P., & Mountford, H. Effects of chemical stimulation of the dorsal hippocampus on learning and performance. *American Journal of Physiology*, 1964, Vol. 207, 1387-1393.

Hamburg, M. D., Best, P. J., & Cholewiak, R. W. Cortical lesion resulting from chemically-induced spreading depression. *Journal of Comparative & Physiological Psychology*, 1968, Vol. 66, 492-494.

Hebb, D. O. *The organization of behavior*. Wiley, New York: 1949.

Hendrickson, C. W., & Pinto-Hamuy, T. Nonretention of a visual conditional heart-rate response under neocortical spreading depression. *Journal of Comparative & Physiological Psychology*, 1967, Vol. 64, 510-513.

Hughes, R. A. Retrograde amnesia in rats produced by hippocampal injections of potassium chloride: Gradient of effect and recovery. *Journal of Comparative & Physiological Psychology*, 1969, Vol. 68, 637-644.

Jung, R., & Hassler, R. The extrapyramidal motor system. In J. Field, H. W. Magoun, & V. E. Hall (Eds.), *Handbook of Physiology*. Vol. 2. Washington, D.C.: American Physiological Society, 1960. Pp. 863-927.

Kesner, R. P., & Doty, R. W. Amnesia produced in cat by local seizure activity initiated from the amygdala. *Experimental Neurology*, 1968, Vol. 21, 58-68.

Koppman, J. W., & O'Kelly, L. I. Unilateral cortical spreading depression: A determiner of behavior at a choice point. *Journal of Comparative & Physiological Psychology*, 1966, Vol. 62, 237-242.

Kukleta, M. Learning in functionally decorticate state and its transfer to normal state. *Journal of Comparative & Physiological Psychology*, 1966, Vol. 62, 498-500.

Kupfermann, I. Is the retrograde amnesia that follows cortical spreading depression due to subcortical spread? *Journal of Comparative & Physiological Psychology*, 1966, Vol. 61, 466-467.

Leao, A. A. P. Spreading depression of activity in the cerebral cortex. *Journal of Neurophysiology*. 1944, Vol. 7, 359-390.

Leao, A. A. P. Further observations on spreading depression of activity in cerebral cortex. *Journal of Neurophysiology*, 1947, Vol. 10, 409-414.

Leao, A. A. P., & Morrison, R. S. Propagation of spreading cortical depression. *Journal of Neurophysiology*, 1945, Vol. 8, 33-45.

Marshall, W. H. Spreading cortical depression of Leao. *Physiological Review*, 1959, Vol. 39, 239-279.

Moelis, I. An evaluation of the effects of spreading cortical depression on motor aspects of performance. Unpublished doctoral dissertation, University of Illinois, 1963.

Ochs, S. The nature of spreading depression in neural networks. *International Review of Neurobiology*, 1962, Vol. 4, 1-64.

Ochs, S. Neuronal mechanisms of the cerebral cortex. In R. W. Russell (Ed.), *Frontiers in physiological psychology*, New York and London: Academic Press, 1966. Pp. 21-50.

Ochs, S., & Hunt, K. Apical dendrites and propagation of spreading depression in cerebral cortex. *Journal of Neurophysiology*, 1966, Vol. 23, 432-444.

Papsdorf, J., Longman, D., & Gormezano, I. Spreading depression: Effects of applying potassium chloride to the dura on the conditioned nicitating membrane response. *Psychonomic Science*, 1965, Vol. 2, 125-126.

Pearlman, C. Similar retrograde amnesia effects of ether and spreading cortical depression. *Journal of Comparative & Physiological Psychology*, 1966, Vol. 61, 306-308.

Ray, O. S., & Emley, G. Time factors in interhemispheric transfer of learning. *Science*, 1964, Vol. 144, 76-78.

Rudiger, W. Interfering subcortical stimulation and cortical spreading depression. *Physiologia Bohemoslovenica*, 1962, Vol. 11, 392-398.

Rudiger, W., & Fifkova, E. Operant behavior and subcortical drive during spreading depression. *Journal of Comparative & Physiological Psychology*, 1963, Vol. 56, 375-379.

Ruscak, M. Incorporation of ^{35}s-methionine into proteins of the cerebral cortex in situ in rats during spreading EEG depression. *Physiologia Bohemoslovenica*, 1964, Vol. 13, 16-20.

Russell, I., & Ochs, S. One-trial interhemispheric transfer of a learning engram. *Science*, 1961, Vol. 133, 1077-1078.

Russell, I. S., & Ochs, S. Localization of a memory trace in one cortical hemisphere and transfer to the other hemisphere. *Brain*, 1963, Vol. 86, 37-54.

Russell, I. S., Ross, R. B., & Strongman, K. T. Memory deficits produced by unilateral spreading depression. Paper presented at American Psychological Association, Los Angeles, September, 1964.

Schneider, A. M. Effects of unilateral and bilateral spreading depression on water intake. *Psychonomic Science*, 1965, Vol. 3, 287-288.

Schneider, A. M. Retention under spreading depression: A generalization decrement phenomenon. *Journal of Comparative & Physiological Psychology*, 1966, Vol. 62, 317-319.

Schneider, A. M. Control of memory by spreading cortical depression: A case for stimulus control. *Psychological Review*, 1967, Vol. 74, 201-215.

Schneider, A. M. Advokat, C., Kapp, B., & Sherman, W. Retrograde amnesic effects of unilateral spreading depression. Paper presented at Eastern Psychological Association, Philadelphia, 1969.

Schneider, A. M., & Behar, M. A chronic preparation for spreading cortical depression. *Journal of the Experimental Analysis of Behavior*, 1964, Vol. 7, 350.

Schneider, A. M., & Ebbesen, E. Interhemispheric transfer of lever pressing as stimulus generalization of the effects of spreading depression. *Journal of the Experimental Analysis of Behavior*, 1967, Vol. 10, 193-197.

Schneider, A. M., & Kay, H. Spreading depression as a discriminative stimulus for lever pressing. *Journal of Comparative & Physiological Psychology*, 1968, Vol. 65, 149-151.

Sperry, R. W. The great cerebral commissure. *Scientific American*, 1964, Vol. 210, 42-62.

Squire, L. R., & Liss, P. H. Control of memory by spreading cortical depression: A critique of stimulus control. *Psychological Review*, 1968, Vol. 75, 347-352.

Tapp, J. T. Reversible cortical depression and avoidance behavior in the rat. *Journal of Comparative and Physiological Psychology*, 1962, Vol. 55, 306-308.

Teitelbaum, P., & Cytawa, J. Spreading depression and recovery from lateral hypothalamic damage. *Science*, 1965, Vol. 147, 61-63.

Teitelbaum, P., & Epstein, A. N. The lateral hypothalamic syndrome: recovery of feeding and drinking after lateral hypothalamic lesions. *Psychological Review*, 1962, Vol. 69, 74-90.

Teitelbaum, P., & Stellar, E. Recovery from the failure to eat, produced by hypothalamic lesions. *Science*, 1954, Vol. 120, 894-895.

Thompson, R. W. Transfer of avoidance learning between normal and functionally decorticate states. *Journal of Comparative & Physiological Psychology*, 1964, Vol. 57, 321-325.

Thompson, R. W., & Enter, R. Shock level and unconditioned responding in rats under sham unilateral, or bilateral spreading depression. *Journal of Comparative & Physiological Psychology*, 1967, Vol. 63, 521-523.

Thompson, R., & Hjelle, L. Effects of stimulus and response complexity on learning under bilateral spreading depression. *Journal of Comparative & Physiological Psychology*, 1965, Vol. 59, 122-124.

Travis, R. P., & Sparks, D. L. The influence of unilateral and bilateral spreading depression during learning upon subsequent relearning. *Journal of Comparative & Physiological Psychology*, 1963, Vol. 56, 56-59.

van Harreveld, A. Compounds in brain extracts causing spreading depression of cerebral cortical activity and contraction of crustacean muscle. *Journal of Neurochemistry*, 1959, Vol. 3, 300-315.

van Harreveld, A., & Ochs, S. Electrical and vascular concomitants of spreading depression. *American Journal of Physiology*, 1957, Vol. 189, 159-166.

van Harreveld, A., & Schade, J. P. Chloride movements in cerebral cortex after circulatory arrest and during spreading depression. *Journal of Cellular & Comparative Physiology*, 1959, Vol. 54, 65-84.

Weiss, T. The spontaneous EEG activity of the mesencephalic reticular formation during cortical spreading depression. *Physiologia Bohemoslovenica*, 1961, Vol. 10, 109-116.

Weiss, T., & Fifkova, E. The use of spreading depression to analyse the mutual relationship between the neocortex and hippocampus. *Electroencephalography & Clinical Neurophysiology*, 1960, Vol. 12, 841-850.

Weiss, T., & Fifkova, E. Bioelectric activity in the thalamus and hypothalamus of rats during cortical spreading EEG depression. *Electroencephalography and Clinical Neurophysiology*, 1961, Vol. 13, 734-744.

Weiss, T., & Fifkova, E. The effect of neocortical and caudate spreading depression on "circling movements" induced from the caudate nucleus. *Physiologia Bohemoslovenica*, 1963, Vol. 12, 332-338.

CHAPTER

9

BRAIN LESIONS AND MEMORY IN ANIMALS

SUSAN D. IVERSEN

I. INTRODUCTION

In approaching the problem of memory, the neuropsychologist has two related tasks: first, to characterize the psychological processes involved, and second, to identify the neurological substrates of such processes. Brain lesions are potentially useful tools for both pursuits.

Induced damage provides one of the most ancient and well-tried techniques for studying the structure and function of the nervous system. It may interest historical connoisseurs to hear that Galen assaulted the frontal lobes of piglets in 170 A.D. Interesting as such studies may be, this writer does not intend to scrutinize the literature from 170–1971 A.D., reviewing all the investigations which have used brain lesions to study memory. Historical comment is made, as many may be unaware of the valuable pre-twentieth century brain lesion studies. Indeed, it often seems that these workers, particularly the pioneers of the 19th Century, were acutely aware of their brief and the limitations of their technique. Ferrier (1876), Brown and Schäfer (1888), Fanz (1907), Bianchi (1922) and Hitzig (1884), in studying the deficits after brain lesions, made determined efforts to describe the changed behavior within the normal psychological framework and, despite less refined neurological and psychological techniques, made highly relevant observations.

In pursuing the problems of localization of function and, in particular, of memory, neuropsychologists have taken nearly 50 years to reattain this level of sophistication. These years were dominated by Karl Lashley, and it would be less than gracious to proceed without some comment on his lasting contribution to this field. It has been fashionable to discredit his work in the recent euphoria which has embraced the evidence for localization of function in the cortex. However, in returning to his writings one cannot but be impressed by the shrewdness of his ideas and concepts of brain function and the wealth of interesting findings, whose significance is only gradually appreciated. Most of this data was collected in the lean years of neuropsychology between 1920 and 1950, and had he lived to experiment with the subhuman primates and behavioral techniques, which he introduced for the succeeding generation of neuropsychologists, he would presumably have modified many of the theories he developed from his rat experiments.

In pursuing a meticulous research program over more than 30 years, Lashley was directed on one hand by the behaviorists postulating that psychological functions were the product of associations of conditioned reflexes. On the other hand were neurologists who saw, in clinical agnosias, a specific loss in such associative processes and suggested that the association cortex adjacent to the primary sensory areas might be the locus of such processes or, in other words, the permanent representation of an engram or memory.

Lashley considered the conditioned reflex as a relevant "psychological element" and sought its substrate. He found that the motor cortex was not vital for the execution of learned response to a sensory stimulus and that although the sensory cortex was necessary for such behavior, every part of the sensory representation on the cortex was equally important. In turning to more complex responses which depend on the association of a variety of sensory inputs and responses, for example, maze learning or conditional reactions, Lashley found that the size of the lesion in the association cortex rather than its locus determined the severity of the loss of habit. A large number of such experiments on the rat led him to postulate that the engram of a habit, conceived as a product of conditioned reflex activity, did not occupy a specific locus in the nervous system. In a review of his work presented in Cambridge in 1950 (Lashley, 1950) he claimed that his series of experiments has discovered nothing directly of the real nature of the engram . . . they do establish limits within which concepts of its nature must be confined, and thus indirectly define somewhat more clearly the nature of the nervous mechanisms which must be responsible for learning and retention.

and indeed it was from a much broader approach to the question of the neural mechanisms involved in learning processes that important lines of research were to develop. Unfortunately, Lashley had started with an inadequate definition of the psychological process involved and sought its substrate, and in general it has proved difficult to pursue neuropsychological problems in such a manner. His findings discounted views that memory occupied an anatomical locus in the CNS and at least exposed the naivete of some of the prevailing physiological theories of memory. Probably because of the overwhelming negation of his results, experimental consideration developed, not as a direct attack upon the question of the memory substrate, but through a reappraisal of the fundamental question of localization of function in the cortex. It is in this more modest direction that advances have been made.

However, in 1950 the results seemed to support his contention that

it is not possible to demonstrate the isolated localisation of a memory trace anywhere within the nervous system. The complexity of the functions involved in reproductive memory implies that every instance of recall requires the activity of literally millions of neurones.

The real problem with memory, as Lashley realized to his cost, is that the process is barely defined psychologically and is accordingly difficult to recognize at either a neurological or cellular level. As psychological analysis proceeds it is possible to differentiate parts of the information processing mechanism which are served by particular neural substrates. It seems possible that such properties could fulfil the requirements of a storage mechanism and in this broader and more logical framework interest in the engram has revived, almost apologetically, in the post-Lashley era.

To a great extent, specific technical developments are responsible for the upsurge of interest in questions of localization and function since the late 1940's. In particular:

1. Experimental animals, and in particular subhuman primates, became more readily available.

2. Lesion techniques were developed and improved by, for example, the uses of subpial aspiration to remove cortical grey matter. This method, unlike earlier knife incisions, made it possible to remove gray matter without producing unwanted damage to the underlying white fibers. The methods for stereotaxic surgery were introduced. These improved techniques together with the use of antibiotics to prevent postoperative infections made it possible to study animals with discrete brain lesions for long postoperative periods.

3. Experimental anatomical studies of the cerebral cortex were undertaken using strychnine neuronography (von Bonin, Garol, & McCulloch, 1942), electrical stimulation (Petr, Holden, & Jirout, 1949), and more traditional staining methods for degeneration (Mettler, 1935; Clark, 1942), in an effort to determine the cortico-cortical and cortico-subcortical interactions of the various cortical areas.

4. Special behavioral tests were designed. The precise details of such tasks were often dictated by controversial issues in learning theory but proved useful in assessing specific psychological functions, for example, delayed response or alternation tasks to study memory, simultaneous discrimination in a Yerkes discrimination box or Wisconsin General Test Apparatus (WGTA) to study discrimination, and operant reinforcement schedules to study appetitive and aversive control of behavior.

5. Clinical cases with localized brain damage were investigated from a psychological rather than a purely neurological point of view, and the findings encouraged similar studies in experimental animals. This has been especially valuable in the case of the temporal lobe where outstanding clinical work has occasioned similar investigations in animals.

With the upsurge of interest in neuropsychological problems, the question of the substrate of memory processes was again considered, but now within the context of studies of human verbal memory and the concomitant theoretical models envisaging short-term processes in the nervous system which eventually give rise to substrates of a more permanent nature. This implied dichotomy between short- and long-term memory processes influenced not only subsequent experimental work on human memory but also pervaded the neuropsychological and physiological experiments from their conception. At a cellular level, transient electrical activity in reverberating circuits was postulated to precede more permanent structural changes and treatment effects such as electroconvulsive shock, and certain drugs, which transiently depress or disrupt the central nervous system, have been used to determine the temporal characteristics of this chain reaction. Such experiments have tended to support a two-process theory of memory and it was therefore reasonable that neurological substrates should be sought for both the short and long term information processing mechanisms as well as for the engram itself.

Memory functions which are easily studied in man in the verbal mode, are experimentally accessible in animals only with indirect methods. Learning is the vehicle by which information can be presented to or retrieved from an animal and, thus, processes such as registration, recall, recognition, and retrieval which may be subjectively or objectively isolated and studied in man, cannot be differentiated with such reliability in animals. One supposes that similar processes occur in the monkey but it is very difficult, having disrupted memory, to find out which of the various parts of the total process is deranged. However, the study of normal memory in man reveals variables which influence the various stages of information processing and storage. Despite the lack of convenient verbal tests in animals, the application of such information begins to broaden our understanding of the defects in memory processing produced by brain lesions.

It might be supposed that it is not of value to use brain lesions to study memory in animals. However, in trying to understand a process there is often no substitute for disrupting the norm. Without lesions, there is very little hope of understanding the neurological circuitry involved in memory.

This review will indicate the progress that has been made in this direction. As studies of the cerebral cortex of the monkey proceeded, the conclusion that localized, functionally significant areas existed became inescapable. Having studied the processing properties of the sensory areas and shown that related areas of the posterior association cortex subserve modality specific discrimination functions, workers have been reconsidering the possibility, that the next stage in the neural processing of information that is, memory, is subserved by other related and localized cortical tissue. Having been reborn within such a logical framework, this idea has become more widely accepted and, once again, considered to be worthy of sustained experimental effort.

However, it is also well to remember that these discoveries were not highly original. The pioneers of the brain lesion techniques in the nineteenth century, irrespective of their doctrinaire position either favoring or challenging ideas of localization of function, investigated almost all the areas of the cortex. Indeed, deficits in memory processing were described in these earlier studies to follow frontal and temporal lesions.

Bianchi (1922) from his experiments and clinical observations concluded that:

Removal of the frontal lobes does not so much interfere with the perceptions taken singly, as it does disaggreate the personality, and incapacitate for serialising and synthesizing groups of representatives. The actual impressions, which serve to revive these groups, thus succeed one another disconnectedly under the influence of fortuitous external stimuli, and disappear without giving rise to associational processes in varied and recurrent succession. With the organ for the physiological fusion which forms the basis of association disappear also the physical conditions underlying reminiscence, judgement, and discrimination, as is well shown in mutilated animals.

Brown and Schäfer (1888) in pioneering brain lesion studies made observations on the effects of bilateral temporal lobe lesions in the monkeys—in one particular animal they reported that:

his memory and intelligence seem deficient. He gives evidence of seeing and hearing and of possession of his senses generally, but it is clear that he no longer understands the meaning of sounds, sights and other impressions that reach him. Every object with which he comes in contact, even those with which he was previously most familiar, appears strange and is investigated with curiosity . . . and he will on coming across the

same object accidentally a few minutes afterwards go through exactly the same
process as if he had entirely forgotten his previous experience.

In both cases, deficits were viewed as impairments of a memory processing
system and not as destruction of an engram, but, in fact, such ideas were
neglected for the next 50 years during the giddy heyday of the search for the
recalcitrant engram. We are now beginning to rediscover some of these deficits.

This review will hope to show, chronologically, how serious study of
memory processes has again become reputable, and the experiments will be
considered within a framework which is fast becoming traditional. This framework holds that areas of the frontal lobes are concerned with short or immediate
memory and the temporal lobes with more permanent storage.

Finally, it will be suggested that both the so-called short and the long-term
memory deficits reflect dysfunction of a single information processing mechanism which precedes permanent storage. An effort will be made to resolve
difficulties and confusions of terminology between the human experimental,
clinical, and animal literature, with a suggestion that between sensory registration
and the final engram, a single memory process operates commiting information
to and retrieving it from storage; a process which (1) is not aptly called immediate or long-term memory is (2) more or less involved, depending on factors such
as the information content, temporal complexity of the incoming information
and levels of interference, and (3) is specifically disorganized by local brain
damage in animals and man in the absence of general intellectual loss.

II. THE ROLE OF THE FRONTAL LOBES
IN MEMORY PROCESSES

Jacobsen (1936) is largely responsible for the revival of interest in this
question. In the 1930's he set out to reexamine many of Lashley's ideas using
monkeys instead of rats as his experimental subjects. He believed in localization
of function by historical conviction and politely justified his experiments by
claiming that the rat may very well be different from the monkey. Lashley had
previously reported that frontal lesions in the rat were no more devastating than
posterior lesions on a variety of sensory/motor and complex maze tasks.
Jacobsen, however, felt that some of the earlier reports of Brown and Schäfer
(1888) and Bianchi (1922) were indicative of highly specific psychological
dysfunction after frontal lesions in the monkey and from the beginning of his
studies he favored an explanation of such deficits in terms of immediate or
short-term memory.

Monkeys with large frontal lobe resections were found to be deficient on
delayed response (Jacobsen, 1936) and alternation tasks, but the acquisition or
retention of conditioned reflexes, discrimination habits, and puzzle box solu-

tions were not affected. The delay tasks should be commented upon because, subsequently, they have been used extensively in neuropsychology, probably more so than any other tests. Jacobsen considered that a critical feature was the delay, and, hence, deficits were interpreted in terms of short term memory. The tests thus became established as measures of short term memory and it has not always been fully recognized that they are, in fact, extremely complicated tasks, including a complex of behavioral parameters in addition to temporal delay. It is now accepted that animals may fail these tasks for many reasons and that failure after a certain brain lesion should not automatically imply the existence of a memory disorder. For example, spatial discrimination is intimately involved in the delayed response task, whereas the ability to inhibit, repeatedly, one response pattern in favor of another is demanded in the alternation task. Indeed, uncritical acceptance of the deficits on such tasks has retarded the development of a theory of frontal lobe function to such a degree that we are only just beginning to advance from Jacobsen's original ideas.

After Jacobsen's results were published it was readily accepted that the frontal lobes were concerned in short-term memory processes. However, as neuropsychological work in primates became more widespread, an increasing number and variety of deficits were reported to be associated with frontal lobe lesions. For example, Harlow and his co-workers tested monkeys with large dorsolateral lesions on a range of complex visual discrimination tasks which involved discrimination reversal (Harlow & Dagnon, 1942) responses to stimuli with multiple sign values (Harlow & Spaet, 1943) and contradictory reactions to similar and to identical stimuli (Settlage, Zable, & Harlow, 1948), and they were found to be deficient. Such findings immediately raised the question of modality specificity in relation to frontal deficits and their relationship to the sensory and discrimination deficits after posterior cortical lesions. At this relatively early stage of the investigation, the contention that the frontal lesions produced specific deficits in memory and discrimination tasks was challenged by studies of Chow, Blum, and Blum (1951) in which they investigated the effects of posterior and anterior cortical lesions, singly or in combination, on a wide range of delay and discrimination tasks. They concluded that

> the data from this and other experiments tend to support the view that the neural substrate which is critical for retention or ready reacquisition of certain habits is organised into discrete centers specific to the functional category. The areas of concentration are supplemented by overlapping fringes of secondary significance. It appears likely that a cortical region may have dual function, i.e., it may be focal for one ability and part of the fringe of another . . . destruction of associative areas (posterior and anterior association cortex) produces effects which are neither an aggregation of discrete symptoms, nor dependent solely on mass of tissue removed.

Clinical findings also failed to support the localization point of view. After lobectomy, leucotomy, or smaller lesions of the frontal lobe, general intellectual loss, affective changes, and sensorimotor deficits were reliably reported, but delayed response and alternation impairments were not seen (Teuber, 1964).

Despite these problems, the monkey experiments continued and the task seemed to be (1) to prove that the frontal discrimination deficits were different from those produced by posterior lesions, (2) to identify the basis of the deficits, and (3) to seek a common unifying principle to explain the apparently different short term memory and discrimination deficits in frontal animals.

As a consequence of further experimentation, it was established that the dorsolateral lesions which resulted in visual discrimination deficits also produced auditory (Weiskrantz & Mishkin, 1958) and tactile discrimination impairments (Iversen, 1967). The finding that a relatively small lesion could produce deficits in three modalities differentiated the frontal discrimination deficits from those following posterior cortical lesions where visual, auditory, and tactile discrimination deficits are associated with three separate and highly localized cortical areas.

Despite this important anatomical difference, it was still possible that both the frontal and posterior deficits reflected sensory discriminative disturbances. Weiskrantz and Mishkin (1958) favored a sensory explanation in discussing the auditory discrimination deficit they had demonstrated after dorsolateral frontal lesions and referred to the anatomical findings of Sugar, French, and Chusid (1948) showing a projection from the primary auditory cortex of the sylvian fissure to the dorsolateral frontal convexity. This view was upheld by Gross and Weiskrantz (1964), when in subsequent experiments it was shown that this auditory deficit was associated with dorsolateral lesions involving the arcuate sulcus, but not with damage to the sulcus principalis. These two selective lesions together constitute the total "dorsolateral" lesion usually studied (Fig. 9-1).

However, others considered it more reasonable to suppose that the frontal discrimination deficits, which are not modality specific or associated with changes in sensory thresholds (Iversen & Mishkin, 1970), reflect a disorder different from those following posterior cortical lesions. The contention that anterior and posterior discrimination deficits differ is also supported by the interesting fact that frontals are less impaired on difficult than on simple discrimination tasks, whereas in posterior animals the opposite is true and the deficit more pronounced on difficult tasks (Chow, 1954), as would be predicted if sensory/perceptual mechanisms are involved. Few workers now doubt that these two groups of discrimination impairments reflect different underlying dysfunction; the question is what is the disorder in the case of frontal monkeys? The reports of frontal discrimination deficits have increased year by year and the discussions of the papers invariably refer to Jacobsen's finding of delayed response and alternation impairments following similar lesions, and to his interpretation in terms of short-term memory loss. In the absence of new ideas, parsimony proved popular, and a great many results were considered to concur, albeit loosely, with Jacobsen's ideas.

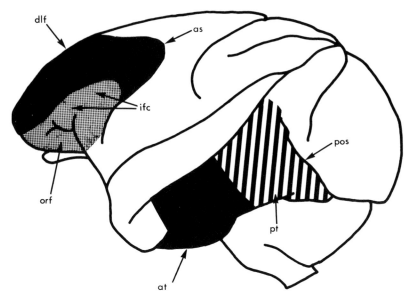

Fig. 9-1. Lateral view of the monkey brain indicating the extent of: dlf, dorso-lateral frontal lesion; orf, orbitofrontal lesion; ifc, inferior convexity of frontal lobe; pos, preoccipital sulcus; pt, posterior temporal lesion; at, anterior temporal lesion.

By the early 1960s it became necessary to accommodate a widely divergent body of data in the memory hypothesis and serious misgivings began to be expressed. Indeed, it seemed to Rosvold and Mishkin (1961), reviewing the field at this time, that no unitary hypothesis which they could advance adequately accounted for all the results. Short term memory difficulty could result in discrimination impairments if the animal failed to retain information from trial to trial, but it seems unlikely that retention would be satisfactory on a difficult simultaneous pattern discrimination but not on certain kinds of simple object discrimination tasks. This kind of synthesis of the data indicated that a memory hypothesis could not explain all the frontal deficits. Mishkin, Rosvold, and their co-workers initiated specially designed object learning set experiments in frontals, and this contention was verified. The experiment was designed so that the animal's preferences were manipulated and controlled by first trial baiting of both objects (half the problems) and first trial no baiting of the remainder. Analysis of the discrimination learning revealed that frontals showed impairment only on object problems when the first response was unrewarded and, therefore, a change of response preference was required for solution. This experiment was developed in various ways and initial preference modified by a variety of prebaiting techniques. The range of results was consistent with the idea that the frontal's difficulty lay in reversing response patterns and not in short term memory—it did not seem reasonable to suppose that an animal could remember perfectly well which was the positive stimulus from the first to the subsequent trials when it was allowed to retain its preference and not when a change was required (Mishkin, 1964).

Shortly afterwards the same workers extended their experiments to include animals with bilateral damage to the frontal cortex lying ventral to the traditional dorsolateral lesion. The effects of the two lesions were compared on a battery of short term memory and discrimination tasks and unexpectedly it was found that the ventral or orbito-frontal lesions resulted in more severe deficits than the dorsal lesions on almost all the discrimination tasks (Fig. 9-2). Only on place reversal (DR was not included) were both groups equally impaired (Fig. 9-2). This result suggested that the discrimination and short term memory deficits might be dissociable to different parts of the frontal cortex, a possibility which had been indicated but not pursued in an earlier study (Gross & Weiskrantz, 1962). With this development, the theory of a frontal lobe memory impairment which had lost its generality and with that its credence, was reborn. It is not relevant to continue a discussion of the frontal discrimination impairments, but for the sake of completeness it might be mentioned that lesions to Walker's cytoarchitectural Area 12 of the frontal cortex (Fig. 9-3), which extends ventrally from about 5 mm below the sulcus principalis to the lateral orbital sulcus and includes the inferior frontal convexity, produces a severe deficit on an auditory go/no go frequency discrimination task and a visual reversal task, without impairing auditory frequency threshold performance (Iversen & Mishkin, 1970). At least on this auditory task the impairment is greater than that produced by either medial orbital or dorsolateral frontal damage (Fig. 9-4). This lesion (called inferior convexity lesion) included cortex which in the past has been variously included in large dorsolateral lesions and damage to which is presumed to have been responsible for the variety of discriminative impairments seen after the traditional dorsal lesion. It remains to be shown that the restricted inferior convexity lesion produced discrimination deficits in all modalities. The equally important question which remains to be solved concerns the basis of such discrimination deficits. Response control and not discriminative capacity appears to be impaired, for, as Lawicka, Mishkin, and Rosvold (1966) have shown, the orbital frontal animal has great difficulty with an auditory discrimination presented as go/no go task, but not if it is presented with a go left/go right response contingency. The orbital animal fails tasks in which trained or innate response bias must be changed. The observed response inflexibility could reflect dysfunction of motor or motivational control or of some relationship between the two. It would seem that these possibilities are not mutually exclusive but that the orbital cortex includes foci modulating both of these responses. Iversen & Mishkin (1970), have reported that although the IC lesion results in a severe go/no go auditory discrimination impairment, a lesion to the remainder of the orbital cortex [designated medial orbital (MO)] which

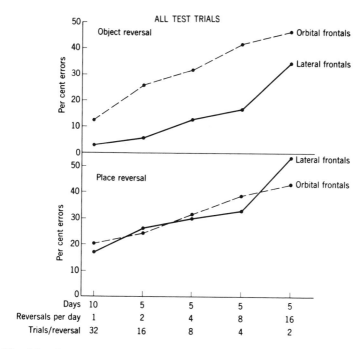

Fig. 9-2. Comparison of dorsolateral and orbital lesions on object reversal (upper graph) and spatial reversal (lower graph). (Reproduced from Mishkin, 1964.)

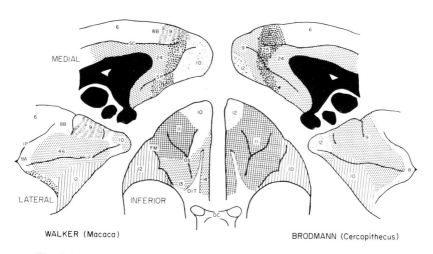

Fig. 9-3. Cytoarchitectural maps of the frontal cortex viewed medially, laterally, and ventrally.

AUDITORY DIFFERENTIATION

(300 versus 2400 CPS)

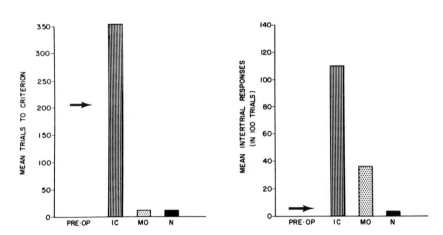

Fig. 9-4. Left: Mean trials to relearn an auditory differentiation task after inferior convexity (IC) and medial orbital (MO) lesions and in control animals. The arrow indicates the mean preoperative learning score. Right: Mean number of intertrial responses on the first five days of post operative testing compared with the number on the five days of preoperative retention testing (arrow).(Reproduced from Iversen & Mishkin, 1970.)

does not impair learning scores on this task (Fig. 9-4) does disturb performance in a manner which may suggest motivational disinhibition. The MO animals were observed to repeatedly open the food box during the intertrial delays, a behavior pattern similar to that reported by Brutowski and Dabrowska (1963) to follow lesions to the medial surface of the frontal lobe in dogs, and ascribed by them to motivational disinhibition. On anatomical grounds, it is not inconceivable that distinct areas of the orbital cortex could modulate motor and hypothalamic systems via their connections with the extrapyramidal and subcortical limbic centers. This provides a convenient point at which to leave the orbital frontal deficit and return to the main purpose of this discussion: memory deficits associated with frontal lesions.

The experiments of Lawicka *et al.* (1966) clarified part of the problem by showing that deficits on certain discriminations involving response control followed orbital but not dorsolateral lesions, as was previously supposed. In demonstrating this she used both go/no go, and go left/go right auditory discriminations and found that while restricted dorsolateral lesions which no longer included inferior convexity tissue did not impair the differentiation (go/no go) task, severe deficits were seen on the go left/go right task. Hence the original confusion dissipated only slowly. A more restricted dorsolateral lesion produces deficits on discrimination tasks but, again, not under all behavioral conditions. In the case of this deficit the go left/go right response pattern in relation to the discriminative cues would seem to be the critical behavioral pattern disorganized by the lesion. Extension of these experiments has shown that restricted dorso-lateral frontal lesions, as indicated in Fig. 9-1, produce DR, DA, and go left/go right discrimination impairments, and the challenge is to find out if this group of deficits reflect a common dysfunction.

Firstly, it is useful to identify any common features of these tasks. In delayed response and alternation, short term intratrial and intertrial delays are striking properties but they also occur in the go left/go right discrimination, as in all other successive or simultaneous discrimination tasks. Another prominent feature of all the three tasks is that they involve spatial information. In the delayed response task, a spatial cue has to be remembered and responded to; in delayed alternation, the animals must remember a spatial position in order to be able to respond to the other position on the next trial, and in the discrimination task the auditory cues elicit responses to either the left or right side of the testing board. It is easy to describe such tasks and claim parsimony in the behavioral strategy required; in fact, it is much more difficult to validate such points. Konorski and Lawicka (1964) have done extensive studies with normal dogs on a great variety of such spatial and nonspatial tasks to evaluate the relative significance of stimulus as opposed to response elements in such performance. The paucity of such fundamental information has not prevented neuro-psychologists from pursuing the frontal lobe problem and the notion of spatial deficits and frontal lesions has received considerable attention recently. The restricted dorsolateral lesion that has been described includes the sulcus princi-palis, cortex dorsally to the midline, and laterally to 5 cm below the princi-palis and area 8 of Brodmann in the limb of the arcuate sulcus (Fig. 9-3). This latter cortex is called the frontal eye field and Kennard (1939) reported some years ago that animals with lesions in this cortex exhibited aberrant visual search behavior indicative of transient hemianopia. This finding has been rep-licated recently (Latto, 1971) using a sensitive perimetry method devised by Cowey (1963) to determine the size, location, and permanence of field defects in monkeys. More recent behavioral work has tended to confirm that this cortex is involved in occulomotor functions, but the most compelling evidence for such a theory comes from stimulation studies in which Robinson and Fuchs (1969) have shown that in the monkey stimulation of neurones in Area 8 produces eye movements of a saccadic nature and from electrophysiological recording experiments of Bizzi (1967) showing that (in the unanaesthetised monkey) neurones in this area discharge only after initiation of eye movements. Teuber (1964) has reported changed visual search behavior in frontal patients and similar impairments have been observed in monkeys with discrete bilateral lesions to area 8 (Latto and Iversen, unpublished results). This cortex projects to the superior colliculus (Kuypers & Lawrence, 1967) which electrophysiological and behavioral work implicates in processes concerned with the detection of events in visual space without being involved in the discriminative processes necessary to identify the sensory content of such events (Sprague & Meikle, 1965; Sprague, 1966; Rosvold, Mishkin & Szwarcbart, 1958). Most of these ideas are novel and lack adequate experimental proof, but evidence is accumulating which implicates Area 8 in the integration of responses to the spatial environment. Reasoning of this kind leads to the suggestion that it is damage to area 8 in the restricted dorsolateral lesion which produces the go left/go right discrimination impairment and, possibly, the delayed response deficit, as both of these tasks are predominantly spatial in nature. The delayed alternation task also involves spatial information, but the animal responds in a regular manner to the two sides; a spatial strategy is required, rather than spatial discrimination on each trial, and the development and maintenance of such a strategy should be strongly influenced by the magnitude of the intertrial delay periods involved. Delayed alternation may therefore be the most relevant of the classical "frontal" tasks in considerations of short term memory.

All of these comments are rather speculative. Can the delayed response and auditory go left/go right deficits be anatomically dissociated from that on the delayed alternation task? This we do not know, as only a limited number of selective dorsolateral lesions have been studied. However, relevent experiments are under way in several laboratories (Goldman & Rosvold, 1970). If this hypothesis proves to be valid, it may be shown that at the end of this dissociation exercise only a small area in the frontal lobe remains which could be specifically related to short term memory processes. The development of this line of research has been unfolded at such length to illustrate how, with a diversity of behavioral tasks and parcellation of a large lesion, an originally simple hypothesis may be lost only to be revived in a more precise form.

We now speculate that the sulcus principalis and its surrounding tissue is involved in short-term memory processing—but what does this term mean? In this respect little advance has been made from Jacobsen's position in 1935. The pursuit of evidence for localization of function has depended to a large extent on well tried behavioral techniques, but in pursuing the basis of a short-term processing deficit a more imaginative behavioral analysis is demanded. The delayed alternation task has been useful, indeed it may be the only test of the traditional battery which is influenced by restricted sulcus principalis lesions. The proof of this statement is wanting but, irrespective of the outcome, it is important to understand the basic behavioral property of this classical test. In discussing frontal deficits in the 1930's, Jacobsen used interesting terms such as defective synthesis, serializing, and organization and, unfortunately, also included the global term "immediate memory." This is the term which had impact, and has perhaps obscured the more dynamic properties of the tests in relation to frontal behavior, although it is well to remember that certainly Jacobsen's ideas were not confused. He states

> Thus while we may grant synthesizing functions to the frontal area our problem now becomes one of stating under what conditions and in what kinds of problems, synthesis or preferably behaviour, is disrupted and ineffectual ... adaptation is inadequate in those situations which require for their solution not only present sensory items but also elements of past experience which can be introduced only through the action of memory.

and yet again

> This then appears to be the peculiar contribution of the frontal association areas, namely, recall of a particular past event which may be only in mediate association with some aspect of the present sensory environment and the integration and organisation of recalled elements with the organism's stable habit systems.

A perusal of the literature reveals that animals with frontal lesions (admittedly of varying size and locus) show abnormal behavior on a wide range of tasks in addition to the delay tasks and spatial discrimination problems involving withholding of a response, referred to earlier. The list may be expanded to include tasks involving a sequential series of responses (Pinto-Hamuy & Linck, 1965), situations in which the ordering of responses is required (Pribram, Ahumada, Hartog, & Ross, 1964; Stamm, 1963), delayed matching from sample (Buffery, 1964), and visual conditional learning (Iversen & Weiskrantz, 1967). Certain common behavior parameters can be identified in the tasks, although it is difficult to describe these characteristics with any degree of precision. For example, short-term delays may be involved, the necessity to retrieve information after a short period of time, the stimulus/response/reinforcement relationships may change regularly and, indeed, repeatedly, ordered responses may be required; and this by no means exhausts the possible elements of parsimony in these tasks.

In discussing the difficulty experienced by frontal patients on paired comparison tasks, Milner has suggested that the discrimination of recency may also play an important role in such situations (Milner & Teuber, 1968). Experiments by Yntema and Trask (1963) are quoted which suggest that items in memory normally carry time-tags which permit the discrimination of the more from the less recent, and frontal lesions could conceivably interfere with such a process. These contentions are supported by experiments showing that frontal performance is greatly improved by certain behavioral manipulations which increase the information value of the relevant stimuli or introduce time markings to impose some structure on the incoming information, thus simplifying storage even for a normal animal. For example, Buffery (1964) reported that in frontal monkeys, impaired postoperative delayed matching from sample of color stimuli improved if novel colored stimuli were introduced into the experiment. Similarly Prisko

(1963) found that frontal patients showed a deficit on a Konorski short-term memory task if colors, light flashes, or click stimuli were used, but showed normal performance if the stimuli were interesting nonsense patterns, each of which was unique. More recently, Pribram and Tubbs (1967) structured the delayed alternation task for frontal monkeys by demanding responses in doublets (e.g., RL delay, RL delay, RL delays, etc.), and reported greatly improved performance. Such results suggest that both frontal monkeys and man have difficulty if the task structure applies pressure to the short-term organization of incoming information but the deficit envisaged does not concur with the traditional idea of short-term memory as a brief impression of the sensory environment which is ultimately transformed into a more permanent trace.

The theory has been verbalized in several ways, for example, in terms of an inflexible noticing order by analogy with the computer simulation model of human problem solving described by Newell, Shaw, and Simon (1958) and, recently, in the more general terms of "proper programming—the passing of the stream of stimulation to which the organism is subject [Pribram & Tubbs, 1967]." Helpful as such theorizing is, it would seem that there is still a long way to go in our understanding of such frontal deficits. For example, is the impairment in "programming" most significant with respect to the organization of information bombarding the organism or with respect to the search strategies the organism may pursue in sampling the sensory environment? Indeed, it is pointless to ask such questions before the interdependence of such processes is established.

It is perhaps premature to claim that one characteristic rather than another determines the frontals failure. We shall only be in a position to attempt this synthesis when animals with selective lesions (and in particular, with discrete sulcus principalis lesions) have been studied on a range of these tasks. However, in view of the fact that disturbed response control, response to motivational contingencies and spatial cues have been convincingly related to nonprincipalis frontal cortex, it would appear that the necessity for ordering or programming of incoming information remains as a distinctive feature of several of the frontal tests which may be sensitive to principalis damage. The dissociation of such a function would be consonant with the traditional view that the frontal lobe has a role in memory processing. Many of the studies by Pribram and his collaborators have pointed to such a theory, although the studies have not yet included animals with lesions to the various parts of the dorsolateral cortex.

The claim for a frontal lobe memory function can only be made if two notes of caution are sounded. First, it remains to be proven that a group of unique memory type deficits are associated with damage to the sulcus principalis and that such deficits are not explicable in terms of a loss of response or motivational control. Second, to date only delayed spatial alternation has been reliably associated with sulcus principalis damage. The other experiments have yet to be done. However, it is possible that the role of the frontal cortex in mnemonic function is not general but modality specific and is, as Goldman and Rosvold (1970) have recently suggested, "concerned with a form of spatial memory."

Thus, in conclusion, it seems possible that a very small part of the frontal cortex is involved in the "synthesizing or serializing" process that Jacobsen postulated. A range of impairments sharing this characteristic have been selected from the frontal literature but many of them have been described only after the traditionally large frontal lesions. Further selective lesion studies will be necessary to discover if this small frontal region is critical for the structuring of incoming information demanded in certain tasks, which we have been encouraged to call short-term memory tests. However, it is fair to point out that although Jacobsen popularized the idea of immediate memory disorders following frontal lesions, he tried to prevent the too ready acceptance of the term with all its implications for psychological and physiological theories of memory.

In using the term immediate memory to designate the defect that follows injury to the frontal areas we do so with little assurance that it is either sufficiently inclusive or descriptively adequate for the phenomena in point. In some respects recognition memory and recall appear to be better suited. It is obvious that use of any of these terms adds little to our understanding of the essential physiological and psychological problems beyond a comfortable feeling of familiarity. For the present operational definition of the functions involved may be a more satisfactory procedure.

Such ideas were not original and Jacobsen was well aware that Bianchi had said it before. Thirty years later we know a little more about the substrate of such processes, practically nothing more about the process itself, but the climate is clement and a little attention to operational definitions may yet bear fruit.

III. THE ROLE OF THE TEMPORAL LOBE
IN MEMORY PROCESSES

The proposal that the temporal lobe is involved in memory processes has long historical and experimental standing and should also be told chronologically. Even so it involves the chronology of at least three parallel lines of research, all involving brain lesions but dictated by different theoretical biases.

1. Studies of the posterior association cortex of the monkey.

2. Studies of the whole temporal lobe, which includes both limbic structures and posterior association cortex in the monkey.

3. Studies of temporal lobe lesions in man.

It is difficult to know which of these progresses should be given priority; together they are converging powerfully to the heart of the matter, but each line of work has benefitted from the existence and stimulation of the others. I have chosen to approach the problem through studies of the posterior association cortex, referring when appropriate to the other lines of research.

Lashley repeatedly demonstrated that visual and other discrimination deficits resulting from lesions to the posterior association cortex of the rat reflected the size of the lesion rather than its locus (1942). He drew similar conclusions from his preliminary work on the monkey (1948). At about this time, subhuman primates became more readily available for behavioral work and Lashley initiated a series of further experiments on the posterior cortex, presumably to substantiate his preliminary results of 1948. Blum, Chow, and Pribram (1950) studied the effect of total temporal, total parietal, and combined temporal-parietal-preoccipital lesions on visual pattern discrimination, patterned string problems, visual conditional learning tasks, and auditory and tactile discrimination tasks. The parieto-temporal lesioned animals were impaired on the visual and somaesthetic tasks, but the temporal animals only on visual tasks and Blum *et al.* (1950) were forced to conclude that visual discrimination deficits were more likely to occur if the prestriate lesions extended into the ventral temporal lobe. At this time, Chow (1951) and Blum (1951) independently pursued the analysis of the visual and tactile deficits after various bilateral posterior cortex lesions. They eventually reported that lesions in the preoccipital region were more likely to produce visual discrimination deficits if the damage extended into the lateral temporal lobe cortex (Chow, 1951) and tactile discrimination deficits if the parietal cortex was involved in the lesion (Blum, 1951). These results were important because they suggested that modality specific foci outside the primary sensory areas subserve sensory discriminative functions. Neither Chow nor Blum were willing to accept that these deficits reflected a purely associative dysfunction or "agnosia," as the lesions resulted in both sensory and discriminative loss. Indeed, they questioned the traditional dichotomy between sensory and discriminative function and it is interesting to note that this problem has been carefully avoided ever since. The historical contribution of these studies was to suggest that modality specific areas existed in the posterior association cortex, but in subsequent studies, despite the reticence of Chow and Blum, it has been tacitly accepted that these deficits are of a "higher associative" nature and their basis has been sought within this framework.

It seems that Lashley's students were uncertain whether to believe their own results in 1951. Chow *et al.* (1951) reported further experiments on the posterior cortex using sensory, discrimination, and short term memory tasks, such as the delayed response. The spectrum of results led them to suggest that "different foci of prime, though not exclusive significance for various functions exist within association areas, together with neuronal pools common to several functional categories."

Despite this reticence on the part of some experimenters, the problem was pursued, and Mishkin and Pribram (1954) and Mishkin (1954) reported that

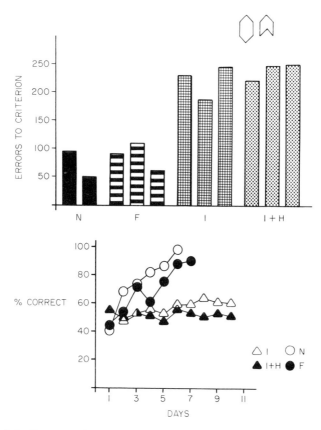

Fig. 9-5. Post operative learning of a pattern discrimination task in normals (N), dorsolateral frontals (F), inferotemporals (I), and animals with more extensive ventral temporal lobe lesions including the hippocampus (I + H). (Reproduced from Iversen and Weiskrantz, 1970.)

bilateral lesions to the ventral temporal lobe cortex extending from the superior temporal sulcus to include the middle and inferior temporal gyri (inferotemporal cortex) impaired the postoperative retention and learning of visual pattern discriminations (Fig. 9-5). Bilateral lesions to the superior temporal gyri, entorhinal cortex, or the hippocampus itself did not produce such an impairment. Subsequent behavioral studies involving electrical stimulation (Chow, 1961), epileptic foci (Stamm & Knight, 1963), and combination lesion studies (Mishkin, 1966), in addition to more recent anatomical studies using the Nauta degeneration technique [Kuypers, Szwarcbart, Mishkin, & Rosvold, 1965 (Fig. 9-6)], have served to establish firmly that localized areas existed in the posterior association cortex concerned with "higher" levels of sensory and discriminative

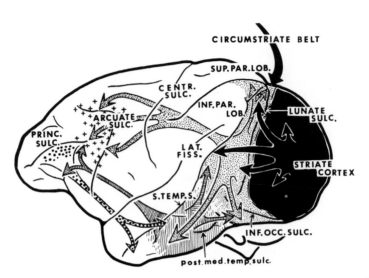

Fig. 9-6. Summary diagram of the visual cortical projections. (Reproduced from Kuypers *et al.*, 1965.)

processes. Cortical areas concerned with visual processing, and presumably analogous to the inferotemporal cortex in the Rhesus monkey and Baboon, have been identified in the cat (Warren, Warren, & Akert, 1961; Hara, 1962) and less reliably in rats (Thompson, Lesse, & Rich, 1963). The auditory (Neff, 1961), tactile (Wilson, 1957), and olfactory (Brown, Rosvold, & Mishkin, 1963) modalities have similar higher processing areas in the posterior associative cortex of the monkey, although these areas have been identified in fewer species, and much less intensively studied.

Animal experiments developed simultaneously with clinical studies of the temporal lobe. At the Montreal Neurological Institute, Penfield and his collaborators were using surgical techniques for the treatment of epilepsy, and large groups of patients became available with localized, defined, surgical removals of the cerebral cortex. As epilepsy is commonly of temporal lobe origin, a substantial patient population sustained left or right temporal lobe lesions, and these clinical cases have proved valuable for those interested in localization of function. Pathological brain lesions in man (commonly tumors, vascular accident, bacterial, or viral infections) invariably produce diffuse damage, which may increase with time in an ill-defined manner. It is therefore often difficult to associate the psychological deficits observed with any particular part of the damage. Epileptic surgical cases do not have such disadvantages, although critics have been quick to point out that in the cases with longstanding seizure histories the organization of the CNS may have been modified over the years as a result of the epileptic dysfunction and, thus, be abnormal at the time of adult surgery. In other words, in these cases the brain organization studied postoperatively may not be the same as that in a normal brain sustaining equal damage. However, although this "reconstitution" argument is frequently used, it attracts scanty experimental support. For example, in considering the effects of brain bisection in humans the 1940 series of Akelaitis (1944) is often quoted as the discordant evidence. He reported that callosal section did not impair interhemispheric relations and it was frequently suggested that his patients had a long presurgical history of epilepsy, and that this condition over the years probably induced cortical reorganization. In fact, Goldstein and Joynt (1969) have recently reexamined one of the patients from this series and report interhemispheric deficits despite the apparent lack of them 25 years before. In this case, insensitive tests proved to be the problem, and not cortical reorganization.

In the mid 1950's, Brenda Milner studied two series of patients with bilateral medial temporal lobe lesions. In one series, Scoville was the surgeon and a direct bilateral lesion was made which was restricted to the medial temporal region and included the hippocampi. The other group were patients of Penfield's from the Montreal Neurological Institute who had sustained unilateral ventro/medial temporal lesions which also included the hippocampus. Electroencephalographic investigation subsequently revealed that the medial temporal structures of the unoperated side of the brain were abnormal and the patients had, in functional terms, bilateral medial temporal lesions. Milner (Scoville & Milner, 1957; Penfield & Milner, 1958) reported that both groups of patients showed extremely severe and specific memory difficulties. Despite the fact that their short term memory, as assessed by observation and by more formal digit span measures, was intact, they appeared unable to form any new memories. One of the patients from the Scoville series, H. M., has been carefully and repeatedly studied over the last twelve years and his mnemonic difficulties have shown little improvement (Milner, Corkin, & Teuber, 1968). The impairment can be demonstrated in the visual, auditory, and tactile modalities in a variety of behavioral situations involving maze learning in the visual (Milner, 1965) and tactile mode (Corkin, 1965), recurring visual (Kimura, 1963) and auditory material (Milner, 1968), paired comparison of simple visual and auditory stimuli presented on the Konorski short term memory paradigm (Prisko, 1963), and delayed matching from sample of visual stimuli (Sidman, Stoddard, & Mohr, 1968). Successful performance on all of the tasks involves storage of information over time, albeit in some cases a relatively short period.

These results raised the interesting possibility that the hippocampus (which was the most prominent structure damaged in both Scoville's and Penfield's cases) is critically involved in memory storage processes.[1] It was

[1] In this review, such patients will be described as having medial temporal lesions, a cautious note reflecting uncertainty as to whether specific hippocampal damage or more generalized deep medial temporal involvement (hippocampus plus entorhinal cortex plus white matter) is critically related to the mnemonic disturbances. Patients with dissociable hippocampal and medial temporal lesions have not been studied.

apparent that the engram itself was not located in the hippocampus or adjacent temporal cortex because the patients who were unable to form new permanent memories after the operation showed only slight retrograde amnesia and could retrieve memories of long preoperative standing. This synthesis of the results is supported by dramatic demonstrations made during the preliminary stages of the operation when electrical stimulation of the cortex is employed to map the critical motor and speech areas in the vicinity of the intended lesion. Penfield noted that stimulation of temporal lobe cortex could evoke highly specific memories from the patient, memories which could still be elicited after the cortex itself had been removed (Penfield, 1965; Penfield & Perot, 1963). In a rather different series of experiments, Bickford, Mulder, Dodge, Svien, and Rome (1958) found that deep stimulation of the temporal lobe in human patients resulted in retrograde amnesia, the extent of which was related to the length of stimulation.

As mentioned earlier, a third line of research concerning the behavioral effects of large temporal lobe lesions in monkeys had been progressing since the mid 1930's. These experiments implicated the hippocampus in emotional behavior, a proposal gradually discredited over the years. Papez (1937) originally suggested that limbic structures of the temporal lobe, notably the hippocampus, fornix, and entorhinal cortex formed major constituents of a circuit involved in emotional balance. These ideas were supported by a group of ill-assorted animal and clinical results, but were reinforced subsequently by the famous studies of Kluver and Bucy (1939) demonstrating that bilateral temporal lobectomy in the monkey resulted in dramatic changes in emotional, appetitive, and discriminative behavior. We now believe that the changes in visual discrimination resulted from damage to the inferotemporal cortex, but at the time it was the emotional and not the visual changes which received attention. The bizarre emotional behavior observed in these animals supported Papez's notions and, in agreement with his theory, it seemed reasonable to suppose that the entorhinal and hippocampal damage included in the lobectomy was responsible for the changed behavior. However, many years and experiments later it became apparent that the amygdaloid complex adjacent to the hippocampus, which had not been included by Papez in his hypothetical circuit, was concerned with the control of emotional responses (Pribram & Weiskrantz, 1957; Weiskrantz, 1956). Such experiments, while undermining the role of the proposed circuit in emotional control, again raised the question of the function of the hippocampus (Pribram & Kruger, 1954).

At this time the clinical findings which have been referred to aroused great interest and experimenters, including many disenchanted with Papez's notions, were encouraged to look for memory disturbances after bilateral hippocampal lesions in animals. These experiments raised the fundamental problem of how to assess long-term storage in animals. Even the most cursory examination of a man's intellectual capability usually reveals any existing memory difficulties, but it is a formidable task to reliably demonstrate a storage deficit in a monkey and still more difficult to establish whether such deficits involve acquisition, storage, or retrieval mechanisms. In order to demonstrate a memory loss, stimulus information is presented to the animal, its reception noted, and its availability after various delays and treatments determined. Verbal reports satisfy these criteria in man with the added bonus that the content of the original impression can be ascertained as well as its mere existence. However, in a monkey such information can only be obtained in learning situations. The task may require recognition of a ○ but this can only be demonstrated if in a discrimination situation the animal learns to respond in the presence of the ○ and not in the presence of another form such as a +. Recognition is assumed to correlate with a certain level of accuracy of response (i.e., the criterion) and memory is assessed in terms of ease of reattainment of the same criterion after specified treatments or delays. These difficulties are increased because animals may only be tested for a limited number of trials each day and the attainment of the criterion may require several days testing and, therefore, depend on long-term storage processes. Such indirect methods create problems of interpretation. For example, if, after a lesion, an animal requires as many trials to relearn a problem as it did preoperatively, one could claim that it had forgotten. But there are several possible interpretations of such a result which are not mutually exclusive. The final long-term storage process could be impaired; information could reach the long-term storage but be inaccessible to retrieval mechanisms; equally, information could be acquired slowly owing to impaired perceptual mechanisms, and, therefore, provide an inadequate engram; perception could however be normal but an increased sensitivity to interference may prevent the information from being stored. This by no means exhausts the possible ways in which memory mechanism could be impaired in these animals and it is entirely conceivable that several mechanisms are simultaneously deranged. Few experimenters take full account of these difficulties and definitive experiments are accordingly few and far between. The best one can hope to do is to design tests which put the pressure on one part of mechanism rather than another, and in considering a spectrum of test performance it may be possible to understand which of the processes is most critically affected by the lesion.

In pursuing the clinical findings, Orbach, Milner, and Rasmussen (1960) devised an ingenious set of behavior tests for the monkey which they felt were behaviorally equivalent to the kinds of situations in which the hippocampal patients showed marked impairments. Monkeys with bilateral medial temporal lesions similar to those in the clinical patients were investigated on: (1) delayed response under various conditions, (2) delayed alternation, (3) visual and tactile discrimination, (4) object discrimination with widely spaced trials interposed with massed trials on irrelevant, visual discriminations, and (5) retention of preoperatively learned discrimination. The results were somewhat disappointing. Delayed alternation performance was impaired, as was visual and tactile discrimination performance, although to a lesser degree. However, there was no impairment on the distraction task (4) which had been designed to mimic the condition in which the clinical patients experienced most difficulty. In discussing their results, the authors commented upon the difficulty of designing an adequate test of animal memory but also considered the possibility that the hippocampus in the monkey subserves a function other than memory, although they did not specify what the function might be:

> It is emphasised that the requirements of the tests applied to man are difficult to adapt to behaviour that is within the repertoire of the monkey. We may have been unsuccessful, and this source of discrepancy may not have been ruled out at the present stage of test analysis. Neither can the possibility be ruled out of species differences in the organisation of temporal allocortical tissue.

The last point seemed to be reinforced over the years as many endeavored and failed to demonstrate specific memory impairments after medial temporal lesions in monkeys (Cordeau & Mahut, 1964; Correll & Scoville, 1967), rats (Isaacson & Wickelgren, 1962; Kimble, 1968), and cats (Flynn & Wasman, 1960). This statement must be qualified in that such tests were designed with certain preconceived ideas about the organization of memory and, in particular, that short-term memory "generally refers to transient 'holding' of information which decays rapidly with time, having formed no permanent trace [Drachman & Ommaya, 1964]." The clinical results were seen to demonstrate impairment of such a process, and, yet, lesioned animals could apparently form a permanent record of information in a variety of situations.

In the early 1960's the experimental work in animals was beginning to appear highly enigmatic as the hippocampus apparently subserved neither emotion nor memory. At this time, the work on the posterior cortex began to converge with the rather discordant clinical and animal studies of the medial temporal structures. The visual discrimination deficit localized by Mishkin and Pribram in 1954 had been extensively studied in the succeeding years in an effort to determine its basis. It had been shown to be modality specific in a classical double dissociation experiment by Wilson (1957) in which it was shown that lesions to the parietal cortex resulted in tactile and not visual deficits, while inferotemporal lesions produced the opposite results. In a series of experiments on inferotemporals, Chow (1952, 1954) found that certain visual discriminations, such as color, brightness, or objects were more easily learned than form discriminations and that preoperative overtraining reduced the severity of the deficit (Orbach & Fantz, 1958). Several experimenters demonstrated the apparent difference between primary sensory deficits following damage to the sensory projection areas and the "higher" or "associative deficits" after temporal cortical lesions (Mishkin & Hall, 1955; Wilson & Mishkin, 1959) although Pasik,

Pasik, Battersby and Bender (1960) have consistently maintained that primary sensory loss resulting from concomitant geniculo-striate damage underlies the inferotemporal visual deficit. However, most people were ready to accept that the deficit reflected impairment of a higher visual processing mechanism and it seemed possible that the storage mechanisms necessary for learning were impaired. At this time, Weiskrantz suggested that, despite obvious differences in lesion site and testing methods, the monkey inferotemporal deficit might be related to the hippocampal impairment seen in Milner's patients. First, the animal tests involve the learning and retaining of visual tasks on the basis of 30 trials per day and their inability to remember today what was learned yesterday would certainly result in slow acquisition. Second, the inferotemporal lesion does not include the hippocampus, but both the animal and clinical lesions include ventral temporal lobe cortex. This cortex has shown enormous enlargement during primate evolution according to the anatomist von Bonin (1941), which may well be accommodated by a progressive ventral migration of cortex in the temporal lobes, and if this is so the similarity between the clinical and animal lesions might be greater than it seems. We were therefore keen to test inferotemporal monkeys on visual memory tasks which (1) avoided the day to day acquisition problem referred to previously and (2) could be presented on testing paradigms similar to the interference situations in which the clinical cases showed the most severe memory difficulties (Iversen & Weiskrantz, 1970).

The test material consisted of object discrimination problems which inferotemporals are reported to be able to learn. Series of such problems of increasing difficulty were presented on the following paradigms.

Experiment 1				
Day 1	Object Problem A	Object Problem B		
Day 2		Object Problem B	Object Problem C	
Day 3			Object Problem C	Object Problem D
Day 4				Object Problem D	Object Problem E

These essentially consisted of learning an object discrimination problem, for example, B, and retaining it either after a 24-hour delay (Experiment 1), or after two successive 24-hour delays (Experiment 2), or after a 24-hour and further short delay (Experiment 3).

Experiment 2

Day 1	Object Problem A	Object Problem B	Object Problem C		
Day 2		Object Problem B	Object Problem C	Object Problem D	
Day 3			Object C Problem C	Object Problem D	Object Problem E
Day 4				Object Problem D	Object Problem E	Object Problem F etc.

Experiment 3

Day 1	Object Problem A	Object Problem B	Object Problem A		
Day 2		Object Problem B	Object Problem C	Object Problem B	
Day 3			Object Problem C	Object Problem D	Object Problem C
Day 4				Object Problem D	Object Problem E	Object Problem D etc.

The principal findings were: (1) that inferotemporals have difficulty in learning the object problems on their first presentation but finally are able to reach criterion of 18/20; (2) that inferotemporals require almost as many trials to relearn the problems when they are represented after a 24-hour delay (Experiment 1, Fig. 9-7) and show little further improvement after another 24 hours (Experiment 2); and (3) that a 24-hour delay is not necessary to produce this retention decrement. A 15-minute delay occupied with new visual learning (Experiment 3) was sufficient to impair retention. Results (2) and (3) were similar to the clinical findings but it did not seem feasible to claim that they demonstrated categorically a memory impairment in view of the fact that the initial acquisition over a relatively short number of consecutive trials was also deficient. If these results were considered to reflect a unitary impairment, it seemed most reasonable to suppose that the basic deficit resulted in slow and inadequate acquisition, which in turn precluded adequate storage. But it proved difficult to dissociate, experimentally, perceptual acquisition and memory. Both

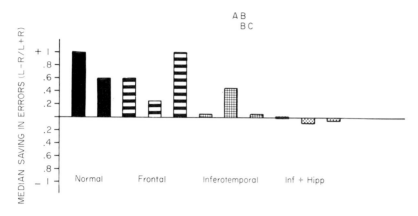

Fig. 9-7. Mean saving score after 24-hour delay on 48 object discrimination problems for individual animals in the four experimental groups N, F, I, and I + H. (Reproduced from Iversen and Weiskrantz, 1970.)

the temporal and normal animals reached the same criterion of acquisition, but the lesioned animals required more trials to do so. However, one may question what an arbitrary criterion of 18/20 represents. Performance at this level does not mean that both groups had acquired the same amount or kind of visual information. For example, if a tin soldier with a red hat, blue trousers, a gun, and six medals is used as an object discriminandum, noticing the red hat will suffice to distinguish this soldier from another with a green hat, red trousers, and no gun or medals, and, indeed, the criterion could be attained on this basis. However, noticing the blue trousers, the gun, and the six medals greatly increases the distinctiveness of the percept and would presumably serve to increase the probability that the impression of this particular object which is stored, has sufficient distinctiveness to resist interference from another very similar soldier. To show impaired storage one would need to demonstrate that temporals learned a problem as easily as controls, and yet showed poor retention. Even then, one could not be sure that during the initial perceptual analysis, occurring at the same rate, the amount or nature of the visual information analyzed by both groups was equally "meaningful" for storage processes, although one could aim to eliminate this difficulty by adjusting criterion levels to equate perceptual processes. However, such an approach lacks theoretical direction.

In the midst of this practical dilemma and consideration of the various indirect ways of trying to resolve the problem, evidence was presented showing that temporals are indeed deficient and abnormal in their perceptual processing abilities, irrespective of what their storage capacity might be. This advance was largely due to Butter who, with others, has reported impaired visual generalization (Butter, Mishkin, & Rosvold, 1965), and equivalence (Butter, 1968) performance in inferotemporal monkeys, which he considers

> not due to a defect in coding perceptual features. Rather, the present findings suggest that their impairment may be due to a defect in sampling or attending to several aspects of stimuli.

At this time it appeared cautious to relate our experimental findings to impaired visual categorization (Iversen & Weiskrantz, 1967). Even so, there remained, in the range of data, indications that storage capacity was deficient irrespective of difficulties in acquisition. In a later series of experiments, for example, the effects of interference and delay on retention were compared, and it was found that in the inferotemporals memory for object problems after visual interference was reduced, despite an insignificant impairment in initial acquisition (Iversen, 1970). More recently we have begun to understand why our data appeared to provide evidence both of impaired visual perception and of memory. The classical inferotemporal lesion extends from near the preoccipital sulcus to within 5 mm of the temporal pole and ventrally from the superior temporal sulcus to include the medial and inferior temporal gyri (Fig. 9-1). In some studies designed to dissociate the primary receiving area from the inferotemporal cortex, Mishkin and his collaborators studied various preoccipital lesions and a careful analysis of the results showed that a small lesion in the preoccipital region which certainly failed to anatomically dissociate the two areas resulted in very severe visual discrimination deficits (Ettlinger, Iwai, Mishkin, & Rosvold, 1968). This observation was painstakingly pursued by Iwai and Mishkin (1967, 1970). Bilateral 5-mm strip lesions were made from the preoccipital sulcus to the anterior pole region and it was found that animals with small lesions in the posterior interotemporal cortex had severe visual pattern discrimination deficits. The immediately anterior lesions did not result in such a severe deficit but lesions yet more anterior in the temporal lobe again produced evidence of an impairment, albeit a less severe one than from the posterior lesion. These results indicated that two foci existed in the traditional inferotemporal lesion and in later studies they have produced evidence that the basis of the visual deficits produced by the focal lesions may be different. The posterior focus severely impairs pattern discrimination which is considered a sensitive test of perceptual analysis or categorization. The anterior focus impairs the concurrent learning of simple object discrimination problems. These foci and deficits are doubly dissociated in that the anterior lesions do not severely impair pattern discrimination nor the posterior lesion impair concurrent learning. It therefore seems likely that the higher levels of perceptual analysis are mediated by posterior temporal lobe cortex and that mechanisms vital for concurrent learning are subserved by related anterior cortex.

The concurrent learning paradigm is a useful behavioral test, as it can be employed as a measure of associative or learning ability but may also serve as a vehicle to compare the rate of acquisition of visual problems varying in perceptual difficulty. If such a range of problems is studied as individual simultaneous discriminations, it is difficult to dissociate testing order effects and learning set effects from the influence of task difficulty. The concurrent learning paradigm circumvents this difficulty by presenting the full range of discriminations within each teaching session. Each problem is presented for the same number of trials during the session, but the trials on any given problem occur singly and distributed among trials on the other problems. Acquisition of a given problem on the basis of isolated, random trials presumably taxes not only discriminative but, probably, more importantly, memory processes. With such a test it might be possible to begin to dissociate perceptual and memory functions. If, for example, perceptually difficult problems were presented, presumably posterior inferotemporals would show severe impairments, while on perceptually simple problems they would be unimpaired. Anterior inferotemporals, on the other hand, should be impaired on the concurrent learning irrespective of the perceptual difficulty of the problems. Obviously one would not expect a clear dissociation, as it is reasonable to suppose that the perceptual and memory processes involved in such a task are not completely independent. Preliminary results using this behavioral technique are promising.

The rate of acquisition of color, brightness, size, contour, pattern, and orientation discriminations has been studied, and it was found that posterior inferotemporal lesions impair only the perceptually most difficult problem pattern (the mirror image tilt discrimination being too difficult for either the temporals or controls). Color, brightness, size, and contour problems were learned equally well by the posterior inferotemporals and the controls. Related results have been obtained in a visual oddity experiment (Iversen & Humphrey, 1971). This task involved the acquisition of a principle— "respond to the odd one" —and not on the ability to remember from trial to trial which of the stimuli is rewarded. All that is demanded is the ability to see the difference between the stimuli and to respond according to the principle. This behavioral method also provides a useful vehicle for studying the acquisition of problems of varying perceptual difficulty. We found in this experiment that the posterior inferotemporals were not impaired in oddity learning per se, but were impaired if the oddity response was guided by a perceptually difficult discrimination such as pattern (Fig. 9-8). On the other hand, animals with large inferotemporal lesions, which impinged on both the posterior and the anterior segments, were impaired in the "principle" learning in both of these experiments. In the concurrent learning tasks, such animals showed impaired acquisition of all the problems and, likewise, in the oddity experiment showed impaired retention and slower acquisition of new problems. However, these learning deficits were also influenced by perceptual difficulty, but this is to be expected as the large lesion included both the anterior and the posterior foci, and not only the selective anterior lesions as in the original Iwai and Mishkin experiment.

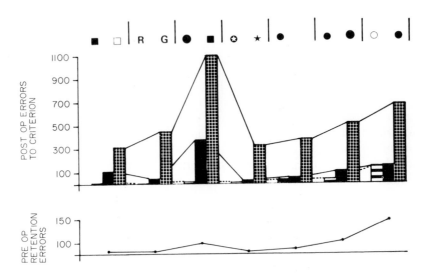

Fig. 9-8. Upper: Post-operative relearning scores on seven oddity problems ranging in perceptual difficulty in controls (stripes), posterior inferotemporals (black), and total inferotemporals (check). Lower: Preoperative retention score profile for all *S*s.

Thus, we now have a brain lesion which impairs learning processes rather than perceptual mechanisms, and presumably such learning is dependent on memory processes. One could imagine that concurrent learning would put a considerable onus on memory process as a discrimination is developed on the basis of isolated, random exposure to the problem, in the context of severe interference from related problems. But do these results correlate with the clinical observation that bilateral medial temporal lesions, including the hippocampus, produce severe memory difficulties? It could be suggested that in the clinical cases the hippocampal damage is not the critical pathology, even if, as has been assumed, it exists bilaterally in H. M. However, this argument is not accepted by the clinicians, especially in view of the fact that a case from the Scoville series which has come to autopsy shows major hippocampal involvement in both hemispheres. If, then, the clinical statements are valid, why have we been apparently unsuccessful in producing memory deficits in animals with bilateral medial temporal damage? Probably because of a rather naive assumption that memory can be measured in animals with simple in/out tests of storage capacity. For example, Mishkin and Pribram included hippocampal lesions in their 1954 studies and found no impairment on the postoperative retention of pattern discriminations tested for 30 trials per day. Orbach *et al.* (1958) using more extensive medial temporal lesions were also unsuccessful with a much wider range of problems—including tactile discriminations and visual discriminations with interference between the isolated trials. Simultaneous tactile discrimination and day-to-day tactile memory tests are insensitive to ventral temporal lobe lesions which include hippocampal damage (Iversen, 1967). However, medial temporal lesions [2] are not without effect in animals and result in deficits on a wide range of tasks including concurrent learning (Correll & Scoville, 1965a), visual matching from sample (Correll & Scoville, 1965b), sequential tasks (Kimble & Pribram, 1963), reversal tasks (Mahut & Cordeau, 1963; Webster & Voneida, 1964; Teitelbaum, 1964), and maze learning (Kaada, Rasmussen, & Kveim, 1961), spatial reversal (Waxler & Rosvold, 1970; Mahut, 1971). In general both in monkeys and rats hippocampal lesions impair the ability of the animal to adjust its behavior when discriminative and reinforcing stimuli in the environment change unpredictably. If the spatial environment or the learning conditions are stable (e.g., discrimination learning) the hippocampal animal is not impaired.

These results have appeared in literature over a number of years and often not as a direct attack on the problem of hippocampal involvement in memory function. Superficially, such tasks are not simply tests of memory (as our AB/BC experiment might be considered to be). On the other hand these tasks do share common features. All demand considerable flexibility at the registration stage and not simply a repeated registration of the identical information, as in a simultaneous discrimination. The information to be registered may change repeatedly, indeed, as often as every trial in the concurrent learning task, and the stimulus/reinforcement contingency may also change repeatedly as in a reversal task. Furthermore, these tasks, with their organized change, also have built into them high levels of pro- and retroactive-interference, and it is equally possible that this is their most crucial property for the hippocampal animal. We know from studies of normal human memory that interference is a major influence on mnemonic efficiency (Broadbent, 1957; Conrad, 1960; Brown, 1964; Keppel & Underwood, 1962). As the medial temporal patients have been studied over the years it has been frequently reported that tests involving built-in interference, such as the visual (Kimura, 1963) and auditory (Milner, 1962) recurring figure tests, complex maze learning in the visual (Milner, 1965) or tactile modality (Corkin, 1965), and paired comparison as in the Konorski type matching task (Prisko, 1963) are particularly difficult for these patients.

However, to return to the main theme of our paper concerning lesions and memory in animals, it may be noted that lesions to the anterior temporal cortex as well as the medial temporal structures result in deficits on concurrent learning

[2] The term medial temporal damage is again used in the absence of direct evidence that the behavioral deficits are related specifically to hippocampal involvement. This reticence is not shared by some experimenters who assume that the hippocampal damage is the source of the impairment despite evidence of involvement of adjacent tissue in their lesioned animals. Selective lesion studies would be difficult but necessary to clarify this point.

which are considered to reflect mnemonic disturbances. On the basis of such results, it seems possible that the anterior inferotemporal cortex is functionally related to the limbic system with respect to memory processes. This hypothesis is worth pursuing in view of recent clinical findings of Corsi (quoted by Milner) indicating that anterior left or right temporal cortex lesions impair performance on material specific memory tasks modelled on the Peterson tests. These deficits are intensified if the hippocampus is included in the lesion and are most severe in the bilateral hippocampal patient, H. M.

The exposition of the hypothesis that the anterior temporal lobe cortex and the medial temporal structures are involved in memory functions, and that there is some agreement between the animal and clinical data, is very much a post hoc exercise. In the lean years while it looked as if there was a major discontinuity in temporal lobe organization in animals and man, the study of a striking visual deficit in temporal lobe monkeys progressed. It seemed that the deficit studied for so many years had as its major element impaired perceptual processes, but further study has revealed an anterior temporal focus which appears to be involved in memory processes, and removal of this cortex produces a deficit which resembles the medial temporal syndrome at least on the concurrent learning task. The functional relationship between the anterior cortex and limbic system should be pursued in animals; it would be interesting to have more precise information about the anterior focus and to know if it is, in fact, the area of cortex classified by Pribram and Kruger (1954) as part of the juxta-allo cortex of the limbic system. It is also becoming clear that the amygdala and hippocampus contribute in different ways to the processes involved in learning and memory (Douglas and Pribram, 1966; Pribram, 1967).

Temporal lobe involvement in memory is now unravelled and nothing has been said about the substrate and location of the memory store; indeed very little can be said. An irreversible lesion is not the technique for studying widespread, short- and long-term modifications in neuronal substrates. Progress has been made since 1950 in delineating the brain structures involved in the highest levels of sensory organization and in processes which are relevant to mnemonic coding. In the discussion, it has been tacitly assumed that the mnemonic organization necessary for laying down memories is impaired by temporal lobe lesions. However, all the results mentioned could equally well be due to impaired retrieval or, indeed, impaired coding and retrieval if both processes are subserved by the same neurological substrates. The dissociation of these possibilities is receiving theoretical consideration (Weiskrantz, 1966), but the practical challenge is even greater, as most of the behavioral techniques are interdependent, as, for example, tests for assessing registration depend on retrieval and vice versa. If progress can be made in the direction of more refined behavioral analysis, resultant insight into the preliminary organizational processes of memory may enable us to recognize the functional characteristics of the engram itself.

IV. SYNTHESIS

The history of the experimental brain lesion as a tool for studying memory has been reviewed and it may now be relevant to search for parsimony between brain lesion studies in animals and man and to examine the memory deficits observed in relation to current models of normal human memory. A few years ago the prognosis for this task was unfavorable. If the behavioral results obtained from frontal monkeys and bilateral medial temporal man were combined, the simple two process model of memory then in fashion was vindicated and it could be claimed that frontal lobe cortex is involved in short-term memory and the temporal lobe in more permanent storage processes. Unfortunately, however, parsimony between animal and clinical studies was wanting and there were several reports in the literature which failed to demonstrate the expected short-term memory defects in frontal man (Ghent, Mishkin, & Teuber, 1962; Teuber & Proctor, 1964; Chorover & Cole, 1966) and an equally large number of animal studies which apparently failed to produce deficits resembling the very severe memory disorders seen clinically after bilateral medial temporal damage.

Experimental lesion studies continued, but at the same time a two process model of memory was applied at the neurophysiological level and it became important to establish both how long was required for a short-term memory to attain permanence and what physically constituted these two memory states. This is not the place to discuss how electroconvulsive shock and other treatments which depress or disrupt the activity of the nervous system have indicated that, at least in one trial learning situation, electrical activity begins to give rise to a more permanent record within a few seconds. Consequently, workers came to think of short-term memory as a transitory process, perhaps mediated by reverberating circuits, which gave rise ultimately to unidentified long-term substrates. The earlier lesions studies predated such speculation and Jacobsen, for example, unaware that short-term memory lasted for only a few seconds, quite accurately discussed the frontal impairments as disturbances of short or immediate memory. On the other hand, the temporal lobe work saw major developments after some of the physiological experiments had become established, and at this conjuncture terminology became confusing. Acquisition type deficits after temporal lobe lesions were now viewed as long-term memory impairments, largely, one supposes, because the workers concerned saw that the training process involved more than a few seconds or minutes and presumed that their experiments were now out of the bounds of short- and into long-term memory.

This confusion was not shared by some of the influential clinical workers studying the temporal lobe. The dramatic memory disturbances observed after bilateral medial temporal lesions in man were correctly inferred to be immediate- or short-term memory disturbances despite their resemblances, at least in practical terms, to the kinds of deficits being studied in temporal monkeys. Contrived tests of long-term memory were used to study temporal lesions and, in particular, hippocampal animals, and the negative results led many to suppose that major discontinuity existed between the temporal lobe of man and monkey, in addition to verbal function. It is possible that these differences in the origin and context of the terminology has hindered the recognition of parsimony, insofar as it exists.

The last few years have seen a great deal of interest and experimentation on these problems, but the results have not, in all cases, clarified the issues. On the one hand, certain semantic problems have been restated and it may now be possible to reconcile the apparent discontinuity between animal and clinical studies of the temporal lobe. But, on the other hand, the results on frontal lobe animals suggesting the existence of memory impairments, have been absorbed into other classifications of the frontal deficit conceived in terms of aberrant response, motivation control, or spatial perception, and it is at present uncertain if there is any independent memory impairment associated with localized anterior cortical damage. Further selective lesion studies of the frontal cortex may satisfy this glaring omission, but during the following discussion other discrepancies will no doubt become apparent which are conceptually and experimentally more challenging.

A Reappraisal of Terminology

In the frontal lobe, the animal experiments suggested that the ability to organize and retrieve information over a short period of time was one of the deficits associated with such lesions. As the time delays in the early experiments involved seconds rather than hours, the term "immediate" was attached to the inferred memory disorder. As Jacobsen (1936) noted, at the time there appeared to be a real distinction underlying the fact that a frontal monkey is able to

> learn and retain sensory-motor habits and visual discrimination but it is unable to remember for even a few seconds under which of two cups a piece of food had been concealed. . . . The present experiments suggest that two discrete processes, mediated through different neurological mechanisms, are being studied. The sensorimotor tasks and visual discrimination tests favour establishment of stable sensory motor habits by repeated trials. On the other hand, the delayed response test makes quite different demands and is suggestive of the kind of events which in Man we characterize as immediate memory.

But even as he attached this description to the observed defect, he was sufficiently uncertain to warrant the comment quoted previously on page 321.

The identification of the process deranged by medial temporal lesions has been no easier to define; indeed, clinical and animal workers have tended to emphasize different aspects of the spectrum of memory disorders seen after this lesion. In the initial studies of Milner it was apparent that the clinical syndrome showed three features which have over the years been characterized more precisely as (1) retrograde amnesia, (2) acquisition deficits, and (3) short-term memory loss in the presence of distraction. The clinical workers originally emphasized (3) and, indeed, one of the original papers was entitled "Loss of recent memory after bilateral hippocampal lesions." The overlap of this terminology with that of the animal frontal literature was not commented upon but may have been responsible for the tendency of animal workers themselves to emphasize characteristic (2) and to view the memory deficits associated with medial temporal lesions as indicative of impaired long-term storage which would thus be clearly differentiated from the immediate memory loss of the frontal syndrome. This seemed especially appropriate in view of the fact that the initial demonstrations of the deficits in man involved day-to-day memory situations and verbal memory tasks (e.g., story repetition) based on repeated trials, which from subjective experience one would suppose involved long-term memory. For example, Patient A of the Penfield and Milner study could not remember what happened during the day; for example

> he sat outside on the gallery the whole of one afternoon and was interviewed by one of us (B.M.) there; yet later that same day he denied ever having been on the gallery . . .

On the other hand, clinical attention focussed on more formal psychological testing situations where

> it is particularly interesting that there has been no impairment of attention or concentration (as measured by digit repetition and mental arithmetic tests), a finding which contrasts markedly with the patient's inability to recall test material after as little as five minutes if his attention has been diverted to something else in the meantime. The change of attention appears to be crucial, since he can retain a three figure number or an unfamiliar word association for many minutes, provided no distractions are introduced.

This fundamental difference in emphasis was responsible for the development of perhaps inappropriate animal tests involving acquisition over repeated trials, in some of which intertrial delays were varied. In retrospect neither delay nor acquisition per se is the most crucial factor for the medial temporal but certain task features demanding flexible organization during the memory storage process. It may therefore be claimed that medial temporal lesions in man are associated with inefficient transfer of information from short-term to long-term memory rather than inadequate long-term storage processes as such. If the range of experiments are examined in this light, it may be possible to find more correspondence between animal and clinical studies than was once supposed. The use of the same terminology may indicate parsimony, but the proof lies in identifying the functional justification for such usage.

Indeed, it is questionable if the temporal characteristics of memory performance are at all helpful in the identification and understanding of the underlying processes. The temporal characteristics of the processes themselves and the stage at which transfer from process to process takes place are probably more variable

than we would like to suppose for the purposes of a simple model. The
relationship between particular tasks and the operating characteristics of such
models have not been delineated and it should be recognized that

> a task in which retention is measured a few minutes after presentation of the item to
> be remembered may well be heterogeneous with respect to the underlying processes,
> and therefore should not be arbitrarily labelled a short term memory test [Milner,
> 1968].

Drachman and Arbit (1966) have also been concerned with the problem of
identifying and naming memory states and consider temporal considerations to
be of minor importance, indeed misleading. They prefer to use "immediate- or
short-term" memory for the process handling attended to, subspan memoranda.
"Long-term" memory refers to all other processes and

> deals both with supraspan memoranda held for long or short intervals and with
> subspan memoranda recalled following the redirection of attention.

Such a proposition differs from the standard models of human memory
where "short-term" has become a temporal classification. Such models do not
attempt to account for the fact that the nature of the memory process operating
at an interval after presentation is determined by the information kind rather
than the delay. The precise terminology is unimportant but it is the "long-term"
process thus defined by Drachman and Arbit which is considered to be severely
impaired by medial temporal lesions.

It is difficult to apply physiological data to models of memory, but such
studies have indicated that it is valid to dissociate a transitory process (c. 20
seconds) which may be called immediate memory. The classical test of this
short-term process is the digit span, a task which (except in isolated dominant
posterior lesions) is not affected by focal brain damage in the absence of general
dementia. However, even at delays as short as 20 seconds, memory impairments
may be seen if variables such as presentation rate, nature of information,
distraction, and ability to rehearse tax the subject. In such cases, what shall we
call the impairment? Not "short" because the temporal characteristic is secondary, but not "long" because an impairment may be detected after short or long
delays. It seems most likely that the manipulations have impaired the transfer of
the information from its transiency to its more permanent state. The terms short
and long are perhaps irrelevant tags to memory disorders, reflecting only the
delays at which deficits may be seen and not the temporal characteristics of the
process which has been impaired. It might even be claimed that transfer functions of this kind are the only parts of the memory process affected by focal
brain damage, for, indeed, once firmly established and in a permanent store,
memories are extremely difficult to destroy, except again in the case of global
cerebral dysfunction.

Unwittingly, it would seem that those who investigate human verbal
memory and provide the models and those who study the disruption of memory

process with brain lesions have both focused on the same aspect of the process—
the short-term to long-term transfer. Few theorists have been interested by
simple digit span except to disrupt it, and Bilodeau (1966) is one of the few
since Ebbinghaus to concern himself with the acquisition properties of long-term
memory.

Perhaps, therefore, it would be valuable to start again at the beginning,
without any preconceptions about terminology, in an effort to identify and
characterize the memory process disordered by frontal and temporal lesions. In
the process it will be proposed that

1. It is very difficult to distinguish experimentally frontal and medial
temporal impairments in animals.

2. The frontal and temporal memory impairments may be loosely identified in simple two-process models of memory. The more sophisticated models of
recent years are largely irrelevant to our present discussion, as the scope of
animal testing does not allow us to study precisely transfer functions, or the
structure of the long-term memory store, or the characteristics of the short-term
trace. If such experiments were possible, many would hope that the remarkable
similarity of frontal and temporal impairments would be shown to be fortuitous,
and that two distinct processes are being affected by the different lesions.
However, if the data is taken at face value, it would seem that at present the
distinction is maintained by little more than historical conviction.

3. The effects of medial temporal lesions in animals and man are similar.

4. The effects of frontal lesions in animals and man are similar (on the
basis of limited evidence).

1. Comparison of Frontal and Medial Temporal Impairments in Animals

If, as an exercise, a list of animal frontal and medial temporal deficits is
made, the similarity is striking (Table 9-1). These lists of impairments represent a
less than complete search of the literature and include experiments on a variety
of species. The behavioral tests used in the studies may bear the same name
although the precise testing conditions differ considerably. Of greater significance is the fact that the lesions between species and, much more importantly,
within a species vary both in size and locus. It will be apparent from what has
been said in the section on the frontal lobe deficits, that there is, at present, no
evidence of independent memory disorders in the frontal lobe, although it is
possible that lesions to the sulcus principalis may give evidence of such a
function. Accordingly, many of the deficits listed as being associated with
frontal lesions were obtained with lesions extending far outside this sulcus
principalis focus and, indeed, the deficits may in fact be due to involvement of
other foci concerned with response control, spatial responses, and so on. However, the validity of the list is amenable to experimentation and all of these tasks
should be examined after appropriate selective lesions, one of which should be
the sulcus principalis. The variability of the temporal/hippocampal lesions is

equally great and it would be of value to examine anterior temporal, medial temporal, discrete hippocampal or amygdala and combination lesions on at least some of the tasks which seem to be significant with respect to memory processes. Having stressed the inherent inadequacy of the data presented, it may be noted that the lists are remarkably similar. This may seem surprising in view of the fact that it has long been assumed and apparently proven that these lesions produce different if not opposite effects on memory processes.

Some of the possible explanations for this coincidence, if true, are uninteresting and disconcerting in so far as they would reinforce critics who consider lesions inadequate and useless tools for studying brain function and, in particular, memory. For example it could be suggested that:

1. The behavioral tests are poor and involve many psychological processes, with the result that despite localization of function, almost any brain lesion results in deficits.

2. A single memory substrate is involved in such tasks, but it is widely distributed in the CNS, and, accordingly, disrupted by damage to any part of the brain.

(1) is a difficult interpretation to undermine because it is difficult to devise valid behavioral tests for animals which measure an isolated psychological process; (2) is not unlike Lashley's interpretation of his memory studies on the rat but will not apply to the monkey results where, using more precise tests, it is found that all lesions simply do not impair performance on the tasks listed in Table 9-1.

What then of the more unlikely hypothesis that frontal and medial temporal lesions produced a similar range of deficits? The frontal cortex appears to be involved in (1) Response control; (2) Motivational control; (3) Memory processes; and (4) Spatial functions, bearing in mind the qualifications expressed earlier. Is it not possible that with the exception of function (4) (related to a highly specific projection to Area 8), a total lesion to the hippocampus results in a similar heterogenous group of deficits. There is no evidence of localization of function within the hippocampus, but anatomy often provides the clues for subsequent dissociation studies. At least with respect to response and motivational control, both areas have the necessary and similar connections; first, both project, in a topographical manner, to the basal ganglia and, second, both project to the "subcortical elements" (Brady, 1958) of the limbic system known to be concerned in motivational behavior. What is lacking in both bases is any clear indication of an anatomical substrate for the indicated memory function. The existing information about the subcortical projections from the sulcus principalis (Johnson, Rosvold, & Mishkin, 1968) is not particularly suggestive. They reported that lesions within the dorsolateral cortex (including discrete sulcus principalis lesions) do not, unlike orbital lesions, show degeneration to the septal nuclei and the lateral hypothalamus, but do show slight degeneration in the hippocampus. The hippocampus itself, via the fornix, provides what is perhaps the most important efferent system from the forebrain, and Penfield speculated about the role of such a projection in memory function when he referred to the "centrencephalic system." However, it is premature to pursue this line of argument before a discrete memory function is dissociated in both frontals and hippocampals from the impairments in response control. In the earlier parts, reference was made to various characteristics of the memory tasks which seem to differentiate them from tasks involving only response or motivational control. They may be summarized as (a) changing stimulus–response–reinforcement contingencies; (b) the trials are not autonomous in the sense that in order to respond accurately access is required to previous information; (c) high interference levels because of (a) and (b).

In view of the speculative nature of such ideas, this is not the appropriate time to dwell on all possible interpretations. Three features of the tasks have been commented upon, which may be common to all of them and which may be important, but it represents no more than an inspired guess. Other common features could no doubt be found which may prove more relevant. The value of pursuing this problem at a theoretical level must await further verification of the similarity between the anterior-medial temporal and dorsolateral frontal deficits. To satisfy this point, the effects of appropriate selective frontal lesions, anterior temporal, and hippocampal lesions should be examined on a wide range of the tasks where this has not already been done and, in point of fact, very little has been done with selective lesions. This will involve an enormous amount of work and only then will it be legitimate to pursue the hypothesis voiced here.

In the absence of such evidence, a good case can be made for a unitary explanation of impairments (1) and (2) in terms of a loss of internal inhibition. Douglas (1967) and Kimble (1968) have both convincingly argued that the most common feature of hippocampal deficits on a range of tasks, some of which have been mentioned already, reflects dysfunction of an inhibition mechanism. They emphasize such a deficit in relation to impairment of extinction of instrumentally and classically conditioned responses, changing response rates in accordance with changed reinforcement schedules, discrimination reversal, distractibility to novel stimuli, passive avoidance, spontaneous and learned alternation, maze learning, DRL performance, and successive discrimination.

In his recent review of the behavioral effects of hippocampal lesions, Douglas (1967) briefly considered the possibility that the effects of hippocampal and frontal lesions were similar but felt that while it was too early to be dogmatic on this point, the divergence of results, particularly on memory tests, encouraged the view that the lesions produced different behavioral effects. Douglas placed most emphasis on the behavioral deficits which he (and Kimble, also 1968) considers to reflect disturbance of an inhibitory process mediated by the hippocampus and, in searching for a unitary theory of hippocampal disorders, was influenced to a large extent by the experiments on rats to somewhat

TABLE 9-1

Effect of Lesion and Behavioral Measure[a]		Frontal Lesion	Hippocampal Lesion
Increase	Locomotor activity	Gross, 1963	Douglas & Isaacson, 1964; Jarrard & Bunnell, 1968; Gotsick, 1969; Jarrard, 1968
Increase	Exploratory behavior	Lindsley, Weiskrantz, & Mingay, 1964	Kamback, 1967b; Leaton, 1968
Increase	Distractibility	Kamback, 1967a	Rogozea & Ungher, 1968
Change	Autonomic responses	Robinson & Mishkin, 1968	Votaw & Lauer, 1963
Impair	Spatial alternation or reversal	Jacobsen, 1936; Mishkin, 1964; Teitelbaum, 1964	Kimble & Kimble, 1965; Teitelbaum, 1964; Mahut & Cordeau, 1963
Impair	Delayed response	Jacobsen, 1936	Correll & Scoville, 1967
Impair	Alternation of two responses	Gross, Chorover & Cohen 1965	Gross, Chorover, & Cohen, 1965
Impair	Discrimination reversal	Gross, 1963; Teitelbaum, 1964; Harlow & Dagnon, 1942	Silveira & Kimble, 1968; Teitelbaum, 1961, 1964; Webster & Voneida, 1964
Impair	Maze learning		Kaada, Rasmussen, & Kveim, 1961; Jackson & Strong, 1969; Kimble, 1963

Impair	Shock avoidance	Pribram & Weiskrantz, 1957; Lichtenstein, 1950	Pribram & Weiskrantz, 1957; Isaacson & Wickelgren, 1962; Niki, 1962; Snyder & Isaacson, 1965
Impair	Go/No Go discrimination	Gross & Weiskrantz, 1962; Brutowski, Mishkin, & Rosvold, 1967	McCleary, 1966
Impair	Matching to Sample	Buffery, 1964; Glick, Goldfarb, & Jarrick, 1960	Drachman & Ommaya, 1964; Corell & Scoville, 1965.
Disrupt	Extinction performance	Butter, Mishkin & Rosvold, 1963	Douglas & Pribram, 1966; Jarrad, Isaacson & Wickelgren, 1964; Niki, 1965; Peretz, 1965; Rabe & Haddad, 1968
Disrupt	Motivational control	Brutowski & Dabrowska, 1963; Brutowski, 1964	Schmaltz & Isaacson, 1966; Jarrad, 1965; Kimble & Coover, 1966; Pizzi & Lorens, 1967
Disrupt	Response control	Rosvold, 1970	Ellen & Wilson, 1963
Disrupt	Sequential responding	Pinto-Hamuy & Linck, 1965	Kimble & Pribram, 1963
Disrupt	Timing behavior	Stamm, 1963; Glickstein, Quigley, & Stebbing, 1964	Clark & Isaacson, 1965; Ellen & Powell, 1962

[a]This list was compiled without consideration of size of lesion, species, or comparability of behavioral measures.

hesitatingly favor the inhibition hypothesis. The present author feels that the more recent Primate experiments strengthen the theory that disturbed memory process may underly one class of the medial temporal and frontal deficits and that any theory must account for such data. Indeed, it is possible that response and motivational control contribute to a general memory process which depends largely on internal inhibition for its operation. The fact that in the frontal lobe response and motivational control and memory processing are anatomically distinct does not negate the proposition because such processes could be functionally integrated through their efferent projections. In the hippocampus, the organization of the fields of neurones and their dendritic fields suggests Olds' (1970) concept of a working memory for coding input/output relationships. Disinhibition [or lack of internal inhibition (Pavlov) as used by Kimble] prevents irrelevant, and, invariably, in animal experiments, nonreinforced events from being recorded. In this sense the hypothesis provides an adequate explanation of the response and motivational impairments seen in the hippocampal and frontal animals although its application is not so apparent to some of the more complex deficits such as delayed matching from sample, where the stimulus, response, and reinforcement relationships are constantly changing. Moreover, Warrington and Weiskrantz (1970) have recently pointed out the preponderence of false positive errors shown by human amnesics (one of which sustains medial temporal damage) on certain memory tasks suggests a disinhibition of material in the memory store rather than a simple paucity of stored information as is usually suggested. In this respect, the medial temporal memory disorders in man may be reconciled with the apparently different "disinhibition" deficits commonly seen in hippocampal rats and monkeys.

The suggestion that the frontal and medial temporal lesions produce the same range of behavioral deficits may seem outrageous but it is not new. A relationship between frontal cortex and limbic structures has previously been suggested on the basis of anatomical evidence (Fulton, 1952; Pribram, 1958) and reviewed recently by Nauta (1964, 1971). Frontal cortex is connected with limbic structures and both project to the same subcortical structures. "This similarity," writes Nauta, "could raise the suspicion that the prefrontal cortex affects the same general brain-stem mechanisms which are also governed by neural discharge from the limbic forebrain. It could even be asked if the available anatomical data do not suggest that the prefrontal cortex is the isocortical representative of the same category of functions that is subserved by the limbic forebrain and its affiliated subcortical structures." Lesion and anatomical studies suggest that both the hippocampus and frontal cortex are part of circuitry necessary if behavior is to be adjusted to a changing internal or external environment.

2. Animal Frontal and Temporal Impairments in Relation to Models of Human Memory

If it is maintained that both frontal and medial temporal lesions disturb a process which organizes and holds information for a limited period prior to the formation of a permanent memory, it may be relevant to examine current models of the memory process to see if these deficits can be related to any clearly defined part of the memory mechanism. Extensive work in the human verbal memory sphere has produced models in which a process of limited duration gives rise to more permanent engram (Broadbent, 1958). These processes are considered to have a different basis and the recent experimental effort has largely concerned the so-called short-term process, a terminology which loosely accommodates a wide range of the temporal and organizational properties of human memory (Brown, 1964). The task is to try to identify the frontal and temporal recording impairments in terms of such models of the memory process. The following diagram remains the most widely accepted model at present

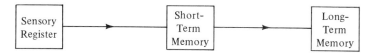

in which a complete representation is held for a very short period (< 200 msec) in the sensory register; a proportion of the information is held and recirculated by the short term mechanism during which time a copying or transfer process initiates the elements of a long-term trace, which strengthens over a certain period of time.

In simple terms, the frontal impairment was seen as an inability to retrieve information from the short-term store soon after its entry, but not as a loss of information, as frontals showed normal cumulative learning of difficult discrimination tasks. Temporal lobe disorders reported in man being characterized by a difficulty in forming long-term memories were seen as being complimentary to the frontal disorder. The failure to demonstrate the anticipated long-term memory impairments in animals was accepted philosophically but, in fact, the temporal lobe acquisition impairments in man are seen to be secondary to the most important fact that information is lost by such patients very shortly after acquisition if any demand is placed upon holding in the presence of distraction, presumably a routine requirement of the normal memory. It therefore seems more apt to call the clinical defects short-term memory disorders which, on account of their severity, preclude almost any permanent or semipermanent storage. In this light, the animal temporal lobe literature may be reexamined and it is found, as discussed earlier, that, in fact, such animals have severe deficits on a range of tasks which demand a high degree of flexibility and information accessibility from trial to trial. Thus, it seems that if information requiring a degree of organization is put into a frontal or medial temporal lesioned animal, it is found to be unobtainable shortly afterwards.

Frontals, it is claimed, suffer a temporary disorganization and, given time, the confusion clears and storage proceeds. But what evidence do we have that this is so? The kinds of tasks used to show the short-term loss and are not extended in time to assess the ultimate storage. This is assumed on the basis of independent evidence of discrimination learning. By contrast, it is not shown that in a simultaneous discrimination task the frontal is unable to retrieve the information shortly after registration. Furthermore, it is interesting to note that despite an impressive list of deficits, hippocampal monkeys learn difficult simultaneous pattern discriminations easily (Mishkin, 1954). Thus, at least in monkeys, frontal and medial temporal lesions do not preclude the memory of repetitive stimulus response correlations but only of highly unpredictable ones. The question is what is the fate of the unpredictable information intake in these lesioned animals? The supposition is that in the frontal, storage would ultimately take place while in the medial temporal, it would not. But proof of this is lacking. Indeed, if, as the models suggest, long-term memories are copied from the short-term store while it is "in action," then, perhaps, one would not expect the frontal to form adequate long-term traces of information handled inadequately in the short-term store. By the same token, the medial temporal gives evidence of inadequate short-term traces, but there is no independent evidence to prove that an abnormal transfer process from short- to long-term memory is any more responsible for the inability to form long-term memories than the inadequate short-term trace itself.

Current models are therefore inadequate for differentiating the frontal and medial temporal impairments. But the original model can be modified to accommodate some of the characteristics of these deficits.

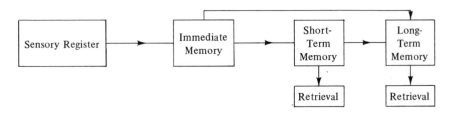

Considering the previous arguments, it is envisaged that the STM process is affected by both frontal and medial temporal damage, but that the STM is not necessarily involved in memory processes. It could be suggested that this process is only brought into action if the quality, quantity, organization, or temporal characteristics of the incoming information overloads the direct route from input to permanent storage. In this way, some very simple immediate memory tests or subspan memory tests, which involve uncomplicated registration and immediate retrieval, may not involve short-term processes such as the ones being discussed here, but only the IM with its independent access to long-term stores. Memory processing of this straightforward nature may be a function of a simple sensory registration/fixation system which is such a basic neurophysiological property of the cortical system that it is only disrupted by massive cerebral damage. Unfortunately, animal tests of such a process have not been developed on account of the practical difficulties involved in "one trial" registration or retrieval. Clinically, such tests are simple to design because of the advantages of verbal instruction, and digit span in the verbal or nonverbal mode is an excellent example. A decrement of digit span performance is seen in the context of general intellectual loss, but relatively rarely after discrete brain lesions. Highly specific defects in the immediate reproduction of short verbal sequences have been reported (Luria, Sokolov, & Klinkowski, 1967; Warrington & Shallice, 1969), but it remains to be demonstrated how such defects differ from subtle perceptual changes affecting the modality involved and whether they are dissociable from aphasia invariably seen, at least to a degree, in such cases.

If the frontal and temporal data we have looked at are considered within such a framework, one wonders on what basis these two classes of deficit may be differentiated, as only a single process would seem to be theoretically demanded between SR and IM and long-term storage. The hypothetical short-term memory box could be expanded to include two processes differing in their temporal involvement and may be in their processing properties. However, this seems unnecessary for is it not possible that both the frontal and temporal lesions are disturbing a unitary process? This may seem an outlandish proposition, but if the deficits associated with frontal and with anterior/medial temporal lesions are examined, it seems difficult to explain the remarkable similarity of the two groups of deficit in any simpler way.

3. Comparison of Animal and Clinical Studies of the Temporal and Frontal Lobes

Animal workers have often mistakenly discussed the clinical temporal lobe data as indicating intact short-term memory and impaired long-term storage. The error of this conclusion and the general confusion of terminology has already been discussed. If we concentrate on a short-term information processing function, it could be claimed that appropriate temporal lobe lesions in animals result in memory difficulties which resemble the nonverbal deficits originally described in medial temporal and right temporal lobe patients.

In the recurring figure task (Kimura, 1963), for example, the patient is asked to memorize a few visual or auditory stimuli, and these are then submerged in a larger series presented in quick succession. As each stimulus appears, the patient has to say whether or not he has been presented with it before. In the Konorski paired comparison task (Prisko, 1963), a visual or auditory stimulus from a series is presented and the immediately following stimulus must be identified as the same or different. Again, there is no way of predicting stimulus response relationships. Similarly, in delayed matching from sample of visual forms as used by Sidman *et al.* (1968), closely similar stimuli occur in quick succession and must be matched across varying delays. In the maze task used in the tactual or visual mode, a variety of responses are possible at each point, and during the learning process a whole series of responses must be chained together in the presence of interference. It would be inappropriate for an animal worker to dwell on clinical results, but in view of the persistent and pessimistic reports of a major discontinuity between monkey and man it is important to note that all the tasks described above, and others with similar characteristics, are sensitive to right temporal lobe or medial temporal damage in man. Furthermore, it seems probable that posterior lesions show primarily perceptual defects, but as the lesion encroaches anteriorly, and particularly into the medial temporal structures, the memory aspects of the tasks are more severely affected (Corsi, quoted by Milner; Warrington & Rabin, 1970). This dissociation of perceptual and memory functions in the temporal lobe cortex is also a feature of the organization of the monkey's brain (Iwai & Mishkin 1970).

Medial temporal animals also fail recurring tasks such as the concurrent learning task, paired comparison tasks, and delayed matching from sample and maze tasks, although it is premature to claim that failure occurs in the three major modalities, as it does, apparently, in medial temporal man.

It is almost certainly true that the involvement of language in man confuses the issue and complicates it far more than by creating an independent verbal hemisphere. Naively, one might suppose that a monkey's brain is like a man's right hemisphere. But a man without his left hemisphere is not equivalent to a monkey, despite that fact that his nonverbal capabilities are intact. Consider, for example, one major discrepancy in the present claim that certain temporal lesions in man and monkeys are equivalent.

Medial temporal monkeys, despite severe deficits on the kinds of memory tasks described, are able to learn simultaneous discriminations in the visual and tactile mode. Such storage may simply not involve the limited capacity short term mechanism, either bypassing it or, alternatively, being processed by a neural circuitry not linked with the hippocampus. Bilateral medial temporal man should be capable of similar limited storage capacity by means of direct access to alternative mechanisms, but H. M. seems unable to form long-term memories—even of repetitive and unchanging information. The reason for this is unclear, but it is at least possible that in man verbal coding mechanisms play a central role in memory processes, even for information which is essentially nonverbal and apparently very difficult to code verbally. Such verbal coding may inevitably be a complex process and thus involve the short-term memory store. Indeed, in a model such as that of Atkinson and Shiffrin (1968) (Fig. 9-9), the short-term verbal store is the only one differentiated in the STM process. This almost total dependence on verbal coding strategies may also explain the rather unexpected finding that H. M. cannot match simple visual and auditory stimuli after 20 seconds—stimuli which one supposed would not involve a recoding process and would therefore be handled by a registration process within the existing immediate memory span.

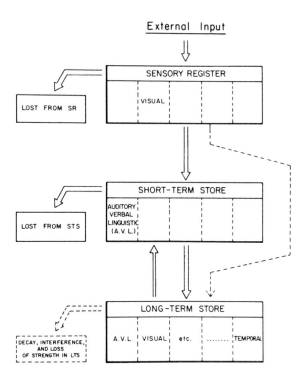

Fig. 9-9. Structure of the memory system. (Reproduced from Atkinson and Shiffrin, 1968.)

In uniquely impaired patients such as H. M. residual memory performance may reflect the properties of the nonhippocampal storage mechanism. The amnesias associated with less discrete temporal lobe pathology may be more indicative of the role of the hippocampus and its associated circuitry in working memory. It is not true to say that all patients with severe amnesias of temporal lobe origin are unable to form new long-term memories—the impairment may be impressively large, as in the case of H. M., but never complete. Recently, Weiskrantz has considered the basis of the amnesias seen after temporal lobe damage and, in his synthesis, has focused on the kinds of information which such patients are able to learn and remember, rather than the many things they cannot remember. As mentioned earlier Warrington and Weiskrantz (1968) have reported that such patients show evidence of learning on the Gollin Test, in which the line drawing of a common object is prepared in five stages of increasing fragmentation. The increasingly complete line drawings are presented until the patient is able to recognize the object. If a series of such line drawings of objects or words is presented, amnesics show evidence of learning and day to day retention, albeit much less than controls. Milner *et al.,* (1968) have reported that Mr. H., the bilateral lateral medial temporal patient, also shows evidence of some learning on this task and on a considerably shortened model of the tactual maze originally used by Corkin (1965).

Weiskrantz suggests that amnesics show intact motor performance and learning in certain situations (such as the Gollin Test) because interference is low in these tasks (albeit for different reasons), and retrieval mechanisms accordingly are facilitated. In pursuing this argument it is claimed that the severe amnesia associated with temporal lobe lesions reflect retrieval rather than acquisition difficulties. In contrast to the widely accepted interpretation and the view put forward in this article, it is suggested that such patients process information into the long-term store but are unable to retrieve it satisfactorily on account of failure to organize the store in the face of normal interference phenomena. The presentation of partial information, as in the Gollin Test, facilitates both learning and retention in amnesics, but Warrington and Weiskrantz (1970) have recently shown that retention in amnesics is also improved if partial information is given at the retrieval stage only and suggest that this retrieval method facilitates the inhibitory mechanism necessary to find the correct item in the long-term store. Undoubtedly, this tenet will be challenged by those who see these memory disorders as a basic difficulty in processing information from the short-term into long-term memory and consider the remnants of performance to be due to facilitation of this "ingoing" mechanism. However, if, as Tulving (1970) suggests, the coding of retrieval cues is a more critical determinant of the properties of short- and long-term memory than the storage of the raw information, there may be no conflict between the so-called storage and retrieval hypotheses. Tests like the Gollin may facilitate such retrieval coding during acquisition and thus enhance the memory of the information, particularly if additional cues are also provided at the time of retrieval. Whether the hypotheses are mutually exclusive remains to be shown, but one supposes that it will not be an easy task to prove that retrieval rather than storage is impaired in the amnesic patient.

However, irrespective of the outcome of such clinical studies, the present thesis of an impairment in the STM process could be sustained. Considering the temporal overlap of the various memory processes, one may suppose that information processing in the long-term mechanism begins to operate as the short-term processing occurs. Consequently, at any subsequent time, retrieval will involve not only access to material still held in STM storage but also access to its representation in long-term memory. In current models there is a retrieval arrow from LTM to STM which may operate as a feedback process during storage or a retrieval mechanism at later times (Fig. 9-9). In this sense, an impairment of the short-term process could equally well influence storage or retrieval. Is it not possible that just as certain kinds of information or information presented in a particular manner appear to be stored in temporal lobe amnesics, so the conditions and the demands of the retrieval mechanism either involve or do not involve a "limited capacity" process like the short-term store and, thus, aid or limit further the mnemonic capacity of amnesics? If this were so, one would expect the retrieval procedures which help amnesics to also facilitate normal performance.

So much for parsimony in the temporal lobe; what about in the frontal lobe? Here the data is even less complete. In man, as in animals, frontal lesions do produce evidence of motivation change, perseveration, and spatial disorientation, but there is a paucity of evidence on selective frontal lesions in relation to these impairments, and one can say little of their dissociation. Milner (1963), in one of the few studies comparing different frontal lesions in man, investigated performance on the Wisconsin Card Sorting Task and found evidence of perseveration of sorting set on this test to be associated with dorsolateral rather than orbital frontal damage. The opposite result would have been predicted on the basis of the monkey experiments. However, the Wisconsin Card Sorting Task is complex and, conceivably, it could be failed for a variety of reasons, a fact which may explain why posterior as well as anterior lesions can produce impairments (Teuber, Battersby, & Bender, 1951). The anatomical evidence on spatial deficits is more coherent. Lesions to Area 8 in both monkey and man produce a range of disorientation and "search" defects which Teuber (1964) has convincingly described as manifesting a basic disorder in the ability to "distinguish those changes in sensory input that result from his own, self produced movements, and those that result from actual movement in the environment."

The next task is to consider the behavioral basis of frontal impairments in man and to ask, as with the animal frontal literature, having demonstrated impairment of response and spatial control, how strong is the independent evidence for a memory defect?

In man, frontal lesions do not impair the delayed response or alternation task, probably because it is difficult to design a test equivalent to that used with animals, but also because such tasks tend to be solved by sophisticated verbal coding strategies. Turning to other tasks used to assess short- and long-term memory, the evidence for a frontal memory impairment in man is not obvious. Indeed, there is direct evidence that frontal patients have exceedingly good short- and long-term memory in certain formal testing situations, added to which clinical psychologists are often adamant that characteristically one simply doesn't see anything resembling amnesia for recent or remote events in frontal patients. Milner (1964) also doubts the validity of describing frontal impairments as straightforward memory defects, pointing out that while frontal patients perform normally on a recurring bird song memory task, if visual nonsense figures are used as the stimuli they show an impairment as severe as that seen after right temporal lesions. This apparent contradiction, and others like it, are difficult to explain unless, as Milner suggests, "the short pause between stimuli or the lively and more interesting character of the birdsong material could compensate for the confusion engendered by the continuous recognition procedure." Bearing in mind the frontal impairment on a tactile recurring figure task, visual and tactile finger mazes, and the paired comparison task employing a few constantly repeated flash and click frequencies and colored lights, it would seem that the frontal is impaired if pressure is put on the STM processing mechanism while it is handling easily confusable material. Either temporal structuring of the task to allow the mnemonic process to handle redundant material or increasing the information content of the material itself may significantly enhance performance. The notion of an impairment in monitoring and organizing the content of the STM does not have to be restricted to sensory input; indeed, there is every reason to suppose that memory processes constantly monitor both internal and externally initiated events. Such a process could also be concerned with the monitoring of reafference, that is, the consequence of the response to input and, extended in this way, the explanation would account for the various spatial, response, and sorting impairments seen after frontal lesions.

If it is reasonable to conceive of a unitary frontal hypothesis in such terms, we may again ask if independent evidence of a memory disorder is required—an inability to monitor the stimulus which has just disappeared, or the response made to it, could very well give convincing evidence of what we would unhesitatingly call a memory defect.

To conclude, let us extend the search for parsimony and ask if frontal lesions in man impair performance on the tasks sensitive to temporal lesions, just as frontal and medial temporal monkeys appear to fail on a substantial number of the same tasks. At a clinical level, this question is as outrageous as it was of the animal literature. There is a strong tradition that frontal and temporal defects differ. The dissociation of various functions within the frontal cortex of man has not progressed as far as in the monkey, and one may suppose that the frontal deficits commonly seen in man share the heterogenuity of the early frontal lesions in the monkey. The literature is sparse and, unfortunately, small frontal lesions are relatively rare. However, be this as it may, it is worth noting that Digit Span performance is not impaired by anterior lesions, but among the human frontal, deficits recognized and quantified are:

1. Maze learning deficits in both the visual and tactual mode.
2. Deficits on recurring figure tasks.
3. Impairment on the paired comparison memory test.

All of these tasks are also failed by patients with appropriate temporal lobe lesions. Even in terms of details, the correspondence is impressive. On recurring figure tasks both groups tend to show high false positive scores. But despite impairment on this task with many of the stimuli, both Mr. H. and the frontals show much better performance if interesting stimuli, such as birdsong, are used

(Milner, 1968). The significance of novelty in relation to frontal deficits has often been noted in the animal literature. Buffery (1964), for example, found that impaired delayed matching from sample performance in frontal monkeys improved considerably if a completely novel set of color stimuli were introduced. Novelty may also be significant in the observation that both frontals and temporals improve on the paired comparison task if a set of unique nonsense line drawings are used as stimuli instead of a limited number of repeated flashes and click stimuli.

There are inconsistencies with this argument, of which I am aware, and, probably even more, of which I am unaware. For example, frontals fail the Wisconsin Card Sorting Task, but it is one task that H. M. does remarkably well on, achieving 4.0 sorting categories compared with a mean of 4.6 sorting categories in combined controls. One supposes that this is a task demanding of short-term memory processes such as we have discussed. Milner has suggested that H. M. succeeds because he forgets the previous sorting strategies and is therefore not confused. But if he can forget in one trial the last sorting strategy and start the next, why does he not forget the relevant strategy from trial to trial?

In many of the reports it is claimed that the frontals and temporals fail the same tasks for different reasons. Indeed, different error patterns are noted and subjective differences in the reaction to the tests. For example, an inability to adhere to verbal instructions is commonly noted in frontals and not in temporal lobe amnesics, where the rigid adherence to instructions stands in marked contrast to the severely impaired retention of test material. The results on the recurring figure tasks is obviously a point of overlap worthy of investigation, where Milner herself suggests that more detailed study of reaction times to recurring stimuli, response strategies, and confidence ratings by subjects may help to differentiate the various groups of brain damage patients showing impairment. However, if the influence of parsimony and the possibility of the lesion encroaching on several foci are recognized, it seems at least possible to the present author that frontal and medial temporal deficits in man are more alike than is generally supposed.

Undoubtedly, it will be considered inappropriate for one without clinical experience to make such obviously erroneous statements about two clinical syndromes which are very easily differentiated in "the field." I have no doubt that my claim of parsimony will not withstand experimental pressure, but it may be hoped that the experiments to dispel the parsimony may define more precisely the nature of the memory defects associated with frontal and temporal lesions.

Finally, do we have any inklings of the neurophysiology mechanisms subserving short-term memory processing such as we have been discussing in relation to frontal and temporal lobe lesions? Here we stoop to rank plagiarism.

Several workers have already noted that the hippocampus and associated structures (including frontal cortex) constitute a major efferent influence on midbrain activating mechanisms which are known to be concerned in arousal and habituation processes (French, 1960). It is not unreasonable to suppose that the processing of incoming information will be dependent on such mechanisms which control the physical properties of sensory transformations and thereby their storage potential. But to speculate further on such matters would be both ill-founded and premature.

REFERENCES

Akelaitis, A. J. A study of Gnosis, Praxia and Language following section of the corpus callosum and anterior commissure. *Journal of Neurosurgery,* 1944, Vol. 1, 94-102.

Atkinson, R. C., & Shiffrin, R. M. Human memory: A proposed system and its control process. In K. W. Spence & J. T. Spence (Eds.), *The psychology of learning and motivation.* New York: Academic Press, 1968 Pp. 89-195.

Bianchi, L. *The mechanism of the brain and the function of the function of the frontal lobes.* (Translation by J. H. MacDonald) Edinburgh: E & S Livingston, 1922, Pp. 348.

Bickford, R., Mulder, D. W., Dodge, H. W., Svien, H. J., & Rome, H. P. (1958). Changes in memory function produced by electrical stimulation of the temporal lobe in man. *Research Publications, Association for Research in Nervous & Mental Disease,* 1958, Vol. 36, 227-257.

Bilodeau, E. A. Retention. In *E. A. Bilodeau (Ed.), Acquisition of skill.* New York: Academic Press, 1966. Pp. 315-347.

Bizzi, E. Discharge of frontal eye field neurons during eye movements in unanaesthetized monkeys. *Science,* 1967, Vol. 157, 1588-1590.

Blum, J. S. Cortical organization in somaesthesis. Effects of lesions in posterior associative cortex on somato-sensory function in Macaca mulatta. *Comparative & Psychological Monograph,* 1951, Vol. 20, 219-249.

Blum, J. S., Chow, K. L., & Pribram, K. H. A behavioural analysis of the organization of the parieto-temporo-preoccipital cortex. *Journal of Comparative Neurology,* 1950, Vol. 93, 53-100.

Brady, J. V. The paleocortex and behavioural motivation. In H. F. Harlow and C. N. Woolsey (Eds.), *Biological and biochemical bases of behaviour.* Madison, Wisconsin: University of Wisconsin Press, 1958. Pp. 193-235.

Broadbent, D. E. Immediate memory and simultaneous stimuli. *Quarterly Journal of Experimental Psychology,* 1957, Vol. 9, 1-11.

Broadbent, D. E. *Perception and communication.* Oxford: Pergammon Press, 1958.

Brown, J. Short term memory. *British Medical Bulletin,* 1964, Vol. 20, 8-11.

Brown, S., & Schäfer, E. A. An investigation into the functions of the occipital and temporal lobe of the monkey's brain. *Philosophical Transactions of the Royal Society of London,* Series B, 1888, Vol. 79, 303-327.

Brown, T. S., Rosvold, H. E., & Mishkin, M. Olfactory discrimination after temporal lobe lesions in monkeys. *Journal of Comparative & Physiological Psychology,* 1963, Vol. 56, 190-195.

Brutowski, S. Prefrontal cortex and drive disinhibition. In J. M. Warren & K. Akert (Eds.) *The frontal granular cortex and behaviour.* New York: McGraw-Hill, 1964. Pp. 242-269.

Brutowski, S., & Dabrowska, J. Disinhibition after prefrontal lesions as a function of duration of intertrial intervals. *Science,* 1963, Vol. 139, 505-506.

Brutowski, S., Mishkin, M., & Rosvold, H. E. Positive and inhibitory motor conditioned reflexes in monkeys after ablation of orbital or dorso-lateral surface of the frontal cortex. In G. P. Honik (Ed.), *Central and peripheral mechanisms of motor functions.* Czechoslovak Academy of Sciences, 1963. Pp 133-141.

Buffery, A. W. H. The effects of frontal and temporal lobe lesions upon the behaviour of baboons. Ph.D. thesis. University of Cambridge, 1964.

Butter, C. M. The effect of discrimination training on pattern equivalence in monkeys with inferotemporal and lateral striate lesions. *Neuropsychologia,* 1968, Vol. 6, 27-40.

Butter, C. M., Mishkin, M., & Rosvold, H. E. Conditioning and extinction of a food rewarded response after selective ablations of frontal cortex in rhesus monkeys. *Experimental Neurology,* 1963, Vol. 7, 65-67.

Butter, C. M., Mishkin, M., & Rosvold, H. E. Stimulus generalization in monkeys with inferotemporal and lateral occipital lesions. In D. J. Mostofsky (Ed.), *Stimulus generalization.* Stanford, California: Stanford University Press, 1965. Pp 119-133

Chorover, S. L., & Cole, M. Delayed alternation performance in patients with cerebral lesions. *Neuropsychologia,* 1966, Vol. 4, 1-7.

Chow, K. L. Effects of partial extirpations of the posterior association cortex in visually mediated behaviour in monkeys. *Comparative Psychological Monograph,* 1951, Vol. 20, 187-217.

Chow, K. L. Visual discrimination following temporal ablations. *Journal of Comparative & Physiological Psychology,* 1952, Vol. 45, 430-437.

Chow, K. L. Temporal ablation and visual discrimination. *Journal of Comparative & Physiological Psychology.* 1954, Vol. 47, 194-198.

Chow, K. L. Effect of local electrographic after discharge on visual learning and retention in monkey. *Journal of Neurophysiology,* 1961, Vol. 24, 391-400.

Chow, K. L., Blum, J. S., & Blum, R. A. Effects of combined destruction of frontal and posterior "associative areas" in monkeys. *Journal of Neurophysiology,* 1951, Vol. 14, 59-71.

Clark, C. V. H., & Isaacson, R. L. Effect of bilateral hippocampal on DRL performance. *Journal of Comparative & Physiological Psychology,* 1965, Vol. 59, 137-140.

Clark, W. E. Le Gros. The visual centres of the brain and their connexions. *Physiological Review.* 1942, Vol. 22, 205-232.

Conrad, R. Very brief delay of immediate recall. *Quarterly Journal of Experimental Psychology,* 1960, Vol. 12, 45-47.

Cordeau, J. P., & Mahut, H. Some long term effects of temporal lobe resections on auditory and visual discriminations in monkeys. *Brain,* 1964, Vol. 87, 177-190.

Corkin, S. Tactually-guided maze learning in man; Effects of unilateral cortical excisions and bilateral hippocampal lesions. *Neuropsychologia,* 1965, Vol. 3, 339-352.

Correll, R. E., & Scoville, W. B. Effects of medial temporal lesions on visual discrimination performance. *Journal of Comparative & Physiological Psychology,* 1965, Vol. 60, 175-181. (a)

Correll, R. E., & Scoville, W. B. Performance on delayed match following lesions of medial temporal lobe structures. *Journal of Comparative & Physiological Psychology,* 1965, Vol. 60, 360-367. (b)

Correll, R. E., & Scoville, W. B. Significance of delay in performance of monkeys with medial temporal lobe resections. *Experimental Brain Research,* 1967, Vol. 4, 85-96.

Cowey, A. A perimetric study of visual field defects in monkeys. *Quarterly Journal of Experimental Psychology,* 1963, Vol. 15, 91-115.

Douglas, R. J. The hippocampus and behaviour. *Psychological Bulletin,* 1967, Vol. 67, 416-442.

Douglas R. J., & Isaacson, R. L. Hippocampal lesions and activity. *Psychonomic Science,* 1964, Vol. 1, 187-188.

Douglas, R. J., & Pribram, K. H. Learning and limbic lesions. *Neuropsychologia,* 1966, Vol. 4, 197-220.

Drachman, D. A., & Arbit, J. Memory and the Hippocampal complex. II. Is memory a multiple process? *Archives of Neurology,* 1966, Vol. 15, 52-61.

Drachman, D. A., & Ommaya, A. K. Memory and the Hippocampal complex. *Archives of Neurology,* 1964, Vol. 10, 411-425.

Ellen, P., & Powell, E. W. Temporal discrimination in rats with rhinencephalic lesions. *Experimental Neurology,* 1962, Vol. 6, 538-547.

Ellen, P., & Wilson, A. S. Perseveration in the rat following hippocampal lesions. *Experimental Neurology,* 1963, Vol. 8, 310-317.

Ettlinger, G., Iwai, E., Mishkin, M., & Rosvold, H. E. Visual discrimination in the monkey following serial ablation of infero-temporal and preoccipital cortex. *Journal of Comparative & Physiological Psychology,* 1968, Vol. 65, 110-117.

Fanz, S. I. On the functions of the cerebrum; the frontal lobes. *Archives of Psychology,* 1907, Vol. 2, 1-64.

Ferrier, D. *The functions of the brain.* London: Smith, Elder, 1876.

Flynn, J. P., & Wasman, M. Learning and cortically evoked movement during propagated hippocampal after discharge. *Science,* 1960, Vol. 131, 1607-1608.

French, J. D. The reticular formation. In J. Field, H. W. Magoun, & V. E. Hall (Eds.), *Handbook of neurophysiology,* Vol. 11. Baltimore, Maryland: Williams & Wilkins, 1960. Pp. 1281-1305.

Fulton, J. F. The frontal lobes and human behaviour. *The Sherrington lectures.* Liverpool, England: Liverpool University Press, 1952.

Ghent, L., Mishkin, M., & Teuber, H. L. Short term memory after frontal-lobe injury in man. *Journal of Comparative & Physiological Psychology,* 1962, Vol. 55, 705-709.

Glick, S. D. Goldfarb T. L., & Jarvik, M. E. Recovery of delayed matching performance following lateral frontal lesions in Monkeys. *Communications in Behavior Biology,* 1960, Vol. 3, 299-303.

Glickstein, M., Quigley, W., & Stebbing W. C. Effect of frontal and parietal lesions on timing behaviour in monkeys. *Psychonomic Science,* 1964, Vol. 1, 265-266.

Goldman, P. S., & Rosvold, H. E. Localization of function within the dorsolateral prefrontal cortex of the rhesus monkey. *Experimental Neurology,* 1970, Vol 27, 291-304.

Goldstein, M. N., & Joynt, R. J. Long term follow-up of a callosal-sectioned patient. *Archives of Neurology,* 1969, Vol. 20, 96-102.

Gotsick, J. E. Factors affecting spontaneous activity in rats with limbic system lesions. *Physiology & Behavior,* 1969, Vol. 4, 587-593.

Gross, C. G. Discrimination reversal after lateral frontal lesions in monkeys. *Journal of Comparative & Physiological Psychology,* 1963, Vol. 56, 52-55.

Gross, C. G. Locomotor activity following lateral frontal lesions in rhesus monkeys. *Journal of Comparative & Physiological Psychology,* 1963, Vol. 56, 232-236.

Gross, C. G., Chorover, S. L., & Cohen, S. M. Caudate, cortical, hippocampal and dorsal thalamic lesions in rats: alternation & Hebb-Williams maze performance. *Neuropsychologia,* 1965, Vol. 3, 53-68.

Gross, C. G., & Weiskrantz, L. Evidence for dissociation between impairment on auditory discrimination and delayed response in frontal monkeys. *Experimental Neurology,* 1962, Vol. 5, 453-476.

Gross, C. G., & Weiskrantz, L. Some changes in behaviour produced by lateral frontal lesions in the Macaque. In J. M. Warren & K. Akert (Eds.), *The frontal granular cortex and behaviour.* New York: McGraw Hill, 1964. Pp. 74-98.

Hara, K. Visual defects resulting from prestriate cortical lesions in cats. *Journal of Comparative & Physiological Psychology,* 1962, Vol. 55, 293-298.

Harlow, H. F., & Dagnon, J. Problem solution by monkeys following bilateral removal of the prefrontal areas. I. The discrimination and discrimination reversal problems. *Journal of Experimental Psychology,* 1942, Vol. 32, 351-356.

Harlow, H. F., & Spaet, T. Problem solution by monkeys following bilateral removal of the prefrontal areas. IV. Responses to stimuli having multiple sign valves. *Journal of Experimental Psychology,* 1943, Vol. 33, 500-507.

Hitzig, E. Zur physiologie des Grosshirns. Arch.f. *Psychiatry und Nervenheik,* 1884, Vol. 15, 270-275.

Isaacson, R. L., & Wickelgren, W. O. Hippocampal ablation and passive avoidance. *Science,* 1962, Vol. 138, 1104-1106.

Iversen, S. D. Tactile learning and memory in baboons after temporal and frontal lesions. *Experimental Neurology,* 1967, Vol. 18, 228-238.

Iversen, S. D. Interference and inferotemporal memory deficits. *Brain Research,* 1970, Vol. 19, 277-289.

Iversen, S. D. & Humphrey, N. K. Ventral temporal lobe lesions and visual oddity performance. *Brain Research,* 1971, Vol. 30, 253-263.

Iversen, S. D. & Mishkin, M., Perseverative interference in monkeys following selective lesions of the inferior prefrontal convexity. *Experimental Brain Research,* 1970, Vol. 11, 376-386.

Iversen, S. D., & Weiskrantz, L. The acquisition of conditional discriminations in Baboons following temporal and frontal lesions. *Experimental Neurology,* 1967, Vol. 19, 78-91.

Iversen, S. D., & Weiskrantz, L. An investigation of a possible memory defect produced by inferotemporal lesions in the Baboon. *Neuropsychologia,* 1970, Vol. 8, 21-36.

Iwai, E., & Mishkin, M. Two inferotemporal foci for visual functions. Paper read at Annual Meeting, American Psychology Association, Washington, D. C., 1967.

Iwai, E., & Mishkin, M. Further evidence on the locus of the visual area in the temporal lobe of the monkey. *Experimental Neurology,* 1969, Vol. 25, 585-594.

Jackson, W. J., & Strong, P. N. Differential effects of hippocampal lesions upon sequential tasks and maze learning by the rat. *Journal of Comparative & Physiological Psychology,* 1969, Vol. 68, 442-450.

Jacobsen, C. F. I. The functions of the frontal association areas in monkeys. *Comparative Psychological Monograph,* 1936, Vol. 13, 1-60.

Jarrard, L. E. Hippocampal ablation and operant behaviour in the rat. *Psychonomic Science,* 1965, Vol. 2, 115-116.

Jarrard, L. E. Behaviour of hippocampal lesioned rats in home cage and novel situations. *Physiology & Behavior,* 1968, Vol. 3, 65-70.

Jarrard, L. E., & Bunnell, B. N. Open field behaviour of hippocampal lesioned rats and hamsters. *Journal of Comparative & Physiological Psychology,* 1968, Vol. 66, 500-502.

Jarrard, L. E., Isaacson, R. L., & Wickelgren, W. O. Effects of hippocampal ablation on runway acquisition and extinction. *Journal of Comparative & Physiological Psychology,* 1964, Vol. 57, 442-444.

Johnson, T. N., Rosvold, H. E., & Mishkin, M. Projections from behaviorally defined sectors of the prefrontal cortex to the basal ganglia, septum and diencephalon of the monkey. *Experimental Neurology,* 1968, Vol. 21, 20-34.

Kaada, B. R., Rasmussen, E. W. and Kveim, O. Effects of hippocampal lesions on maze learning and retention in rats. *Experimental Neurology,* 1961, Vol. 3, 333-335.

Kamback, M. C. The effect of prefrontal lesions of food deprivation on response for stimulus change. Exp. Neurol, 1967, Vol. 18, 478-484. (a)

Kamback, M. C. Effect of hippocampal lesions and food depreviation on response for stimulus change. *Journal of Comparative & Physiological Psychology,* 1967, Vol. 63, 231-235. (b)

Kennard, M. A. Alterations in response to visual stimuli following lesions in the frontal lobe of monkeys. *Archives of Neurological Psychiatry,* 1939, Vol. 41, 1153-1165.

Keppel, G., & Underwood, B. J. Proactive inhibition in short-term retention of single items. *Journal of verbal Learning & verbal Behavior,* 1962, Vol. 1, 153-161.

Kimble, D. P. The effects of bilateral hippocampal lesions in rats. *Journal of Comparative & Physiological Psychology,* 1963, Vol. 56, 273-283.

Kimble, D. P. The Hippocampus and internal inhibition. *Psychological Bulletin,* 1968, Vol. 70, 285-295.

Kimble, D. P., & Coover, G. D. Effects of hippocampal lesions on food and water consumption in rats. *Psychonomic Science,* 1966, Vol. 4, 91-92.

Kimble, D. P., & Kimble, R. J. Hippocampectomy and response perseveration in the rat. *Journal of Comparative & Physiological Psychology,* 1962, Vol. 3, 474-476.

Kimble, D. P., & Pribram, K. H. Hippocampectomy and behaviour sequences. *Science,* 1963, Vol. 139, 824-825.

Kimura, D. Right temporal lobe damage. *Archives of Neurology,* 1963, Vol. 8, 264-271.

Kluver, H., & Bucy, P. C. Preliminary analysis of functions of the temporal lobes in monkeys. *American Medical Association Archives of Neurological Psychiatry,* 1939, Vol. 42, 979-1000.

Konorski, J., & Lawicka, W. Analysis of errors by prefrontal animals on the delayed response test. In J. M. Warren and K. Akert (Eds.), *The frontal granular cortex and behaviour.* New York: McGraw Hill, 1964. Pp. 271-286.

Kuypers, G. J. M., & Lawrence D. G. Cortical projections to the red nucleus and the brain stem in the rhesus monkey. *Brain Research,* 1967, Vol. 4, 151-188.

Kuypers, G. J. M., Szwarcbart, M. K., Mishkin, M., & Rosvold, H. E. Occipitotemporal cortico-cortical connections in the Rhesus monkey. *Experimental Neurology,* 1965, Vol. 11, 245-262.

Lashley, K. S. The problem of cerebral organization in vision. *Biological Symposium,* 1942, Vol. 7, 301-322.

Lashley, K. S. The mechanism of vision. XVIII. Effects of destroying the visual "associative areas" of the monkey. *Genetic Psychology Monograph,* 1948, Vol. 37, 107-166.

Lashley, K. S. In search of the Engram, *S.E.B. Symposium,* 1950, Vol. 4, 454-482.

Latto, R. Visual field defects after frontal eye-field lesions in monkeys. *Brain Research,* 1971, Vol. 30, 1-24.

Lawicka, W., Mishkin, M., & Rosvold, H. E. Dissociation of impairment on auditory tasks following orbital and dorsolateral frontal lesions in monkeys. Congress Polish Physiological Society Lectures, symposia abstracts of free communications. p. 178. Lublin. Pol. Physiol. Soc. Ed., 1966.

Leaton, R. N. Exploratory behaviour in rats with hippocampal lesions. *Journal of Comparative & Physiological Psychology,* 1965, Vol. 59, 320-325.

Lichtenstein, P. E. Studies of anxiety. II. The effects of Lobotomy on a feeding inhibition in dogs. *Journal of Comparative & Physiological Psychology,* 1950, Vol. 43, 419-427.

Lindsley, D. F., Weiskrantz, L., & Mingay, R. Differentiation of frontal, inferotemporal and normal monkeys in a visual exploratory situation. *Animal Behavior,* 1964, Vol. 12, 525-530.

Luria, A. R., Sokolov, G. N., & Klimkowski, M. Towards a neurodynamic analysis of memory disturbances with lesions of the left temporal lobe. *Neuropsychologia,* 1967, Vol. 5, 1-11.

Mahut, H. Spatial and object reversal learning in monkeys with partial temporal lobe ablations. *Neuropsychologia,* 1971, Vol. 9, 409-424.

Mahut, H., & Cordeau, J. P. Spatial reversal deficit in monkeys with amgdalohippocampal ablations. *Experimental Neurology,* 1963, Vol. 2, 426-434.

McCleary, R. A. Response modulatory functions of the limbic system: Initiation and suppression. *Progress in Physiological Psychology,* 1966, Vol. 1, 209-272.

Mettler, F. A. Corticofugal fiber connections of the cortex of Macaca mulatta. The occipital region. *Journal of Comparative Neurology,* 1935, Vol. 61, 221-256.

Milner, B. Laterality effects in audition. In V. B. Mountcastle, (Ed.), *Interhemispheric Relations and Cerebral Dominance.* Baltimore: The Johns Hopkins Press, 1962. Pp. 177-195.

Milner, B. Effects of different brain lesions on card sorting. *Archives of Neurology,* 1963, Vol. 9, 90-100.

Milner, B. Some effects of frontal lobectomy in man. In J. M. Warren & K. Akert (Eds.), *The frontal granula cortex & behaviour.* New York: McGraw Hill, 1964. Pp. 313-331.

Milner, B. Visually-guided maze learning in man: effects of bilateral hippocampal, bilateral frontal and unilateral cerebral lesions. *Neuropsychologia,* 1965, Vol. 3, 317-338.

Milner, B. Corkin, S. & Teuber, H. L. Further analysis of the hippocampal amnesic syndrome: 14-year follow-up study of H. M. *Neuropsychologia,* 1968, Vol. 6, 215-234.

Milner, B., & Teuber, H. L. Alteration of perception and memory in man: reflections on methods. In L. Weiskrantz (Ed.), *Analysis of behavioural change.* New York: Harper & Row, 1968. Pp. 268-375.

Mishkin, M. Visual discrimination performance following partial ablations of the temporal lobe. II. Ventral surfaces vs. hippocampus. *Journal of Comparative & Physiological Psychology,* 1954, Vol. 47, 187-193.

Mishkin, M. Perseveration of central sets after frontal lesions in monkeys. In J. M. Warren and K. Akert (Eds), *The frontal granular cortex and behaviour.* New York: McGraw Hill, 1964. Pp. 219-237.

Mishkin, M. Vision beyond the striate cortex. In R. W. Russell (Ed.), *Frontiers in physiological psychology.* New York: Academic Press, 1966. Pp. 93-119.

Mishkin, M., & Hall, M. Discrimination along a size continuum following ablation of the inferior temporal convexity in monkeys. *Journal of Comparative & Physiological Psychology,* 1955, Vol. 48, 97-101.

Mishkin, M., & Pribram, K. H. Visual discrimination performance following partial ablation of the temporal lobe. I. Ventral vs. lateral. *Journal of Comparative & Physiological Psychology,* 1954, Vol. 47, 14-20.

Nauta, W. J. H. Some efferent connections of the prefrontal cortex in the Monkey. In J. M. Warren and K. Akert (Eds.), *The frontal granular cortex.* New York: McGraw Hill, 1964. Pp. 397-407.

Nauta, W. J. H. The problem of the frontal lobe: A reinterpretation. *Journal of Psychiatric Research,* 1971, Vol. 8, 167-187.

Neff, W. D. Neural mechanisms of Auditory Discrimination. In W. A. Rosenblith (Ed.), *Sensory communication.* Cambridge, Mass.: M.I.T. Press, 1961. Pp. 259-278.

Newell, A., Shaw, J. C., & Simon, H. A. Elements of a theory of human problem solving. *Psychological Review,* 1953, Vol. 65, 151-166.

Niki, H. The effects of hippocampal ablation on the behaviour in the rat. *Japanese Psychological Research,* 1962, Vol. 4, 130-153.

Niki, H. The effects of hippocampal ablation on the inhibitory control of operant behaviour in the rat. *Japanese Psychological Research,* 1965, Vol. 7, 126-137.

Olds, J. The behavior of hippocampal neurons during conditioning experiments. In Whalen, R. E., Thompson, R. F., Verzeono, M., & Weinberger, N. M. (Eds), *The neural control of behavior.* New York: Academic Press, 1970. Pp. 257-293.

Orbach, J., & Fantz, R. L. Differential effects of temporal neo-cortical resections on overtrained and nonovertrained visual habits in monkeys. *Journal of Comparative & Physiological Psychology,* 1958, Vol. 51, 126-129.

Orbach, J., Milner, B., & Rasmussen, T. Learning and retention in monkeys after amygdala-hippocampus resection. *Archives of Neurology,* 1960, Vol. 3, 230-251.

Papez, J. W. A proposed mechanism of emotions. *American Medical Association Archives of Neurological Psychiatry,* 1937, Vol. 38, 725-743.

Pasik, T., Pasik, P., Battersby, W. S., & Bender, M. B. Factors influencing visual behaviour of monkeys with bilateral temporal lobe lesions. *Journal of Comparative Neurology,* 1960, Vol. 115, 89-102.

Penfield, W. Speech, perception and the uncommitted cortex. *Pontifaciae Academiae Scientarum, Scripta varia,* 1965, Vol. 30, 319-347.

Penfield, W., & Milner, B. Memory deficit produced by bilateral lesions in the hippocampal zone. *American Medical Association Archives of Neurological Psychiatry,* 1958, Vol. 79, 475-497.

Penfield, W., & Perot, P. The Brain's record of auditory and visual experience – A final summary and discussion. *Brain,* 1963, Vol. 86, 595-696.

Peretz, E. Extinction of a food reinforced response in hippocampectomized cats. *Journal of Comparative & Physiological Psychology,* 1965, Vol. 60, 182-185.

Petr, R., Holden, L. B., & Jirout, J. The efferent intercortical connections of the superficial cortex of the temporal lobe. (Macaca mulatta) *Journal of Neuropathology & Experimental Neurology,* 1949, Vol. 8, 100-103.

Pinto-Hamuy, T., & Linck, P. Effects of frontal lesions on performance of sequential tasks by monkeys. *Experimental Neurology,* 1965, Vol. 12, 96-107.

Pizzi, W. J., & Lorens, S. A. Effects of lesions in the amydalo-hippocampo-septal system on food and water intake in the rat. *Psychonomic Science,* 1967, Vol. 7, 187-188.

Pribram, K. H. Comparative neurology and the evolution of behaviour. In A. Rowe & G. G. Simpson (Eds.), *Behaviour & Evolution.* New Haven, Connecticut: Yale University Press, 1958.

Pribram, K. H. The limbic system, efferent control of neural inhibition and behaviour. *Progress in Brain Research,* 1967, Vol. 27, 318-336.

Pribram, K. H., Ahumdan, A., Hartog, J., & Ross, L. A progress report on the neurological processes disturbed by frontal lesions in primates. In J. M. Warren and K. Akert (Eds.), *Frontal granular cortex and behaviour.* New York: McGraw Hill, 1964. Pp. 28-55.

Pribram, K. H., & Kruger, L. Functions of the "olfactory brain." *Annals New York Academy of Science.* 1954, Vol. 58, 109-138.

Pribram, K. H., & Tubbs, W. E. Short-term memory, parsing, and the primate frontal cortex. *Science,* 1967, Vol. 156, 1765-1767.

Pribram, K. H., & Weiskrantz, L. Comparison of effects of medial and lateral cerebral resections on conditioned avoidance behaviour of monkeys. *Journal of Comparative & Physiological Psychology,* 1957, Vol. 50, 74-80.

Prisko, L. H. Short-term memory in focal cerebral damage. Unpublished doctoral thesis, McGill University, 1963.

Rabe, A., & Haddadd R. K. Effect of selective hippocampal lesions on acquisition, performance, and extinction of bar pressing on a fixed ratio schedule. *Experimental Brain Research,* 1968, Vol. 5, 259-266.

Robinson, B. W., & Mishkin, M. Alimentary responses to forebrain stimulation in monkeys. *Experimental Brain Research,* 1968, Vol. 4, 330-366.

Robinson, D. A., & Fuchs, A. F. Eye movements evoked by stimulation of frontal eye fields. *Journal of Neurophysiology,* 1969, Vol. 32, 637-648.

Rogozea, R., & Ungher, J. Changes in orientating activity of cat induced by chronic hippocampal lesions. *Experimental Neurology,* 1968, Vol. 21, 176-186.

Rosvold, H. E. The prefrontal cortex and caudate nucleus: A system for effecting correction in response mechanisms. In C. Rupp (Ed.), *Mind as a tissue.* New York: Harper & Row, 1968.

Rosvold, H. E., & Mishkin, M. Non sensory effects of frontal lesions on discrimination learning and performance. In D. Delfraysne (Ed.), *Brain mechanisms and learning.* Blackwell Scientific Publications, 1961. Pp. 555-567.

Rosvold, H. E., Mishkin, M., & Szwarcbart, M. K. Effects of subcortical lesions in monkeys on visual discrimination and single alternation performance. *Journal of Comparative & Physiological Psychology,* 1958, Vol. 51, 437-444.

Schmaltz, L. W., & Isaacson, R. L. Retention of a DRL 20 schedule by hippocampetomized and partially neodecorticate rats. *Journal of Comparative & Physiological Psychology,* 1966, Vol. 62, 128-132.

Scoville, W. B., & Milner, B. Loss of recent memory after bilateral hippocampal lesions. *Journal of Neurology, Neurosurgery, & Psychiatry,* 1957, Vol. 20, 11-21.

Settlage, P., Zable, N., & Harlow, H. F. Problem solution by monkeys following bilateral removal of the prefrontal areas: VI Performance on tests requiring contradictory reactions to similar and to identical stimuli. *Journal of Experimental Psychology,* 1948, Vol. 38, 50-65.

Sidman, H., Stoddard, L. T., & Mohr, J. P. Some additional quantitative observations of immediate memory in a patient with bilateral hippocampal lesions. *Neuropsychologia,* 1968, Vol. 6, 245-254.

Silveira, J. M., & Kimble, D. P. Brightness discrimination and reversal in hippocampally lesioned rats. *Physiology & Behavior,* 1968, Vol. 3, 625-630.

Snyder, D. R., & Isaacson, R. L. Effects of large and small bilateral hippocampal lesions on two types of passive avoidance responses. *Psychological Report,* 1965, Vol. 16, 1277-1290.

Sprague, J. M. Visual, Acoustic and Somaesthetic deficits in the cat after cortical and midbrain lesions. In D. P. Purpura & M. Yahr (Eds.), *The thalamus.* New York: Columbia University Press, 1966. Pp. 391-414.

Sprague, J. M., & Meikle, T. H. The role of the superior colliculus in visually guided behaviour. *Experimental Neurology,* 1965, Vol. 11, 115-146.

Stamm, J. S. Function of prefrontal cortex in timing behaviour of monkeys. *Experimental Neurology,* 1963, Vol. 7, 87-97.

Stamm, J. S., & Knight, M. Learning of visual tasks by monkeys with epileptogenic implants in temporal cortex. *Journal of Comparative & Physiological Psychology,* 1963, Vol. 56, 254-260.

Sugar, O., French, J. D., & Chusid, J. G. Corticocortical connections of the superior surface of the temporal operculum in the monkey (Macaca mulatta) *Journal of Neurophysiology,* 1948, Vol. 11, 175-185.

Teitelbaum, P. A study of hippocampal function in the rat. Ph.D. Thesis. McGill University, 1961.

Teitelbaum, P. A comparison of effects of orbitofrontal and hippocampal lesions upon discrimination learning and reversal in the cat. *Experimental Neurology,* 1964, Vol. 9, 452-462.

Teuber, H. L. The Riddle of the frontal lobe in Man. In J. M. Warren and K. Akert (Eds.), *The frontal granular cortex and behaviour.* New York: McGraw Hill, 1964. Pp. 410-441.

Teuber, H. L., Battersby, W. S., & Bender, M. B. Performance of complex visual tasks after cerebral lesions. *Journal of Nervous & Mental Disease,* 1951, Vol. 114, 413-429.

Teuber, H. L., & Proctor, F. Some effects of basal ganglia lesions in subhuman primates and Man. *Neuropsychology,* 1964, Vol. 2, 185-193.

Thompson, R., Lesse, H., & Rich, I. Pretectal lesions in rats and cats. *Journal of Comparative Neurology,* 1963, Vol. 121, 161-171.

Tulving, E. Short- and long-term memory: Different retrieval mechanisms. In K. H. Pribram and D. E. Broadbent (Eds.), *Biology of memory.* New York: Academic Press, 1970. Pp. 7-9.

von Bonin, G. On Encephalometry. *Journal of Comparative Neurology,* 1941, Vol. 75, 287-314.

von Bonin, G., Garol, H. W., & McCulloch, W. S. *Biology Symposium,* 1942, Vol. 7, 165.

Votaw, C. L., & Lauer, E. W. Blood pressure, pulse and respiratory changes produced by stimulation of the hippocampus of the monkey. *Experimental Neurology,* 1963, Vol. 7, 502-514.

Warren, J. M., Warren, H. B., & Akert, K. Learning by cats with lesions in the prestriate cortex. *Journal of Comparative & Physiological Psychology,* 1961, Vol. 54, 629-632.

Warrington, E. K., & Rabin, P. A preliminary investigation of the relation between visual perception and visual memory. *Cortex,* 1970, Vol. 6, 87-96.

Warrington, E. K., & Shallice, T. The selective impairment of auditory verbal short-term memory. *Brain,* 1969, Vol. 92, 885-896.

Warrington, E. K., Weiskrantz, L. New method of testing long-term retention with special reference to amnesic patients. *Nature,* 1968, Vol. 217, 972-974.

Warrington, E. K., & Weiskrantz, L. Amnesic syndrome. Consolidation or retrieval. *Nature,* 1970, Vol. 228, 628-630.

Waxler, M. & Rosvold, H. E. Delayed alternation in monkeys after removal of the hippocampus. *Neuropsychologia,* 1970, Vol. 8, 137-146.

Webster, D. B., & Voneida, T. J. Learning deficits following hippocampal lesions in split-brain cats. *Experimental Neurology,* 1964, Vol. 10, 170-182.

Weiskrantz L. Behavioural changes associated with ablation of the amygdaloid complex in monkeys. *Journal of Comparative & Physiological Psychology,* 1956, Vol. 49, 381-391.

Weiskrantz, L. Experimental studies of Amnesia. In C. W. Whitty and O. L. Zangwill (Eds.), *Amnesia,* London & Washington, D. C.: Butterworths, 1966. Pp. 1-36.

Weiskrantz, L. & Mishkin, M. Effects of temporal and frontal cortical lesions on auditory discrimination in monkey. *Brain,* 1958, Vol. 81, 406-414.

Wilson, M. Effects of circumscribed cortical lesions upon somaesthetic and visual discrimination in the monkey. *Journal of Comparative & Physiological Psychology,* 1957, Vol. 50, 630-635.

Wilson, M., & Mishkin, M. Comparison of the effects of inferotemporal and lateral occipital lesions on visually guided behaviour in monkeys. *Journal of Comparative & Physiological Psychology,* 1959, Vol. 52, 10-17.

Yntema, D. B., & Trask, F. P. Recall as a search process. *Journal of Verbal Learning & Verbal Behavior,* 1963, Vol. 2, 65-74.

CHAPTER

10

AN ANALYSIS OF SHORT-TERM AND LONG-TERM MEMORY DEFECTS IN MAN

ELIZABETH K. WARRINGTON

and

L. WEISKRANTZ

I. INTRODUCTION

The study of pathology can illuminate not only the structures that are critical for certain capacities, but also can lead to inferences about the organization of those capacities in the nonpathological state. In the field of memory disorders, such inferences have most often been concerned with sequences of events underlying normal memory, as, for example, with hypotheses about "consolidation." But pathology can also help us to fractionate normal phenomena into independent processes (Weiskrantz, 1968, Chapter 14), and that is the main concern of this chapter. In brief, it attempts to examine the extent to which disorders of short-term memory and long-term memory in man can be analysed into dissociable components.

The literature on amnesic phenomena is now vast, but fortunately a number of reviews are available (Whitty and Zangwill, 1966; Talland, 1965). Rather than attempt yet another review, we have selected those observations that appear to be directly relevant to the question just raised. Nor have we concerned ourselves with the possible differences between amnesic disorders due to differing etiologies. For example, "the amnesic syndrome"–characterized by a severe disorder of day-to-day memory with normal intelligence, perceptual skills, and other cognitive functions–can result from temporal lobe surgery, alcoholism, or encephalitis. Perhaps the finer manifestations of these different etiologies could be distinguished, although we ourselves have not yet succeeded in doing so. Nor, it follows, do we discuss the question of the critical anatomical structures involved in the amnesic syndrome, which has been discussed elsewhere by others, although we do refer to preliminary anatomical observations regarding short-term memory disorders.

It is impossible to dissociate two phenomena without considering the properties of each of them, and much of this chapter is an attempt to analyze and characterize short-term and long-term disorders. To arrive at conclusions about the nature of memory defects, it is important to ask whether information that is "forgotten" is stored but inaccessible, whether it has failed to consolidate, or whether information has been misclassified. The answer to such questions depends, in turn, on an examination of those circumstances that allow normal or nearly normal retention in amnesic patients, and such an examination can throw light not only on the theoretical basis of normal memory processing, but also might lead to suggestions for therapeutic approaches to the alleviation of the disorders themselves. Finally, although this chapter is about human disorders, we briefly attempt to relate to each other the results of human and animal investigations of long-term memory.

II. THE AMNESIC SYNDROME

A. Short-term Memory in Amnesic Patients

It has long been observed that the span of apprehension is normal in amnesic subjects (Zangwill, 1946; Williams & Smith, 1954; Rose and Symonds,

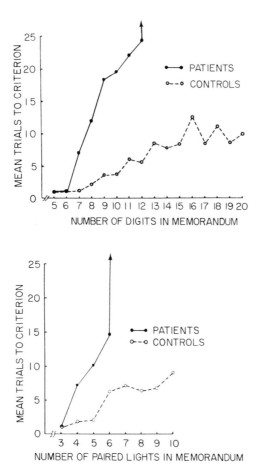

Fig. 10-1. Immediate memory for digits and pairs of light stimuli. (Reprinted with permission from Drachman and Arbit, 1966.)

1960). In one of the first quantitative studies, Drachman and Arbit (1966) showed that amnesic subjects have a normal immediate memory span for both digits (auditory) and the spatial position of pairs of lights (visual), but were impaired in learning sequences beyond their span (see Fig. 10-1). Visual span of apprehension for random digits has also been reported to be normal (Warrington & Weiskrantz, 1968b). Although no deficit in immediate memory span tasks has been demonstrated, it is possible that more sophisticated techniques would show a deficit where simple span measures do not. Wickelgren (1968), using a probe technique, tested short-term recognition memory for single-digit and three-digit numbers in one amnesic subject (H.M.). He found that the decay functions approximated reasonably well to a single exponential decay curve, with a decay rate well within the range of normal subjects.

The evidence of normal immediate memory span in amnesic subjects supports the validity of the distinction between short- and long-term memory. This distinction has been strengthened by the discovery that certain verbal memory tasks have two components, one labile (S.T.M.), and the other stable (L.T.M.) (Glanzer & Cunitz, 1966; Peterson & Peterson, 1959; Waugh & Norman, 1965). Many of these techniques involve recall after a short delay during which rehearsal is prevented by a second distracting task. One striking and reliable experimental finding in normal subjects is that subspan verbal items, such as three words or three consonants, are forgotten very rapidly, an asymptote being reached after a delay of some twenty or thirty seconds if rehearsal is prevented by an intervening task. Is it the case that with this short-term forgetting paradigm the performance of amnesic patients would be impaired? The question is pertinent, as it is often claimed that amnesic subjects forget as soon as their attention is distracted (Milner, 1959; Talland, 1965) and that they are only able to bridge a delay by continuous rehearsal (Milner, 1966; Sidman, Stoddard, & Mohr, 1968). Baddeley and Warrington (1970) compared the performance of six amnesic subjects and six matched normal control subjects on an adaptation of the Peterson short-term forgetting task using delays ranging from 0–60 seconds. There was no difference between amnesics and controls at any delay (see Fig. 10-2). That both groups have the same asymptote is difficult to explain in terms of current theory; nevertheless, it is clearly the case that over these short intervals amnesics are not more susceptible to distraction than normal subjects.

On free recall tasks, in which a word list presented once is recalled in any order, there is a strong serial position effect that can be shown to comprise a stable long-term component and a more labile short-term component. The former is represented by the primacy effect, the latter by the recency effect—the higher probability of recall of the last 4–5 items of the list; the recency effect is no longer present if recall is delayed for 20–30 seconds by an intervening task. This technique was also used by Baddeley and Warrington (1970) in their investigations of amnesic subjects. On the initial serial positions of the immediate recall task the amnesic subjects were impaired, although their recency effect was normal (Fig. 10-3). That is, the long-term component of the task was impaired, whereas the short-term component was normal. These results support the interpretation of free recall tasks in terms of two components and extend the generality of the claim that verbal short-term memory is normal in amnesic subjects.

These experiments on short-term forgetting described so far have, without exception, involved verbal stimuli. Although no entirely satisfactory nonverbal immediate memory span task has yet been devised, short-term forgetting for

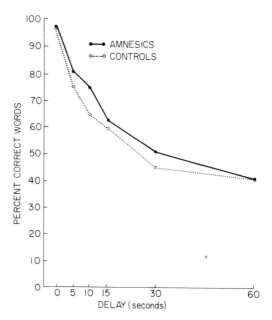

Fig. 10-2. Retention of three words after varying intervals during which rehearsal was prevented. (Reprinted with permission from Baddeley and Warrington, 1970.)

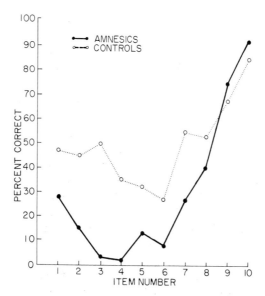

Fig. 10-3. Serial position curve for immediate free recall. (Reprinted with permission from Baddeley and Warrington, 1970.)

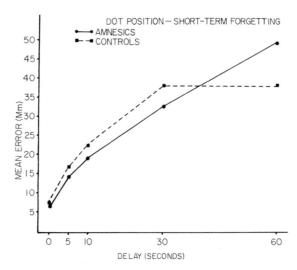

Fig. 10-4. Recall of position of single dot after varying intervals, during which rehearsal was prevented. (Reprinted with permission from Warrington and Baddeley. In preparation).

supposedly nonverbal stimuli has been studied in normal subjects, and these methods have been adapted for investigations of amnesic subjects. These tasks for the most part involve presenting a single stimulus and testing recall or recognition after a delay. To the extent that single rather than multiple stimuli have been used, these tasks are not strictly comparable with verbal short-term forgetting experiments discussed above, and it must be borne in mind that single verbal items are not forgotten over the time periods used in these experiments (Glanzer & Cunitz, 1966). The findings to date with amnesic subjects are somewhat conflicting. Prisko (1963) was the first to use such methods. Two stimuli in the same sense modality (clicks, tones, flashes, shades of red) were presented successively with delays of up to 60 seconds. One amnesic patient (H.M.) showed rapid forgetting, and normal subjects no forgetting. Similarly, Sidman *et al.* (1968) used a delayed matching-to-sample technique (elliptical stimuli) and reported that H.M. rapidly forgot over a period of 30 seconds, whereas two normal children did not. As the normal subjects showed no decrement with time, there is some doubt as to whether the tasks should be described as reflecting S.T.M. processes. Wickelgren (1968) tackled the same problem using recognition of tones and found, in contrast, a rapid decay function in control subjects and, also, that H.M.'s performance on this task was normal. The recall of the position of a single dot illuminated on a screen was tested in a group of six amnesics and six matched controls by Warrington and Baddeley (in preparation). Using intervals of up to 60 seconds during which there was an intervening task, the amnesics showed no greater decline with delays up to 30 seconds, and showed a slight but insignificant deficit at 60 seconds (Fig. 10-4). On balance it would seem that the short-term forgetting of stimuli not readily verbalizable is within the normal range, as is the short-term forgetting of verbal items.

B. Anterograde Amnesia

Defective learning and retention of on-going events is the central component of the amnesic syndrome. There have been many clinical descriptions and a number of useful reviews are readily available (Talland, 1965; Zangwill, 1966; Milner, 1966). Further descriptions will not be given here, but it is worth stressing the global nature of the defect, the impairment being seen in all sense modalities. Quantitative studies are now available which have examined the performance of amnesic subjects on a wide range of tasks including verbal learning, verbal recall, and facial recognition, all of which may be so markedly defective that it is difficult to demonstrate any learning or retention at all. This list is far from exhaustive and the data are relatively well known; therefore it seems appropriate to focus on more positive aspects of learning and retention in amnesic subjects.

The anterograde defects in amnesic patients are not so absolute as either their behavior in daily life or on some formal learning experiments would suggest. H.M. was unable to achieve any learning on a 28-choice point maze but he could learn, at a very slow rate, a shortened version of the task (Milner, Corkin, & Teuber, 1968). Moreover, under these conditions he showed evidence of retention over a week, as he was able to relearn, still very slowly, with some "savings."

Similarly Drachman and Arbit (1966) found that amnesic subjects were able to learn strings of digits exceeding the span at a much slower rate than normal, although with even longer strings (over ten) they were unable to learn the series (Fig. 10-1). It is clear that the task difficulty is relevant and with relatively "easy" learning tasks amnesic patients may learn at a much lower level of efficiency, while on harder tasks their defect has the appearance of being absolute.

Starr and Phillips (1970) confirmed this finding in another amnesic subject who was taught a series of short mazes to the criterion of five correct trials. Relearning was tested two weeks later. The amnesic patient required both more learning and more relearning trials than the control subject, but, nevertheless, significant savings on relearning were recorded.

The first claim of a real exception to the global nature of the defect was seen in motor skills. Milner (1962), in an early report of the patient H.M., reported that he succeeded in learning a mirror drawing task, improving his performance both in terms of errors and time over a three-day period, beginning

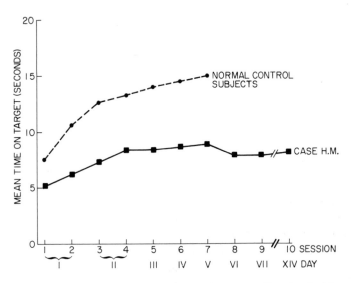

Fig. 10-5. Rotary pursuit learning and retention. (Reprinted with permission from Corkin, 1968.)

each new session at the level he had attained at the end of the previous day. Learning and retention over twenty-four hours was clearly demonstrated, but in the absence of control data it is not certain whether his learning progressed at a normal speed. Some years later Corkin (1968) investigated three motor skills, rotary pursuit, bimanual tracking, and tapping, in H.M. and an appropriate control group. Again H.M. showed learning and retention of the skill for over twenty-four hours; in fact, on one of the tasks, rotary pursuit, complete retention was shown after four days. Normal subjects, however, learned these tasks more quickly and achieved a higher level of performance (see Fig. 10-5). Since H.M. was less good on two control tasks, a reaction time measure and a rank ordering task, his inferior performance on the skills tasks was attributed to nonspecific factors unrelated to his memory defect. Matched control subjects would be necessary before one could agree that "motor skills learning takes place independently of the hippocampal region" (Milner, 1968). An intriguing observation has been reported of a patient, M.K. (Starr & Phillips, 1970), who was able to learn to play a new melody on the piano. On the following day, although he could not recall having learned the melody, he was able to play the whole piece when "prompted" with the first few bars.

Relatively efficient learning and day-to-day retention has now been demonstrated for certain kinds of pictorial and, more importantly, verbal material. A technique involving the presentation of partial information, either fragmented pictures or fragmented words, was used by Warrington and Weiskrantz (1968a)

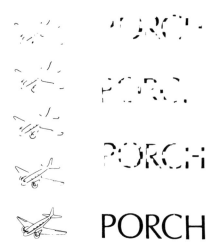

Fig. 10-6. Examples of fragmented picture and word. (Reprinted with permission from Warrington and Weiskrantz, 1968a.)

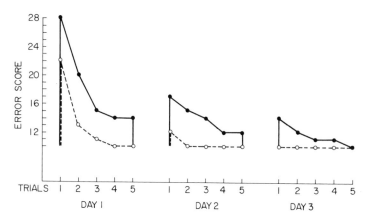

Fig. 10-7. Learning and retention of fragmented pictures. Solid lines, amnesic subjects; dotted lines, normal controls. (Reprinted with permission from Warrington and Weiskrantz, 1968a.)

(Fig. 10-6). Subjects were shown the most incomplete version first, then successively more complete versions until there was correct identification. On subsequent trials normal subjects, and amnesic patients improved their performance until all items were recognized in their most incomplete form. In the original study the amnesic patients were able to learn and show evidence of day-to-day retention (Fig. 10-7). This finding has since been repeated: H.M. was given only one learning trial and after an interval of one hour showed significant savings (Milner *et al.*, 1968).

An interpretation in terms of spared "perceptual" learning in addition to spared motor learning can be discounted. In the first place, in the original study using fragmented drawings, the improved performance by patients was restricted to the specific material to which the subjects had been exposed and was not, therefore, a general improvement in perceptual recognition or a nonspecific practice effect. Second, in a subsequent investigation (Weiskrantz & Warrington, 1970a) it was shown that learning and retention occurred when the partial information was in the form of the initial letters (not fragmented) of the word. Lists of eight words were presented repeatedly in this way until all words were correctly identified from the first two letters. Subjects were taught to a criterion of two errorless trials and retention was tested by the same procedure after one hour. Amnesic patients required rather more trials to learn than the control group but showed significant savings on retention. This is clearly a verbal learning task in which the "perceptual" aspect of the task is minimized. Here, then, is another example of a task on which amnesic subjects can be taught to the same criterion as normal subjects. The question whether those tasks on which amnesics show a varying degree of day-to-day retention is merely related to task difficulty or whether there is some common distinguishing factor will be discussed below.

C. Retrograde Amnesia

The long periods of retrograde amnesia for memories antedating the onset of illness by months or even years is one of the most puzzling features of the amnesic syndrome. The little that is known about retrograde effects in amnesic patients is entirely based on anecdotal and observational data. This is not because it has been a neglected aspect of the amnesic syndrome but, rather, reflects the obvious difficulties in devising quantitative and systematic methods of investigation. Assessment of remote memories in old people and in patients with head injuries has proved equally intractable.

Individual case reports describing the amnesic syndrome have appeared in the neurological literature for nearly 100 years. A recent review by Talland (1965) makes it clear that retrograde amnesia for events preceding the illness is a constant feature of the syndrome. On careful questioning it can be demonstrated that these patients have a very faulty memory for public events and personal experiences before the onset of their illness. There are obvious difficulties in estimating the duration of retrograde effects with any precision, and these estimates have ranged, in individual cases, from a few months (Rose & Symonds, 1960) to many years (Warrington & Weiskrantz, 1968a). H.M., the well-studied Montreal patient, was reported in 1968 (12 years after he had become amnesic) to have a somewhat diminished retrograde amnesia which "manifests itself mainly as a confusion in the order of events occurring during the year or so preceding his operation" (Milner, 1968.) While findings from animal experiments using E.C.S. and other treatments may be interpreted in terms of a consolidation theory of memory, it is hardly plausible to account for retrograde amnesia for such long periods of time in similar terms.

Amnesia after intracarotid injection of sodium amytal has been recorded in patients during the course of investigations for their suitability for surgical treatment. The action of the drug is very short and it is only possible to do simple, brief memory tests. Retrograde amnesia (for the recall of two pictures presented immediately before the injection) was an inconstant feature, not occurring in all eighteen patients showing anterograde effects, and it was always reversible (Milner, 1966). It would be of great interest to establish the temporal extent of these retrograde effects. Bickford, Mulder, Dodge, Svien, and Rome (1958) claimed that the duration of retrograde amnesia, assessed during electrical stimulation via deep electrodes in the temporal lobe, varied with the length of stimulation. With a stimulus of one second, the retrograde amnesia was for only the preceding few minutes; with ten seconds stimulation, memory for the preceding weeks was faulty. The retrograde amnesia under these conditions was clearly reversible, which is consistent with sodium amytal studies.

What, then, is the relevance of these sparse experimental findings to the amnesic syndrome? First, it would seem to suggest that memories are not "lost" but unavailable, and, second, that recent memories are more vulnerable than early memories. Severe amnesic states usually occur in patients with static lesions or lesions increasing in severity. The amnesic syndrome, at least in the well-studied cases, shows little or no recovery. Therefore the issue of whether the very long periods of retrograde amnesia represent unavailable memories may not be resolved.

Although the duration of retrograde amnesia is thought to be very variable and, in some cases, very long, the fact that it can be estimated at all suggests that there is, indeed, some vulnerability of more recent memories, but, clearly, some more objective method of assessment is required.

The feasibility of using questionnaire techniques to obtain quantitave data of "very" long-term memory was demonstrated by Warrington and Silberstein (1970) and thought to justify compiling retrospective questionnaires relating to past public events. Details of the construction of this questionnaire together with results of over 300 normal subjects ranging in age from 40 to 80 years are reported by Warrington and Sanders (1971). In short, 9 equivalent sets of questions relating to events of particular years, sampled over a 40-year period, were compiled and subjects were given both a recall and a recognition form of the questionnaire. Sanders and Warrington (1971) tested five amnesic subjects on these questionnaires and the mean percent correct responses for each "year" for the amnesic group are shown in Fig. 10-8, together with the scores of two hundred normal subjects (mean age, 60 years). It can be seen that the amnesic patients are markedly impaired on both versions of the test; even on the multiple

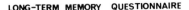

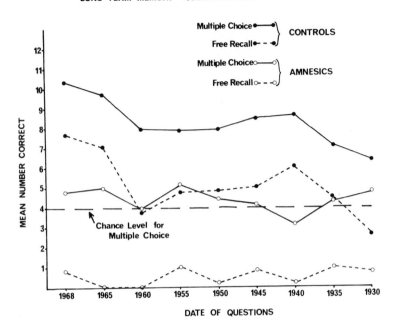

Fig. 10-8. Results of long-term memory questionnaire.(Reprinted with permission from Sanders and Warrington, 1971.)

choice version their performance hardly deviates from chance. Though this questionnaire spans 40 years, there is no indication that more remote events are better recalled or recognized. It seems plausible that if one were to test recall of even more remote events, amnesic patients would still be impaired.

Is, then, the reported vulnerability of recent events an artefact of clinical observations? In a study of normal subjects, Warrington and Sanders (1971) found that the older subjects, contrary to current teaching, were no more impaired on recent events (the preceding year) than on remote events, yet they frequently claimed to recall their early days well. It is possible that individuals, both subjects and experimenters alike, single out individual events which, through rehearsal or some other mechanism, become more "memorable" (Coons and Miller, 1960; Williams, 1969). Leaving these speculations aside, it is suggested that the duration of retrograde memory defects in the amnesic syndrome may have been underestimated and the defect may be present for the subject's entire experience. If this were so, it will be seen below that a unitary functional disorder could account for both retrograde and anterograde effects in the amnesic syndrome.

Language and perceptual skills acquired in childhood have repeatedly been shown to be intact in amnesic patients (Talland, 1965; Milner *et al.*, 1968). Yet these skills clearly require learning, and their maintenance implies some form of memory. In this context, it is of interest to consider if new stimulus material can be learned by amnesic patients. Typically, "new" learning tasks for adult subjects require new and sometimes temporary associations between old items of information. Nonsense syllables were originally devised to test "new" learning, but there is considerable evidence that such learning is strongly influenced by their associative connotations. Nevertheless, we used the technique of partial information in the form of fragmented letters to test nonsense syllable learning in amnesic patients.

Three lists of six nonsense syllables were prepared with two incomplete and one complete version of each syllable. Three amnesic patients and three control subjects were tested, one list being learned on each of three successive days. Subjects were all tested to the criterion of two errorless trials, or to a maximum of fifteen trials. The normal subjects were able to learn nonsense syllables presented by this method of partial information, though rather less efficiently than with fragmented real words. The amnesic patient group improved their performance over the first five trials, and then showed no further learning for the remaining ten trials; in no amnesic was the criterion of two errorless trials achieved.

While these findings might appear to support the view that there is a distinction between learning of "new" and "old" material, there is an alternative interpretation. Some of the individual fragmented letters of the nonsense syllables could be equally a fragment of more than one letter: P-F, R-K, etc. In these instances the partial information was not effective in eliminating incorrect interfering responses. This interpretation will be discussed in detail in the following section.

In a further attempt to assess "new" learning based on novel relationships among familiar items, we tested memory for incongruities on the McGill anomalies task. In this task the subject is required to find the incongruous feature in a complex cartoon-type drawing. The amnesic subjects were told the correct answer to all items they could not solve. Two amnesic patients were tested on 32 items and retested immediately, both showing significant "savings" on the second trial. One of these patients was available for retesting after an interval of three days and again recalled a significant number of items which were not solved on the initial test. A third amnesic patient (temporal lobe case) was on two separate occasions given 5 trials of 20 items, being told the correct answer to every item she failed to identify. Numbers of correct items during learning and retention for the two comparable set of items are shown in Table 10-1. Learning was relatively rapid and there was significant saving on retention after two and four days' interval, respectively.

TABLE 10-1
Learning and Retention of Anomalous Pictures for One Amnesic Subject

	Learning trial no.					Retention
	1	2	3	4	5	
20 items Set M	6	11	17	17	19	16 (2 days)
20 items Set N	8	13	15	19	18	17 (4 days)

These are very preliminary data which require confirmation and extension under standardized test conditions with a control group. If the observations are confirmed and it is accepted that this task involves "new" learning, then it could be argued that neither are old memories necessarily spared, nor "new" learning necessarily impossible.

D. Nature of the Defect

The most clearly stated interpretation of the amnesic syndrome has been formulated by Milner (1966, 1968) in terms of a consolidation defect. Giving weight to the virtual absence of learning of new material, or, at most, learning at a very rudimentary level, together with the preservation of old memories and an adequate short-term memory trace, she suggests that "there is a failure to store information beyond the immediate present." Alternative formulations offered by Milner are "the hippocampal region is essential for the acquisition of new information" and "the essential defect is one of consolidation, so that no stable learning can take place." Consistent with these, but not necessarily equivalent, is "what seems to be impaired is transition from short-term to long-term memory." However, recently there has been an accumulation of findings which raise the possibility of an alternative interpretation.

In an attempt to examine the decay characteristics of the forgetting curve in amnesic subjects (which did not succeed because, in the conditions of the experiment, insufficient learning was achieved by the amnesic group to equate them with the control group), Warrington and Weiskrantz (1968b) noted, nevertheless, certain qualitative differences between the control group and the amnesic group. Not only was the normal relationship between recall and recognition not found in the amnesic group but, importantly, there was a high intrusion rate on the recall task which increased with longer intervals. Surprisingly, many (50 percent) of these false-positives were intrusions from earlier lists, some of which had been learned the previous day. This is clearly an example of proactive interference and evidence that at least some information is being stored for relatively long periods of time and that it has sufficient strength to interfere with new learning. This observation has since been confirmed by Starr and Phillips (1970), and Baddeley and Warrington (1970). At the very least, these findings would not be predicted by consolidation theory.

The difficulties encountered in examining forgetting in amnesic subjects have been tackled by the method of "partial information." Weiskrantz and Warrington (1970b) used this method in the form of fragments of words to teach amnesics to a strict criterion, which can be achieved relatively rapidly, and measured retention after one hour, twenty-four hours, and seventy-two hours. Four measures were recorded: (1) a perceptual score, (2) trials to learn, (3) trials to relearn, and (4) a savings score. The amnesic group were normal on the perceptual score but significantly impaired on the other three measures (summing the results for all three retention intervals). It was argued that the more rapid forgetting in the amnesic group was not a trivial consequence of slower learning (Fig. 10-9). It is not obvious why, in terms of the consolidation hypothesis, material which has been adequately learned over several trials should be subject to more rapid forgetting.

Why then do amnesic patients learn and retain verbal material using this method of partial information when similar items are unavailable using conventional methods? If it were not merely a favorable technique for all subjects, amnesics and controls alike, then the special or unique properties of this task would have to be considered in the interpretation of the syndrome. In a study designed to manipulate different methods of learning and retention independently, Warrington and Weiskrantz (1970) obtained evidence that the retrieval procedure is more relevant than the learning procedure and that the method of retrieval itself was critical in determining the amnesics' performance on retention tasks. Two experiments were reported: in the first, the partial information method of learning was used and, in the second, a conventional word learning task (reading a word list three times) was used. In each experiment retention was tested (after a filled delay of one minute) by different methods of retrieval. Learning by the method of partial information did not improve retention except when retrieval was also tested by the method of partial information (Table 10-2). Of some interest is the finding that information in long-term memory was available, even after learning by conventional methods, when a favorable retrieval method was employed (Table 10-3). Retrieval by recognition was superior to retrieval by recall in the control group but not in the amnesic group, which is consistent with the earlier finding of their relatively greater deficit on recognition than recall. Furthermore, retrieval by partial information was superior to retrieval by recall in the amnesic group. An analysis of variance was computed and the interaction term, groups × retention conditions, was significant, indicating that there was a differential effect of retention conditions in the two groups. These findings refute the hypothesis that retention tested by partial information is particularly favorable as a retrieval method for all subjects,

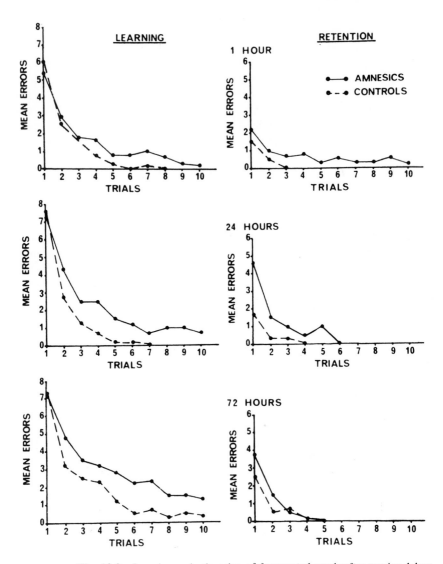

Fig. 10-9. Learning and relearning of fragmented words after varying delays. (Reprinted with permission from Weiskrantz and Warrington, 1970b.)

and they provide further evidence that it is inappropriate to characterize the amnesic syndrome as a failure of registration or consolidation.

One special property of retrieval by partial information is that the subject can eliminate incorrect false-positive responses. The choice of possible responses is restricted by the partial information provided. The number of alternatives

TABLE 10-2
Retention Scores After Learning by Method of Partial Information

	Controls $N = 6$	Amnesics $N = 6$
Recall	48%	14%
Recognition	94%	59%
Fragmented words	96%	94%

TABLE 10-3
Retention Scores After Rote Learning

	Controls $N = 8$	Amnesics $N = 4$
Recall	13.0	8.0
Recognition	18.7	10.5
Fragmented words	11.1	11.5
Initial letters	16.0	14.5

which would "match" or "fit" the fragmented words must be very limited, if not unique, and in the case of initial letters of words the number of alternatives is finite and can be counted. Indeed, it has been shown that the number of alternatives that can be formed from the same first three letters in a five-letter word is a significant variable for both amnesic and control subjects (Weiskrantz and Warrington, 1970).

The opportunity for rejecting incorrect responses would be important if either long-term memory information were not appropriately classified or if there were too many items of stored information (i.e., if information in storage is either not inhibited or not dissipated in a normal fashion). The high incidence of prior list intrusions in amnesic subjects is consistent with either hypothesis. Classification processes operate in amnesic patients apparently no less effectively than in normal subjects. Four experiments were reported (Warrington and Weiskrantz, 1971) in which organization processes were examined in six amnesics and matched control groups. No qualitative differences in their performance emerged that indicated altered organization or classification of either perceptual or mnemonic information in the amnesic patients. On one task involving semantic clustering, the effect of "cueing" (that is, prompting by the category name) was clear-cut in the amnesic group (Table 10-4), indicating not only that information is classified in semantic categories but also the restriction of response alternatives in a very different manner is beneficial to amnesic patients. In a more recent study, Baddeley and Warrington (in preparation) found that amnesics showed better recall of both acoustically clustered and

TABLE 10-4
Mean Numbers of Words Recalled With Free and "Cued" Recall

	Free recall				"Cued" recall			
	2	4	6	12	2	4	6	12
No. of categories per list								
Controls $N = 8$	6.5	5.4	6.5	4.8	7.8	8.3	9.3	7.6
Amnesics $N = 5$	2.2	1.6	1.2	1.4	4.6	4.6	5.6	4.4

semantically clustered lists than of comparable control lists. The view that the amnesic syndrome results from a failure to inhibit or dissipate stored information (Warrington and Weiskrantz, 1970) gains strength from these negative findings.

Thus, there is now evidence that memory is relatively well preserved in amnesic subjects on two types of task: motor learning and testing by partial information. Is there a common factor linking performance on these apparently dissimilar tasks? One property of motor skills is that retention appears to be remarkably unaffected by interference effects in general (Adams, 1967) and, in particular, proactive interference has not yet been demonstrated (Duncan and Underwood, 1953). It therefore may be the case that both types of task, not necessarily for the same reason, are resistant to proactive interference. Day-to-day memory (which is particularly disastrous in amnesic patients) may require that previous events be "forgotten" or suppressed, and the inability to do so in the amnesic subject might produce "confabulations" or other responses analogous to prior-list intrusions recorded in formal verbal learning experiments.

E. Comparison of Human and Animal Experiments

The long-standing discrepancy between the results of clinical studies of anterograde amnesia following medial temporal (including hippocampus) damage in man and animal experiments implicating homologous regions now seems capable of resolution. Efforts have been unsuccessful to produce a "failure of consolidation" in animals with lesions intended to be homologous to those imposed by Scoville in man (Scoville and Milner, 1957). For example, Orbach, Milner, and Rasmussen (1960) found no defect in medial bitemporal monkeys on a discrimination learning task in which widely spaced trials were filled with massed trials involving irrelevant discriminations. There was only a mild impairment on the retention of postoperatively acquired tasks. Butler (1969) also found that monkeys with medial temporal lesions, while they learned visual discrimination tasks more slowly than controls, showed normal retention of the acquired tasks over twenty-four hours. The forgetting curves of monkeys with neocortical plus hippocampal damage for simple visual problems appear to be normal if acquisition performances are matched and if there is minimal interference in the intervals between learning and retesting (Weiskrantz, 1970). Kimble and Pribram (1963) found that bilateral hippocampectomized monkeys were unimpaired on discrimination learning tasks with intertrial intervals of six minutes. In fact, rats with hippocampal damage can learn certain tasks, for example two-way active avoidance (Isaacson, Douglas, and Moore, 1961), even faster than controls.

This is not to say that hippocampal damage is without effect in animals, but that the findings are most readily interpreted in terms of disinhibitory phenomena. Hippocampal rats or monkeys are less likely than controls to stop doing something that is either punishing or nonrewarding. For example, they are slower to extinguish responses in a variety of discrimination, runway, and other operant situations. They are slower to acquire discrimination reversals. They tend to be undistractable by novel stimuli under some conditions, and show a diminished level of spontaneous alternation and a deficit in acquiring learned alternations. They are also deficient in passive avoidance situations. Reviews of the relevant studies can be found in Douglas and Pribram (1966) and Kimble (1969). One recent study by Kimble and Kimble (1970) has shown that even though hippocampectomized rats reach a formal level of criterion learning of a brightness discrimination just as quickly as controls, they nonetheless display longer runs of "hypotheses"; similarly, in extinction, hypotheses persist much longer than in controls.

Thus animals with damage to hippocampal and neighboring tissue display, it could be argued, an inability to eliminate (or suppress) information, rather than an inability to retain information in long-term storage. The jump from the animal studies to our findings in man, which have led us to stress excessive false positive responses and excessive proactive interference, is not difficult to make. Indeed, some recent studies of monkeys with temporal lobe damage reveal abnormal interference phenomena that are prominent in discrimination learning and retention.

Two types of paradigm that are very rich in interference have produced specific deficits in temporal lobe monkeys. Iversen and Weiskrantz (1964, 1970) studied the retention of simple visual problems which were interspersed between large numbers of other visual problems, and found very poor savings over twenty-four hours. Iversen (1970) has reported that visual-discrimination retention deficits in monkeys with combined inferotemporal and hippocampal damage were disproportionately enhanced when the animals had to learn new visual problems in the interval between learning and retention testing.

Another interference-rich situation is "concurrent" or "serial" discrimination learning, in which the trials from several problems are interspersed during acquisition. Using this paradigm, Correll and Scoville (1965) reported a deficit with medial-temporal operated monkeys (hippocampus plus neighboring structures, including neocortex). Iwai and Mishkin (in press) and Cowey and Gross

(1970) have also found that monkeys with anterior inferotemporal lesions (restricted to neocortex) have a deficit on a concurrent discrimination learning task, and this lesion can be dissociated in its effects from one posteriorly placed in the temporal lobe. It still remains to be seen whether the anterior neocortical lesion can be dissociated from a hippocampal lesion. It also remains unclear whether the temporal lobe interference phenomena in monkeys are restricted to the visual modality or are multimodal, as in man. Orbach *et al.* (1960) reported a "mild" tactile learning and retention impairment in their medial temporal-operated monkeys, but Iversen (1967) found normal tactile scores in an inter-ference-rich situation. Mahut (personal communication) recently has found both tactile and visual spatial reversal impairments in hippocampal-operated monkeys. Clearly, more work remains to be done before the question of modality specificity can be resolved.

In both the human and subhuman experiments, therefore, we can point to responses that intrude inappropriately and to an undue prominence of inter-ference phenomena. In both, good retention over long intervals can be demon-strated in favorable circumstances. What appears clinically to be a "failure of consolidation" in man can be accounted for in terms of interference phenomena, whereas it is very difficult to account for those phenomena in terms of a failure of consolidation.

III. SHORT-TERM MEMORY DEFECTS

One of the main sources of evidence that short-term memory and long-term memory are not explicable in terms of a single unitary memory system is the dissociation of S.T.M. and L.T.M. in amnesic subjects. This view would be greatly strengthened if selective impairment of short-term memory could be established as the result of a different anatomical lesion.

A. Impairment of Short-term Memory

The inability to repeat verbal stimuli, including letters and digits, has been recorded in patients with left-hemisphere cerebral lesions as a relatively isolated disability (Wernicke, 1874; Goldstein, 1948; Dubois, Hécaen, Angelergues, Maufras du Chatelier, and Marcie, 1964; Konorski, Kozneiwska, & Stepien, 1961; and Geschwind, 1965). Patients with left hemisphere lesions have been reported to have a poor digit span (McFie, 1960) and this finding has been confirmed more recently (Newcombe, 1969; Warrington and Rabin, 1971). Luria, Sokolov and Klimkowski (1967) reported two patients in whom the main symptom was an inability to repeat a series of phonemes, words, or digits presented auditorially. The deficit was interpreted in terms of memory impair-ment without attempting to differentiate between short- and long-term memory.

Warrington and Shallice (1969) reported a detailed investigation of a single patient (K.F.) in whom there was a profound inability to repeat verbal material. They considered the proposition that this repetition defect, which could equally well be described as a reduced verbal span, was one of impaired verbal short-term memory. Repetition of strings of one to four numbers, letters, and words was examined. K.F. was able to recall only one item reliably; beyond that, performance was directly related to the number of items in each string, the proportion of items correct decreasing with increasing string length (Table 10-5). Two alternative explanations of his disability were examined: first, that his reduced span was secondary to impaired auditory perception and, second, that it was due to impaired motor speech function. They interpreted his normal performance on tasks of rapid identification of "key" stimuli as compelling evidence that faulty auditory perception was not responsible for his deficit. On tests of matching and recognition which require no verbal response, his performance was no better than with recall, indicating that speech production was not critical. They therefore argued that the capacity of the short-term memory store was severely reduced.

In further studies of the same patient, short-term forgetting was investigated using the Peterson technique. Recall of multiple items (words or letters) was tested with no delay and with varying filled intervals. The normal decay functions were not observed. More striking was the finding that short-term forgetting of single letters was abnormally fast (Warrington and Shallice, 1972), since, with the 0-delay condition, his performance was unimpaired (Fig. 10-10). This latter finding of adequate recall with no delay, and very rapid forgetting with short delays, adds strong support to the view that his defect can indeed be attributed to impaired verbal short-term memory.

B. Modality Specificity of Short-term Memory

The experiments with K.F. described so far all used auditory presentation of verbal stimuli. The question arises as to whether the same results would be obtained using visual presentation. K.F.'s ability to recall visually presented

TABLE 10-5

Immediate Recall of Numbers, Letters, and Word Strings of Increasing Length

	String length	1 item	2 items	3 items	4 items
Numbers	No. of items correct	20/20	28/40	37/60	37/80
	No. of strings correct	20	12	6	1
Letters	No. of items correct	19/20	21/40	26/60	22/80
	No. of strings correct	19	7	2	0
Words	No. of items correct	20/20	29/40	32/60	33/80
	No. of strings correct	20	13	4	1

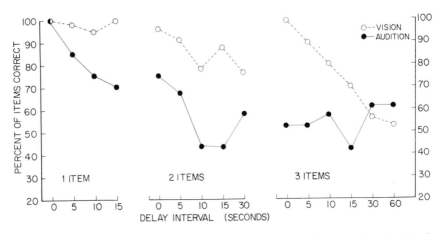

Fig. 10-10. Recall of letters after varying intervals, comparing visual and auditory presentation (Reprinted with permission from Warrington and Shallice, 1972.)

strings of digits and letters (at a one per second rate) was recorded (Warrington and Shallice, 1969). It was found that his performance, though below normal, was superior to his recall after auditory presentation; his visual span of apprehension was superior to his auditory span, although the reverse is the case in normal subjects. This case is not unique. Luria *et al.* (1967) reported a verbal memory defect in two patients in whom the main symptom was an inability to repeat auditorially presented verbal items, though there was relatively little impairment with visual presentation of the same verbal material. The modality specificity of this defect is emphasized by contrasting the short-term forgetting of auditorially and visually presented letters in a Peterson type task. Apparently normal decay functions are obtained over delays of up to 60 seconds with visual presentation, whereas there is a greater decrement with auditory presentation (see Fig. 10-10) (Warrington and Shallice, 1972).

There is, thus, some evidence that auditory short-term memory defects can occur without a defect in visual short-term memory. This position would be more secure if the converse could be shown, namely, impaired visual short-term memory with intact auditory span. One variety of perceptual disorder appears relevant to the visual span of apprehension.

Simultanagnosia, the impairment of interpretation of pictures and difficulty in reading, has been described in terms of a limitation of simultaneous form perception (Kinsbourne and Warrington, 1962). Single visual stimuli such as digits and letters were accurately reported, but simultaneous presentation of two stimuli resulted in failure to report one of them. The visual span of apprehension in unselected patients with unilateral cerebral lesions was examined in terms of a defective visual short-term memory hypothesis (Warrington and Rabin, 1971). Briefly, it was found that visual spans of apprehension for random digits and letters, for sequences approximating to English, and for nonsymbolic line stimuli were impaired in patients with left hemisphere lesions (anatomical considerations are discussed further below). It was argued that this defect could not be accounted for in terms of visual field defects, generalized language impairment, or letter recognition difficulties, and that it was more plausible to implicate a visual short-term memory deficit. This conclusion must be tentative until further critical experiments have been completed.

C. Anatomical Considerations

While the interpretation of impaired auditory and visual span in terms of defective short-term memory cannot be secure without group studies in the case of auditory span, and further experimental investigation in the case of visual span, the anatomical correlates of these two syndromes are reasonably well established. Geschwind (1965) reviewed the available anatomical data in published cases in which there was a specific auditory repetition defect and concluded that the fasciculus arcuatus of the left hemisphere (a "tract which runs from the posterior superior temporal region, arches round the posterior end of the sylvian fissure and then runs forward in the lower parietal lobe, eventually to reach the frontal lobe") was the critical locus. Dubois *et al.* (1964) cite the

TABLE 10-6
Visual Span: Mean Percent Correct in Patient Groups

Groups	Random digits	Random letters	2nd order letters	4th order letters	Lines
Control $N = 20$	80	69	90	92	56
Right $N = 27$	74	68	88	92	55
Left $N = 39$	55	50	73	77	43
R. anterior $N = 8$	81	78	88	93	53
L. anterior $N = 16$	63	56	80	87	49
R. temporal $N = 12$	74	66	91	94	61
L. temporal $N = 10$	54	50	78	73	44
R. Posterior $N = 7$	65	65	85	88	49
L. posterior $N = 13$	44	41	62	62	35

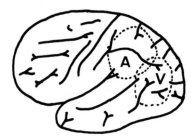

Fig. 10-11. Provisional anatomical foci for auditory (A) and visual (V) short-term memory deficits.

supramarginal and angular gyri of the left hemisphere and Luria *et al.* (1967) reported two such patients with lesions of the left temporo-parietal region. In the patient reported by Warrington and Shallice (1969), a left parietal subdural haematoma was evacuated some days after a motor cycle accident in which he sustained a left parieto-occipital fracture. The site of maximal damage, confirmed during a craniotomy thirteen years later for the treatment of epilepsy, was in the posterior parietal region (Warrington *et al.,* 1971). There is, thus, considerable agreement that damage to the left posterior parietal region is invariably present in patients with defective auditory span. In the group study of visual span (Warrington and Rabin, 1971), the left hemisphere group was significantly impaired relative to the right hemisphere group. Subdividing the groups according to site of lesion within the hemisphere, the left posterior subgroup (patients with parietal, occipital, or parieto-temporal lesions) was significantly worse than the right posterior subgroup and the left nonposterior cases (see Table 10-6). This finding is consistent with the earlier clinical reports of an association between limited simultaneous form perception and a lesion of the left anterior occipital lobe verified at autopsy (Kinsbourne and Warrington, 1963). The provisionally identified anatomical foci are shown in Fig. 10-11.

D. Short-term Memory Deficits and their Relationship
with Long-term Memory

The existence of a patient with a selective impairment of auditory short-term memory can be used to provide information about the relationship between long- and short-term memory systems. No generalized memory defect is clinically observable in patients with reduced auditory span or reduced visual span. It might be argued that, as these deficits are modality-specific, in everyday life compensation via the intact modality might be masking some impairment of long-term memory. Though no quantitative data are available in patients with reduced visual span on long-term memory tasks, this point was specifically investigated in the patient (K.F.) with a severely reduced auditory span (Warring-

TABLE 10-7
Free Recall Scores for Each Serial Position

Serial position	1	2	3	4	5	6	7	8	9	10
No. correct	15	10	7	7	7	10	12	9	9	25
Percent correct	50	33	23	23	23	23	40	30	30	83

ton and Shallice, 1969; Shallice and Warrington, 1970). On two tasks of verbal learning, both of which involved only auditory presentation, his performance was within normal limits. More important, on a free recall task, in which the ten stimulus words were presented once and recovered under conditions of immediate recall, the long-term component was entirely normal as judged from the serial order effect (see above), while the short-term component was markedly reduced. The number of words recalled over the ten serial positions was roughly constant except for the first and tenth serial position (see Table 10-7). Thus, the recency effect is limited to one serial position, which again supports the hypothesis of a much reduced S.T.M. capacity. These findings, thus, are the converse of those obtained in amnesic patients who have been shown to have normal S.T.M. and defective L.T.M. It would appear that K.F. has normal L.T.M. in spite of impaired S.T.M. These two types of syndrome, considered together, provide strong evidence for a double dissociation of function; that is, there are two memory systems (if not more), S.T.M. and L.T.M., which are able to operate independently.

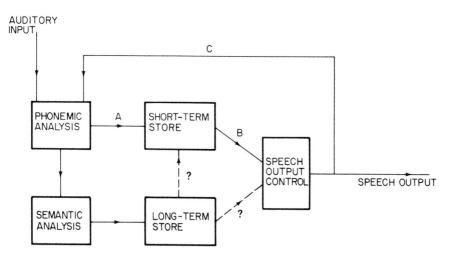

Fig. 10-12. Suggested model for information processing in auditory verbal memory. (Reprinted with permission from Shallice and Warrington, 1970.)

It is of some interest to consider these findings in relation to current theoretical models. It is possible that the commonly accepted flow diagram in which information must be transferred from S.T.M. to L.T.M. may be inappropriate. Shallice and Warrington (1970) proposed a model for processing information in auditory verbal memory tasks in which there is independent input into the two systems, S.T.M. and L.T.M. (see Fig. 10-12).

IV. CONCLUSIONS AND SUMMARY

This chapter has concentrated on two types of memory disorders in man: the amnesic syndrome, and specific deficits of short-term memory. The amnesic syndrome has been well-documented and reviewed in the past, and hence the present account emphasizes recent experimental studies and attempts to bring closer together the work of laboratory experiments and clinical studies. The possibility of specific deficits of short-term memory has only recently been put forward, and such data as are available are reviewed.

Patients with the amnesic syndrome who characteristically are severely impaired on long-term memory tests, can have normal short-term verbal memory as assessed by immediate memory span and short-term forgetting tasks. The evidence regarding nonverbal short-term memory is still ambiguous, but such few reports that exist of abnormally rapid decay functions may have utilized tasks that were primarily long-term memory tasks.

The retrograde amnesic aspects of the amnesic syndrome have not been studied carefully because of the obvious difficulties in doing so with precision, but the results of a questionnaire technique for testing memories of public events suggest that the duration of the retrograde memory defects in amnesic patients may have been seriously underestimated, and that remote events are no better recalled or recognized than recent events.

The anterograde amnesic aspects of the amnesic syndrome are not so absolute as either the patients' behavior in daily life or in conventional formal learning experiments would suggest. Learning and retention not only of motor skills, but also of pictorial and verbal material, have been found with a method of "partial information." Long-term retention over days or weeks can easily be demonstrated. The success of the partial information method does not depend on its merely being a simple test for all patients: the amnesic patients are differentially helped by it. The beneficial effect of the method is seen primarily at the time of testing for retention, and can be demonstrated even with conventional methods of learning, provided the method of partial information is used to test retention. In addition, in formal free recall tests amnesic patients make an impressive number of "false positive" responses, among them items from tests given hours or days earlier.

The amnesic syndrome, therefore, does not appear to reflect, as is commonly assumed, a "failure of consolidation" in long-term memory. The partial information method, by its nature, limits false positive responses, and the hypothesis offered here is that the amnesic syndrome is primarily due to an excess of interference among stored items. This interpretation is consistent with the results of a large body of animal experiments on the effects of hippocampal and medial temporal lobe lesions, which also point to a decrease of inhibition and excessive interference.

Patients suffering from an auditory verbal "repetition" defect have a severely shortened auditory "immediate memory span." The defect is not due to an impairment of auditory perception or motor speech function. Such patients also show abnormally rapid short-term forgetting of single letters and pairs of letters, even though performance is normal with "zero" delay. In contrast, on a variety of long-term memory tasks their performance is normal; in particular, they are normal on free recall tasks. A patient with a reduced auditory span can demonstrate longer visual digit and letter spans, which is the reverse of the relationship in normal subjects. Moreover, short-term forgetting for visual material shows less decrement than for auditory material.

In addition, impairment of visual short-term memory may occur in patients with "simultanagnosia." Such patients have normal auditory spans, but are impaired in reporting multiple visual stimuli although their reports of single stimuli are normal. A group of patients with left posterior pathology has been identified with defective visual span of apprehension for digits, letters, sequences approximating to English, and nonsymbolic line stimuli; the impairment cannot readily be accounted for in terms of field defects, language impairment, or recognition difficulties.

Tentatively, therefore, it can be suggested that a visual short-term memory disorder can be identified, and that it is dissociable from the auditory short-term memory disorder. Preliminary evidence is presented concerning the critical anatomical foci in the left hemisphere of the two defects.

The results as a whole have a bearing on a number of aspects of normal memory mechanisms. Among these are:

1. As short-term and long-term memory deficits can be disturbed independently, it is possible that the commonly accepted flow diagram in which information must be transferred from S.T.M. to L.T.M. is inappropriate.

2. There are strong reasons for postulating the existence of modality-specific short-term memory systems.

3. The method of partial information, because it enables one to control and perhaps even eliminate false positive responses, provides a new approach to the study of interference phenomena.

4. The embarrassing and long-standing discrepancies between animal and human lesion experiments involving medial temporal lesions may now be capable of resolution and, if so, one can draw inferences about the normal role of anatomical systems that can be generalized from animals to man, and vice versa.

REFERENCES

Adams, J. A. *Human memory*. New York: McGraw-Hill, 1967.

Baddeley, A. D., & Warrington, E. K. Amnesia and the distinction between long and short-term memory. *Journal of Verbal Learning & Verbal Behavior,* 1970, Vol. 9, 176-189.

Baddeley, A. D., & Warrington, E. K. Acoustic and semantic coding in amnesic patients (in preparation).

Bickford, R., Mulder, D. W., Dodge, H. W., Svien, H. J., & Rome, H. P. Changes in memory function produced by electrical stimulation of the temporal lobes in man. *Research Publications Association for Research in Nervous and Mental Disease,* 1958, Vol. 36, 227.

Butler, C. Is there a memory impairment in monkeys after inferior temporal lesions? *Brain Research,* 1969, Vol. 13, 383-396.

Coons, E. E., & Miller, N. E. Conflict versus consolidation of memory traces to explain retrograde amnesia produced by E.C.S. *Journal of Comparative & Physiological Psychology,* 1960, Vol. 53, 524-531.

Corkin, S. Acquisition of motor skill after bilateral medial temporal lobe excision. *Neuropsychologia,* 1968, Vol. 6, 255-265.

Correll, R. E., & Scoville, W. B. Effects of medial temporal lesions of visual discrimination performance. *Journal of Comparative & Physiological Psychology,* 1965, Vol. 60, 175-181.

Cowey, A., & Gross, C. G. Effects of foveal prestriate and inferotemporal lesions on visual discrimination by rhesus monkeys. *Experimental Brain Research,* 1970, Vol. 11, 128-144.

Douglas, R. J., & Pribram, K. H. Learning and limbic lesions. *Neuropsychologia,* 1966, Vol. 4, 197-220.

Drachman, D. A., & Arbit, J. Memory and hippocampal complex, II. *Archives of Neurology,* 1966, Vol. 15, 52-61.

Dubois, J., Hécaen, H., Angelergues, R., Maufras du Chatelier, A., & Marcie, P. Etude neuro-linguistique de l'aphasie de conduction. *Neuropsychologia,* 1964, Vol. 2, 9-44.

Duncan, C. P., & Underwood, B. J. Retention of transfer in motor learning after 24 hours and after fourteen months. *Journal of Experimental Psychology,* 1953, Vol. 46, 445-452.

Geschwind, N. Disconnection syndromes in animals and man–Part II. *Brain,* 1965, Vol. 88, 585-644.

Glanzer, M., & Cunitz, A. R. Two storage mechanisms in free recall. *Journal of Verbal Learning & Verbal Behavior,* 1966, Vol. 5, 351-360.

Goldstein, K. *Language and language disturbance*. New York: Grune & Stratton, 1948.

Isaacson, R. L., Douglas, R. J., & Moore, R. Y. The effect of radical hippocampal ablation on acquisition of an avoidance response. *Journal of Comparative & Physiological Psychology,* 1961, Vol. 54, 625-628.

Iversen, S. D. Tactile learning and memory in baboons after temporal and frontal lesions. *Experimental Neurology,* 1967, Vol. 18, 228-238.

Iversen, S. D. Interference and inferotemporal memory deficits. *Brain Research,* 1970, Vol. 19, 277-289.

Iversen, S. D., & Weiskrantz, L. Temporal lobe lesions and memory in the monkey. *Nature,* 1964, Vol. 201, 704-742.

Iversen, S. D., & Weiskrantz, L. An investigation of a possible memory defect produced by inferotemporal lesions in the baboon. *Neuropsychologia,* 1970, Vol. 8, 21-36.

Iwai, E., & Mishkin, M. Two inferotemporal foci for visual functions. *Experimental Neurology* (in press).

Kimble, D. P. Possible inhibitory functions of the hippocampus. *Neuropsychologia,* 1969, Vol. 7, 235-244.

Kimble, D. P., & Kimble, R. J. The effect of hippocampal lesions on extinction and 'hypothesis' behavior in rats. *Physiology & Behavior,* 1970, Vol. 5, 735-738.

Kimble, D. P., & Pribram, K. H. Hippocampectomy and behaviour sequences. *Science,* 1963, Vol. 139, 824-825.

Kinsbourne, M., & Warrington, E. K. A disorder of simultaneous form perception. *Brain,* 1962, Vol. 85, 461-486.

Kinsbourne, M., & Warrington, E. K. The localizing significance of limited simultaneous form perception. *Brain,* 1963, Vol. 86, 697-702.

Konorski, J., Kozneiwska, H., & Stepien, L. Analysis of symptoms and cerebral localization of audio-verbal aphasia. *Excerpta Medica, International Congress Series,* 1961, No. 38. 22.

Luria, A. R., Sokolov, E. N., & Klimkowski, M. Towards a neurodynamic analysis of memory disturbances with lesions of the left temporal lobe. *Neuropsychologia,* 1967, Vol. 5, 1-10.

McFie, J. Psychological testing in clinical neurology. *Journal of Nervous & Mental Disease,* 1960, Vol. 131, 383-393.

Milner, B. The memory defect in bilateral hippocampal lesions. *Psychiatry Research Reports,* 1958, Vol. 11, 43-58.

Milner, B. Les troubles de la mémoire accompagnant des lésions hippocampiques bilatérales. In *Physiologie de l'Hippocampe.* Series Colloques Internationaux, Paris: Centre National de la Recherche Scientifique. Pp. 257-272.

Milner, B. Amnesia following operation on the temporal lobes. In C. W. M. Whitty and O. L. Zangwill (Eds.), *Amnesia.* London and Washington, D. C.: Butterworths, 1966. Pp. 109-133.

Milner, B. Preface: Material specific and generalized memory loss. *Neuropsychologia,* 1968, Vol. 6, 175-179.

Milner, B., Corkin, S., & Teuber, H. L. Further analysis of hippocampal amnesic syndrome: 14 year follow-up study of H. M. *Neuropsychologia,* 1968, Vol. 6, 215-234.

Newcombe, F. *Missile wounds of the brain: A study of psychological deficits.* London and New York: Oxford University Press, 1969.

Orbach, J., Milner, B., & Rasmussen, T. Learning and retention in monkeys after amygdala-hippocampus resection. *Archives of Neurology,* 1969, Vol. 3, 230-251.

Peterson, L. R., & Peterson, M. J. Short-term retention of individual verbal items. *Journal of Experimental Psychology,* 1959, Vol. 58, 193-198.

Prisko, L.-H. *Short-term memory in focal cerebral damage.* Unpublished Ph.D. thesis, McGill University, 1963.

Rose, F. C., & Symonds, C. P. Persistent memory defect following encephalitis. *Brain,* 1960, Vol. 83, 195-212.

Sanders, H. I. and Warrington, E. K. Memory for remote events in amnesic patients. *Brain,* 1971, Vol. 94, 661-668.

Scoville, W. B., & Milner, B. Loss of immediate memory after bilateral hippocampal lesions. *Journal of Neurology, Neurosurgery, & Psychiatry,* 1957, Vol. 20, 11-21.

Shallice, T., & Warrington, E. K. Independent functioning of verbal memory stores: a neuropsychological study. *Quarterly Journal of Experimental Psychology,* 1970, Vol. 22, 261-273.

Sidman, M., Stoddard, J. P., & Mohr, J. P Some additional quantitative observations of immediate memory in a patient with bilateral hippocampal lesions. *Neuropsychologia,* 1968, Vol. 6, 245-254.

Starr, A., & Phillips, L. Verbal and motor memory in the amnesic syndrome. *Neuropsychologia,* 1970, Vol. 8, 75-88.

Talland, G. A. *Deranged memory.* New York: Academic Press, 1965.

Warrington, E. K., & Baddeley, A. D. Short-term forgetting of spatial position in amnesic patients (in preparation).

Warrington, E. K., Logue, V., and Pratt, R. T. C. The anatomical localisation of selective impairment of auditory verbal short-term memory. *Neuropsychologia,* 1971, Vol. 9, 377-387.

Warrington, E. K., & Rabin, P. Visual span of apprehension in patients with unilateral cerebral lesions. *Quarterly Journal of Experimental Psychology,* 1971, Vol. 23, 423-431.

Warrington, E. K., & Sanders, H. I. The fate of old memories. *Quarterly Journal of Experimental Psychology,* 1971, Vol. 23, 432-442.

Warrington, E. K., & Shallice, T. The selective impairment of auditory verbal short-term memory. *Brain,* 1969, Vol. 92, 885-896.

Warrington, E. K., & Shallice, T. Neuropsychological evidence of visual storage in short-term memory tasks. *Quarterly Journal of Experimental Psychology,* 1972, Vol. 24, 30-40.

Warrington, E. K., & Silberstein, M. A questionnaire technique for investigating very long-term memory. *Quarterly Journal of Experimental Psychology,* 1970, Vol. 22, 508-512.

Warrington, E. K., & Weiskrantz, L. A new method of testing long-term retention with special reference to amnesic patients. *Nature,* 1968, Vol. 217, 972-974. (a)

Warrington, E. K., & Weiskrantz, L. A study of learning and retention in amnesic patients. *Neuropsychologia,* 1968, Vol. 6, 283-291. (b)

Warrington, E. K., & Weiskrantz, L. Amnesic syndrome: consolidation or retrieval? *Nature,* 1970, Vol. 228, 628-630.

Warrington, E. K., & Weiskrantz, L. Organisational aspects of memory in amnesic patients. *Neuropsychologia,* 1971, Vol. 9, 67-73.

Waugh, N. C., & Norman, D. A. A primary memory. *Psychological Review,* 1965, Vol. 72, 89-104.

Weiskrantz, L. *Analysis of behavioral change.* New York: Harper & Row, 1968.

Weiskrantz, L. Visual memory and the temporal lobe of the monkey. In R. E. Whalen (Ed.), *The neural control of behavior.* New York: Academic Press, 1970. Pp. 239-256.

Weiskrantz, L., & Warrington, E. K. Verbal learning and retention by amnesic patients using partial information. *Psychonomic Science,* 1970, Vol. 20, 210-211. (a)

Weiskrantz, L., & Warrington, E. K. A study of forgetting in amnesic patients. *Neuropsychologia,* 1970, Vol. 8, 281-288. (b)

Wernicke, C. *Der aphasische Symtomenkomplex.* Brieslau: Cohn & Weigert, 1874.

Whitty, C. W. M., & Zangwill, O. L. *Amnesia.* London and Washington, D. C.: Butterworths, 1966.

Wickelgren, W. A. Sparing of short-term memory in an amnesic patient: implications for strength theory of memory. *Neuropsychologia,* 1968, Vol. 6, 235-244.

Williams, M. Traumatic retrograde amnesia and normal forgetting. In G. A. Talland and N. C. Waugh (Eds.), *The pathology of memory*. New York: Academic Press, 1969. Pp. 75-80.

Williams, M., & Smith, H. V. Mental disturbance in tubercular meningitis. *Journal of Neurology, Neurosurgery, & Psychiatry,* 1954, Vol. 17, 173-182.

Zangwill, O. L. Some qualitative observations on verbal memories in cases of cerebral lesion. *British Journal of Psychology,* 1946, Vol. 37, 8-19.

Zangwill, O. L. The amnesic syndrome. In C. W. M. Whitty and O. L. Zangwill (Eds.), *Amnesia.* London and Washington, D. C.: Butterworths, 1966. Pp. 77-91.

CHAPTER

11

WHAT HAVE THE ANIMAL EXPERIMENTS TAUGHT US ABOUT HUMAN MEMORY?

DONALD A. NORMAN

I. ON ANIMAL AND HUMAN STUDIES

There are curious discrepancies between the structure of memory implied by the studies in this book and the structure proposed by recent theories of human memory. The most complete descriptions of the operations of memory have come from the behavioral studies of humans rather than from the studies of physiological mechanisms. To this date, the numerous physiological studies have failed to tell us much about the structural mechanisms. What happens when a person acquires, retains, and then retrieves information?

In this chapter I review the structures proposed by students of human memory and comment on the gap between the human and animal literature. Although it is easily argued that there are so many differences between animal and human brains that we should not expect correspondences (especially when the animal is a rat or goldfish), nonetheless, it seems strange that so little contact appears to have been made between those studying human and animal memory structures. Of course, almost all the human work derives from studies of verbal material, a type of material which is somewhat irrelevant for application to animal studies. Certainly everybody would be happier were animal and human found to be similar—perhaps with the animal system being simpler or smaller or lacking some features of the human's. The same technical vocabulary is applied to animal and human processes: attention, and short-term and long-term memory. Why do these same words mean different things to different people?

Our knowledge of the structure of human memory comes primarily from the studies of perception, pattern recognition, and short-term and long-term memory performed by the modern student of human information processing. These behavioral studies have allowed us to make a number of concrete statements about the structural organization and composition of the various systems that comprise human memory. The modern theories follow the flow of information through the different stages of processing performed by the peripheral and central nervous system as the incoming signals are first transformed by stimulus analyzing mechanisms and then are analyzed, interpreted, attended to, and stored in both temporary and permanent storage systems. Although there now exist many theories of information processing—some verbal descriptions, some mathematical formulations, some computer models—most of these theories agree with one another on the general structure that is proposed. They differ primarily in the details of their assumptions. Students of human memory claim that their picture is justified from the extensive behavioral studies that have been performed on normal human subjects. Moreover, the few studies that have been made of patients with specific neurological difficulties do seem to fit into the picture that has been constructed (for example, see the Chapter by Warrington and Weiskrantz, this volume).

The theoretical structures which I discuss for humans are reviewed in more detail and with more justification in the texts by Neisser (1967) and Norman (1969). In this chapter, whenever I state theories or results without giving references or credits, I am relying on the fact that they are already given in either or both of these books. Specific assumptions and justifications and the details and more complete assumptions, justifications, and predictions of the models can be found in the book *Models of Human Memory*, edited by Norman (1970), and in each of the volumes of the series edited by Spence and Spence (1967, 1968) and Spence and Bower (1970).

II. MODELS OF HUMAN MEMORY

There are several ways in which the theorist can go about constructing his picture of the memory system. In the sections that follow, I describe two related approaches. One approach is to try to follow the processing of information from the point where it is first perceived, through its temporary storage in a short-term memory system and more permanent storage in other memory systems, and through the stages of selective attention and retrieval of the stored information. This approach requires that the entire system which processes information be analyzed, for each part affects the others: memory plays only one of the many roles which are required. I call this approach the study of *Human Information Processing* (see Section II,A).

The second approach is to start with the general problems of retrieving material from any large scale storage system and to develop the structures necessary to make these processes work, always keeping in mind the observations of human behavior, so that the result will be consistent with the experimental findings. I call this the *Information Sciences Approach to Memory* (see Section II,B).

Yet another approach to the study of human memory (which will not be discussed in this chapter) is to modify the findings, techniques, and theories of learning. The distinction between the study of learning and the study of memory is very slight, so that the classification of an experimental study as one pertaining to memory rather than to learning is often more an exercise in semantics than anything else. Thus, it is only natural that the theories of learning should play an important role in the development of theories of memory. Usually the models and results of studies which are based on learning theory are concerned primarily with the experimental conditions that control the observed behavior, with the acquisition factors (learning) rather than forgetting (memory), and with descriptive models (proactive and retroactive factors) rather than structural models (see Deutsch, 1960, pp. 1–16). There is a discrepancy here between the way the information processing theorist does experiments and constructs theories and the way that the more traditional learning literature goes about it. This is not the place to argue whether one is right and the other wrong, but it is important to note that although they appear to talk about the same concepts, and although they may even use the same words, they are talking about completely different aspects of theorizing.

In the sections that follow I first present the theoretical structures which have been described by the recent workers in the field of human memory, followed by a discussion of experimental implications. I concentrate primarily on those aspects of experimentation which have implications for students of both human and animal processes. In addition, special emphasis is placed on those features of experiments which have been found to be important when working with humans, yet which are often not reflected in the techniques and procedures of experiments on animals.

A. The Human Information Processing Approach

The practitioners of this approach describe the path of the incoming signal as it proceeds through deeper and deeper levels of processing by the nervous system. A number of different stages have been identified: sensory transduction and analysis, sensory information storage, feature extraction, pattern recognition, short-term memory, selective attention, long-term memory, and retrieval. Most of the emphasis on studies of short-term memory (also called primary memory and active storage) stems from this approach, and the theories and experiments borrow heavily from the theoretical and experimental techniques of sensation, detection, and perception.

In general, these studies have led to the following picture. First there is a sensory information storage system (now assumed to exist in all sense modalities) which maintains an image of the sensory input for some several hundred milliseconds. This is followed by a pattern recognition process which, in turn, is either accompanied or preceded by such stimulus analyzing mechanisms as contour enhancement, line and movement detectors, and spectrum analyzers. Then, the physical stimulus is identified with some previously learned item (i.e., transformed from a physical image into a psychological one), and this identified item is maintained temporarily in a short-term memory (STM).

Usually the STM is assumed to have a very limited capacity. There is disagreement over whether the capacity of STM is measured in the number of items it can contain or in the number of seconds it lasts, but in either case the capacity is small. The capacity in items is assumed to be somewhere between 5 and 10; the duration in seconds is assumed to be somewhere between 10 and 30. Even if material in STM does decay in time, it is usually acknowledged that storage of information is severely affected by the presentation of new information. Thus, the ability to maintain material in STM depends strongly upon what else the human is doing at the moment. These properties are going to be important when we start the discussion of the animal literature.

We are on weaker ground when we discuss the next levels of storage. Obviously, everything that is presented to the human is not forgotten. Thus we invoke a further system—long-term or secondary memory (LTM)—which is assumed to store some of the items from STM. The properties of this LTM are not well known. Moreover, the breakdown of the memory structures into the simple dichotomy of short- and long-term systems is rather arbitrary. There is an embarrassing shortage of experimental evidence to justify this simple division. Recently, a few studies have been performed to follow the storage of material beyond the first 5 minutes after presentation to see if other, intermediate memories must be invoked. It is here, in fact, that we need most the physiological evidence about the nature of the initial activation of memory processes and the stages that occur before or during consolidation. In human work, we can probably identify the initial activation of the memory structures with STM and the final consolidated traces with LTM. At least one worker in the field insists that physiological evidence requires us to add a fourth type of memory, an intermediate-term memory between STM and LTM (Wickelgren, 1970).

Note that the specification of the logical properties of the memory system can be made accurately and usefully without any concern for the actual physiological mechanisms by which these occur. In the analysis of the human studies we need to know such properties of short-term memory as its storage capacity and the way that decay processes occur. It is completely irrelevant for many purposes whether these processes come about through electrical or chemical activation of neurological circuits, through reverberating circuits, synaptic potentials, or the release of inter-synaptic chemicals. Nor does it matter where the short-term memory is located—it could be in the big toe for all that we care. We care about function, not location nor the details of the ways it is implemented. This is not to say that these facts are not interesting or important, but they comprise the description of the hardware of the operation, matters that can be entirely independent of the way that the system and the software are implemented. It is critically important, of course, that the operations required by the physiological and logical requirements be compatible with one another. Moreover, some knowledge of the implementation might help one to take a plausible guess at the logic.

Again, although processing theories do not care whether human permanent memory comes about through localized storage or through patterns of information scattered throughout the brain, or whether the structure is molecular, chemical, or caused by the growth or activation of new synaptic mechanisms, the time course by which this final consolidation takes place is important for all of us. Moreover, it is extremely important that the organizational properties of material stored in memory and the properties of the retrieval process be found to be compatible with the physiological mechanisms.

B. The Information Sciences Approach

A second approach to the study of memory is to start by considering the general problems of retrieving material from any large scale storage system, realizing that all systems, be they of animal, man, or machine, must share the same basic considerations and logical constraints. This approach is relatively new and is dominated by talk of organization, mnemonics, list structures, markers, and content addressable storage systems. Some of the developments brought about by this approach to the problem have important implications on the physiological structure of the memory system. This approach differs from the other by its emphasis on the organizational structure of memory. The information processing studies are backed with much experimental evidence, but no one yet knows how to collect the proper evidence on information structures. Thus, this second approach is very theoretical.

Much of the work which results from this approach to the study of human processes owes much to the study of artificial systems of automata, the most common example, of course, being the large scale digital computer. This is a touchy subject, and it is very important to note the nature of the comparison between the processes of man and of machine. No sensible person claims that the human brain is anything like a computer. Rather, the argument is that we can learn something about memory processes by studying the general principles of storage and retrieval involved in any system which stores large quantities of information. All systems which attempt to process and store large quantities of information—whether natural or man-made—must have certain basic principles in common.

This is an appropriate place to expand somewhat on these statements, lest they be misunderstood here as they seem to be misunderstood elsewhere. There are two different arguments. First, the theorist who uses an analogy from the mechanisms of computers is usually told that he is making the same error of logic that guided his predecessors who cited as analogies to the brain whatever was the most recent technological advance—levers, pneumatic tubes, complex gear trains, telephone switchboards, analog and digital computers, and, now, holograms. The critic, however, loses sight of the fact that we have indeed learned something from each analogy. Usually the man who puts forth the analogy does so only to make some point, usually a point that remains valid long after the analogy is forgotten. In fact, the only person who appears to take the analogy seriously appears to be the critic.

Second, the increase in our knowledge about technology is almost invariably accompanied by an increase in our understanding of the general properties of many different scientific problems. The recent developments in computer technology have also spawned new mathematics, new understanding of the principles of knowledge, of computability, and of automata in general. We have learned about the types of storage and communication that must occur in order to maintain and retrieve large amounts of information, to solve problems, and to work on several tasks simultaneously. These basic principles hold whether the analysis is of a system that is a computer or man, analog or digital, serial or parallel, single or multiple processor, abstract or real.

The most important fact concerning the use of any large capacity storage system is that retrieval problems cause the most difficulty. When millions or billions of items are stored in a memory, some system must be imposed upon their organization or else nothing would ever be found except by sheer accident. A misplaced book in a large library might as well not exist at all. Systematic search is out of the question. Thus, it is important that an efficient organizational structure be imposed so that an efficient path among the stored items can be followed to get to the desired material. Moreover, as we shall see, it is probably essential that there be some sort of content addressable structure. That is, it should be possible to get to a particular piece of information directly by the contents of the information: the address structure of memory must be so constructed that access to stored material can be achieved directly by knowing the nature of the material which is being sought.

Content addressable storage systems are not easy to construct. It is possible to make believe that they are understood by talking about an input "resonating" with the critical areas of memory, or of a sensory input being "directed" to the relevant structures, but it is quite a different matter to describe exactly the physiological or chemical processes that actually implement the system. Most physiological studies of possible molecular or synaptic mechanisms neglect the facts imposed by the extremely large size of the memory of which we are talking and the rather rapid access (sometimes measured in fractions of seconds) that is involved. Most schemes of molecular coding do not explain how they could take place at the speeds at which both storage and retrieval are possible.

Most physiological schemes avoid the problem of selectivity. It is easy to see how all of memory might be searched in parallel or how specific sensory codes might activate specific brain locations, but the trouble is that too much will be stored or retrieved at any one time. Although everything may indeed be connected to everything else in the memory structure, usually only the one critical item of interest is retrieved. This selectivity is an extremely important feature of human memory.

III. SENSORY ADDRESSABLE STORAGE

One important area of concern to the worker in human memory is the nature of the mechanism which recognizes and interprets sensory information. A wide variety of experimental techniques is involved, from studies of the role of a masking stimulus on tachistoscopically presented visual material to studies on the speed of searching and identification of material presented to the subject. Sometimes we test the scanning of lists held in memory (the experiments of Sternberg, 1966, 1967); sometimes we test the scanning of a list presented before us (the experiments of Neisser, 1963); sometimes we ask whether one item which has been presented has physical identity with an item presented earlier (is A the same as A or B?); sometimes we study how increasing delays between presentation of the items to be compared causes a test for physical identity to be replaced by a test for name identity (is A the same as a or b?) (see the experiments of Posner, Boies, Eichelman, and Taylor, 1969).

The initial interpretation of the incoming signal takes place very rapidly. This must be done with the aid of the long-term memory system, for that is where the rather arbitrary rules that link the visual and acoustical waveforms with their agreed upon meanings must be stored. Thus, although normal experiments on recall usually demonstrate a prolonged and difficult retrieval of memories, in these perceptual studies we find rather rapid and easy access to memories. This fact has important implications for the memory structure.

The immediacy with which we recognize old situations and well-learned material coupled with a rapid feeling of strangeness and novelty when exposed to new events says that the sensory nature of the event must govern the access and at least part of the structure of memory. Here is a situation in which a search strategy cannot apply. Moreover, any attempt to use the meaning of the signal as an aid to discovering the relevant memory locations must be incorrect, for that only begs the issue of how the meaning comes to be known.

At some stage in the analysis process we must go from the sensory representation to the stored meaning, and this must come about by means of the memory system. Of all the discussions I have seen of this problem, only one which has the access and structure of memory based on the sensory representation of the signals themselves seems to make any sense. Thus, when a signal comes in, the sensory mechanisms get to work on it, enhancing the image, extracting contours, colors, frequencies, movements, and critical features. Then, these features determine the relevant location of the memory system that is to be used to decode the item. Moreover, the location is selected even if the signal is a novel one. How do you know that a situation is novel? How do you know so quickly with mantiness that you do not know the meaning of the word "mantiness?" You could not have scanned all of memory to discover that the new experience or word was not there. No, presumably you looked where the sensory image said that the information ought to be, and found nothing there.

IV. ORGANIZATION OF MEMORY

The manner in which the memory structure is interconnected with itself is of primary importance. Every serious attempt to show the possible mechanisms of the memory system ends up discussing the connections between items of information. From the very first philosophical discussions of memory to the most modern computer-oriented theories, the primary feature of the long-term memory system is its organizational structure.

Different items of information in the memory system are related to each other. Some people prefer to call these relationships associations, others call them bonds, some call them networks, and others markers, nodes, pointers, or links. Regardless of the names, the basic concepts are all similar. In retrieving information, one follows the path laid down by these associations through the network of stored information, until, finally, the desired information is retrieved. Just how one actually follows through the network is not known. Even the very basic question of how one recognizes when the correct answer has been retrieved has not been studied. This last point is extremely important. If you know the answer for which you are looking, then you wouldn't need to look. But if you don't know the answer, then how can you recognize it when you find it? I have been able to think of only one way in which this testing can be done (Norman, 1968); that is by testing each answer as it is retrieved by the memory search and testing to see whether it is consistent with the question—the exact scheme I proposed suggested that you had reached the correct point if you could use as your query of the memory system both the original question and the possible answer. You were successful whenever the question led to the answer and, more important, the answer led back to the question.

These types of observations, coupled with many more different studies of memory—see the chapters by Reitman (1970), Kintsch (1970), Shiffrin (1970), and Quillian (1968)—tell us that the study of the mechanisms of acquisition and of storage cannot really be separated from the study of mechanisms used in retrieval. The retrieval aspects must include ways of getting into the memory structure, of guiding the search path through the memory, and of testing and making decisions on the retrieved information. All aspects are so intermingled that it may be impossible to separate these different aspects of retrieval from one another.

The preceding arguments have several different implications for the physiological mechanisms of memory. One implication concerns the manner of getting access to stored information and the type of mapping from sensory representation to memory storage representation that must exist. This, in turn, says something about the physiological relationship that might hold between short- and long-term memory. Finally, we can say something about the associative nature of memory.

If we can get direct access to information from the sensory form of the input, then there must exist a relatively clean mapping of sensory features into the memory. Although we might expect the sensory representation to undergo a considerable amount of processing before it is used to get access to stored information—for example, through stimulus analyzing mechanisms of several orders of complexity, including hypercomplex detectors, if necessary—we still would hope to find the sensory addressable storage system visible in the neuroanatomy of the memory and sensory structures. Furthermore, we know from experiments on memory and attention that incoming information is often retained for only a very short amount of time (that is, only in short-term memory) even though it had to have access to long-term structures in order to identify it properly. By this and similar arguments, one is led to conclude that short- and long-term memory are intimately related to one another. One possible relationship that can account for much of the experimental findings is to have them both correspond to different modes of excitation of the very same memory structures (Norman, 1968). Thus, short-term memory might reflect the temporary excitation of the permanent structures of long-term memory. The answer to the speculation on whether short- and long-term memories are phys-ically distinct or simply result from different ways of using the same structures can come only from physiological studies. Indeed, the nature of the limitation on short-term memory is not known, and, again, only a study of the actual physiological mechanisms would appear to be capable of stating why there is such a small, limited capacity.

The study of the associations that occur in memory offers yet another area of research that is waiting for information from physiological investigations. It is possible, of course, that the associations are stored in the same fashion as the memory information itself, so that they cannot be interpreted until we know the physiological code for storage. But they might also get reflected in the biological and chemical structures of the memory. In this case, the structures would change as new information was acquired, offering some hope that their nature might be discoverable.

V. EXPERIMENTAL CONSIDERATIONS

A. Methods of Test

1. The Human Literature

One important experimental tool comes from the distinctions among the various methods of testing memory, for example, between the results of recall and recognition tests. In a recall situation, the subject is given some clues and is asked to retrieve a specific item: "What was the list of words I showed you?" "What is my name?" In a recognition test the subject is shown a test item and asked whether or not he recognizes it: "Was the word houseboat on the list I showed you?" Both methods test the same underlying memory structure (an assumption, of course, but one that has some logic and some experimental evidence behind it), but in quite different ways. The types of cues that are given are extremely important in the recall situation, for it is assumed that here the subject must trace out the trail through his memories until he finds the item that he seeks. In recognition there need be no search for the item, only a check to see whether it was presented earlier. The important measures of performance are both the false and the correct recognition rates, for the errors are as useful in interpreting the structure of the memory system as are the correct responses. Recognition studies tap a completely different aspect of the memory system than do recall studies, for no extensive search process appears to be necessary. Studies of the nature of false recognitions give us useful clues to the study of the relationships among stored items (see Bjork, 1970, and Kintsch, 1970).

2. The Animal Literature

Where do we find such neat distinctions in experimental techniques in the animal literature? Nowhere. Different investigators use different experimental techniques and get different results, but nowhere does there appear to be the same type of structuring of experimental techniques that one finds in human studies. As far as I can tell, experiments which involve maze learning and bar pressing, discriminations and reversals, stepping off platforms and avoidance and escape procedures, mix up the various types of memory tests in different amounts. It should not be difficult to devise a battery of tests that range from something similar to recall to something similar to recognition, with maybe a few new aspects of retrieval that are unique to animal studies thrown in besides. But the important thing would seem to be that the same animals (if possible) and the same physiological manipulations be tested by the same experimenter in a wide variety of tests. The conclusions from a single type of behavioral test are incomplete and can be misleading.

Many of the physiological descriptions of the memory system which result from studies using ECS, drug, and spreading depression techniques strike the person who studies human memory as crude and naive discussions of the complexities of memory. (This assessment is quite independent of the fact that we can probably be accused of using crude and naive discussions of physiological mechanisms.) Many of the physiological manipulations used in experiments seem to be rather nonspecific in the ways that they attack neurological structures. Granted that a particular drug may affect only specific classes of neurological mechanisms, it is obviously absurd to conclude that the drug affects only very specific memories, leaving all the rest unaltered. Due to the closely intermingled structure of storage, retention, and retrieval, it is not clear how one can claim that a physiological manipulation affects one aspect and not the others. The worker in human memory would like to see a whole battery of tests applied to the study of memory deficits caused by physiological manipulations. What aspects of memory are affected, what are left unchanged? Do the manipulations affect recall of information, recognition of information, or both?

B. Rehearsal by Humans

One very important behavioral strategy used by human subjects is that of rehearsal. In the usual verbal studies, rehearsal means a deliberate repetition of the material contained in STM. Rehearsal of verbal material is usually assumed to be a type of "inner speech" and its properties do seem to reflect the acoustic nature of spoken speech. Rehearsal of motor activities appears to be an imaginary reenactment of the relevant motor movements, although there may be no actual motor activity involved. Rehearsal of verbal material appears to be a reasonably slow, serial process. Only one item can be rehearsed at any instant of time. Between 6 and 30 items can be rehearsed per second; the presently popular estimate is around 10. This rehearsal does two things. One, it allows an image to be retained in STM indefinitely. Two, it helps transfer the information to a more permanent storage system. These properties of rehearsal are often thought to be consistent with other properties of the STM system. The extreme sensitivity of the STM system to interference from newly presented material or distracting events may really reflect the single-natured properties of the rehearsal system. Thus, it might be that material in STM decays with the passage of time unless rehearsed and that there is a limit to the number of items that can be kept active by rehearsal. These two properties—a time-decay STM and an item-dependent capacity of the rehearsal process—are compatible with many observations of the properties of the STM system.

There is much less knowledge about the storage of nonverbal or motor events (see Posner, 1966, 1969; Posner, Lewis, & Conrad, in preparation; Bower & Spence, 1969). It is tempting to speculate that much the same processes are involved there, as well. Rehearsal in this case would denote a repetition of the motor movements involved (see, for example, Hebb, 1968). Note that there is no logical reason why the process of thinking need involve movement of any part of the motor system. The notion that some kind of micromovement will occur during thinking or rehearsal appears to be carried over from the oldest traditions of stimulus-response theory. But in terms of more modern concepts, rehearsal might simply be a repetition of the mental program with complete suppression of all the actual input-output commands. Real motor movements might very well occur during rehearsal, but, logically, they need not necessarily do so.

C. Rehearsal by Animals

What this means, of course, is that animals might also have rehearsal mechanisms similar to ours for motor movements. Thus, if an animal had a STM much like that of a human, he might very well engage in a rehearsal of its latest actions. If the possibility exists, it is extremely important to devise tasks which will prevent him from rehearsal after the presentation of the task on which he later is to be tested.

The favorite way of eliminating rehearsal with humans is to have the subject do some interfering task, such as to count backwards as rapidly as possible by threes; this appears to be very effective in blocking rehearsal of verbal material. This technique does not stop motor rehearsal. It is also a difficult technique to use with animals. In human studies it has turned out to be very important to make the rehearsal-preventing task one that truly prevents rehearsal of the material to be retained. Having a human subject run on an activity wheel will not prevent him from rehearsing a series of digits. Having a human count backwards by threes may not prevent him from rehearsing a finger maze (see Peterson, 1969).

In animal studies of STM, it would seem to be important to try to replicate some of the human studies (e.g., Peterson & Peterson, 1959) including rehearsal-prevention activities. Thus, to study the immediate memory an animal might retain for an avoidance task, he should be placed in the training situation for a controlled number of trials (hopefully very small in number) and then immediately be given a distracting task—either a completely different experiment or even another series of different avoidance tasks. In this way it would be possible to examine the behavior of animals in a similar fashion to that of humans. It would be possible to compare the influence of the amount, type, and duration of the intervening situation on the retention of the first task in a manner analogous with studies of human memory on the effect of the number of intervening items upon ability to retain information. Once rehearsal is controlled, it becomes possible to say something about the effect of time upon retention. Obviously the animal experimenter is going to have difficulties doing these experiments. Moreover, unless he uses animals who, like their human counterparts, are so well trained on the class of experiments that they are doing that all they need to remember about the new task is which of the many possible variations of the situation it is, then the experiment will be subject to such criticisms as that the "rehearsal-preventing" task is simply causing positive or negative transfer (depending upon which way the results come out). Paralyzing the animal with curare in order to stop his rehearsal by stopping all his motor activity will prove nothing to information theorists, although it might to more traditional psychologists. Remember, we believe that mental rehearsal need not involve actual movements.

It is extremely important that animal studies not be contaminated with the learning of the experimental situation or learning-to-learn phenomenon. It is important to emphasize this again. In human studies, simple instructions are sufficient to let the subject know that the important task for him is to remember, for example, one or more three-digit numbers or three-consonant syllables. With animals, it must be clear that the subject is familiar with the basic experimental situation and simply needs to know, for example, which lever is the critical one, which response leads to avoidance or escape, or which tube contains the sugar water. The animal should be so well trained on the class of experiments that acquisition is as close to one-trial learning as is possible. To my knowledge, the only experiments on animals that have tried to mimic the human experiments in this way are the platform experiments used in ECS studies. But none of these experiments have considered the possibility of animal rehearsal. Thus, rehearsal in these situations will vary with the peculiar way in which animals are handled between the training and the later test.

It is quite true that no one has demonstrated that animals can indeed rehearse. It may be considered heretical for me even to suggest this possibility. But I don't mind being a heretic. After all, up to a few years ago there was a rather unbelievable reluctance on everyone's part even to admit that humans could rehearse. Given the important role that rehearsal has been shown to play in human memory, might it not also be important in animals, if only in a vestigial fashion?[1]

In the few animal experiments that have been performed with concern for the various variables known to affect human memory, the results have been instructive. The best studies known to me are those using a delayed matching-to-sample task in the monkey (Etkin and D'Amato, 1969; a number of experiments and a good review can be found in Jarrard and Moise, 1971). These studies do get results very similar to those reported for human subjects. The main differences which appear would seem to result from differences between the human verbal rehearsal processes and whatever processes the animal uses as a substitute. The results I have seen indicate that some sort of mediating process does occur in animals. Whether this be rehearsal or some other process can probably best be determined through an examination of the effect of interfering tasks on the memory. Those tasks which interfere most severely with memory would be expected to be those which occupy the same internal processes that the animal uses for his rehearsal strategies.

VI. THE STRUCTURE OF MEMORY

The memory system is tightly interconnected with itself. Stored concepts, images, and ideas are all associated with one another. The acquisition of new information requires that the new be inserted properly into the cross-referencing of the old. The retrieval of information may sometimes require lengthy interactions among the stored information, but it is also guided by schemes that

---

[1] Several of my colleagues who have read an earlier draft of this paper have commented that they have observed activity of their animals which looks very much like rehearsal. It is not uncommon, I am told, for an animal to be "going through the motions" of the response in the intervals between one reinforcement and the next trial, as well as after the experiment, in the home cage. An experienced animal caretaker is reported to have remarked that she could always tell what schedule a pigeon had been on simply by watching its behavior in the home cage. Certainly the experiments on delayed reaction look very much like experiments in short-term memory, complete with such rehearsal-like activity as maintenance of body orientation. I find little difference between the activity of an animal which performs "a series of attacks on the barrier in the direction of the lighted door" in an experiment on delayed reaction and the activity of a human subject who keeps repeating the stimulus sequence to himself in an experiment on short-term memory (the quotation is from Woodworth and Schlosberg, 1954, p. 605).

allow immediate access to a concept or new sensory event through sensory or content addressable storage schemes. Immediate access to a starting location in the memory can tell us whether we have any knowledge of the topic or input signal: it cannot tell us the full interpretation of that input, however, for interpretation requires the retrieval of relations and this comes only by tracing through the various paths of memory.

The fact that sensory inputs have immediate access to long-term mechanisms says nothing about whether these inputs will get stored. There is much evidence from behavioral and physiological studies that it requires time and effort to store something. The human behavioral studies say that newly acquired information must be fit into the organization scheme of memory. The physiologists say that stages of consolidation must occur. All agree that some short-term memories may fade away leaving little or no trace. To get a permanent storage requires time.

All these discussions appear to be compatible with the literature on the physiological basis of human memory. There are a number of studies on various amnesias and aphasias caused by concussions, brain wounds, surgery, and lesions resulting from diseases and malnutrition. These studies corroborate the distinctions between short-term and longer-term memories, and among storage, retrieval, and acquisition of information. In almost all such cases, there is always good and ready acquisition of old, permanent memories. Amnesiac patients eventually recover their speech habits and motor skills (assuming no damage to the motor controls and systems which are necessary to speak, write, and move about). It has generally been believed that they tend to forget events which occurred just prior to their disability (Barbizet, 1970) and, in some of the more interesting cases, appear to have great difficulty in inserting recently experienced material into their long-term memories. Their LTM system works, for they still talk and read and write. Their STM system works, for they can hold a conversation, answering sensibly the questions put to them. But the acquisition of new information is severely hampered, so that a conversation will not be remembered. The interesting interplay between the ability to get at previously acquired information in LTM while failing to insert new information is a potentially valuable source of physiological information about the nature of memory (Talland, 1965, 1968; Talland & Waugh, 1970).

Study of these patients is very difficult, for the damage is usually caused by rather severe injuries to the CNS and one is never clear exactly what structures are involved. In addition, motivational aspects clearly become important (to say nothing of the problems of confabulation). These difficulties are especially severe with aphasic and Korsakoff syndrome patients. Occasionally, however, rather clean cases come to light, and these are often rather informative (see Corkin, 1968; Milner, Corkin, & Teuber, 1968; Scoville, 1968; Sidman, Stoddard, & Mohr, 1968; Teuber, Milner, & Vaughan, 1968; Wickelgren, 1968).

A good review of the analysis of short- and long-term memory deficits is provided by the chapter in this volume by Warrington and Weiskrantz. Their studies provide some interesting new explorations of the multifaceted structure of human memory. Here we find evidence that memory disorders of amnesiac patients may not always be well-ordered in time. (Presumably, the memories of patients with brain damage caused by surgery or by lesions differ from the retrograde amnesias produced by blows on the head, documented by Barbizet, 1970.) Evidently, the apparent difficulties that some patients have in acquiring new material (patients suffering from the Korsakoff syndrome or patients such as HM, who had bilateral mesial temporal-lobe excision) may result from excessive interference among memories rather than from a true difficulty in acquisition. This would indicate that the difficulties were primarily those of getting access to the new material, not of actually acquiring it. One could speculate that the neurological deficits impair the organizational processes, but sufficient data are not yet available for any serious proposals at this stage. Moreover, the existing data show that some organizational factors still operate with these patients, so it is clear that the eventual explanation of the deficit must be a reasonably sophisticated one.

Studies of one patient with an abnormally small STM but apparently normal LTM raise questions about the existing theories of memory that imply STM is a necessary stage in the processing of new material. Such an assumption is a basic part of my own theories, so I welcome future exploration of this patient. Fortunately for my theoretical position, these patients do not lack STM; rather, they simply have one of reduced size. Moreover, the impairment seems to be present only for auditory material, not for visually presented material.

The kinds of evidence reported by Warrington and Weiskrantz would seem to be in exactly the form in which the animal investigations can be used most profitably. Studies of memory impairments can provide valuable clues to the organization of memory that will not be found in the behavioral studies of the normal, intact human. If the techniques of animal experimentation can be made to match the level of sophistication of human experimentation, then a whole new source of data is open to us, for with animals we can obtain control and measurement of physiological functions that are impossible (or unethical) to obtain from humans.

Studies of human memory behavior are reasonably compatible with the implications about memory which can be drawn from the study of patients with neurological deficits. The big gap in our knowledge is between the results learned from the studies on humans and the results from studies of animals. So far there has been little contact between the workers in these different areas. In this chapter I have tried to explore some of the reasons for this lack of contact. By explaining my own biases and interests I hope that I have managed to indicate some of the reasons for our differences in techniques and theoretical positions.

All areas of research must eventually come together if ever we hope to understand the structure of memory.

REFERENCES

Barbizet, J. *Human memory and its pathology.* San Francisco: Freeman, 1970.

Bjork, R. A. Repetition and rehearsal mechanisms in models for short-term memory. In D. A. Norman (Ed.), *Models of human memory.* New York: Academic Press, 1970.

Bower, G. H., & Spence, J. T. (Eds.) *The psychology of learning and motivation.* Vol. 3. New York: Academic Press, 1969.

Corkin, S. Acquisition of motor skill after bilateral medial temporal-lobe excision. *Neuropsychologia,* 1968, Vol. 6, 255-265.

Deutsch, J. A. *The structural basis of behavior.* Chicago, Illinois: University of Chicago Press, 1960.

Deutsch, J. A. (Ed.) *Physiological basis of memory.* New York: Academic Press, 1972.

Etkin, M., & D'Amato, M. R. Delayed matching-to-sample and short-term memory in the capuchin monkey. *Journal of Comparative and Physiological Psychology,* 1969, Vol. 69, 544-549.

Hebb, D. O. Concerning imagery. *Psychological Review,* 1968, Vol. 75, 466-477.

Jarrard, L. E. (Ed.) *Cognitive processes of nonhuman primates.* New York: Academic Press, 1971.

Jarrard, L. E., & Moise, S. L. Short-term memory in the monkey. In Jarrard, L. E. (Ed.), *Cognitive Processes of nonhuman primates.* New York: Academic Press, 1971.

Kintsch, W. Models for free recall and recognition. In D. A. Norman (Ed.), *Models of human memory.* New York: Academic Press, 1970.

Milner, B., Corkin, S., & Teuber, H. -L. Further analysis of the hippocampal amnesic syndrome: 14-year follow-up study of H. M. *Neuropsychologia,* 1968, Vol. 6, 215-234.

Minsky, M. (Ed.) *Semantic information processing.* Cambridge, Massachusetts: MIT Press, 1968.

Neisser, U. Decision time without reaction-time: experiments in visual scanning. *American Journal of Psychology.* 1963, Vol. 76, 376-385.

Neisser, U. *Cognitive psychology.* New York: Appleton-Century-Crofts, 1967.

Norman, D. A. Toward a theory of memory and attention. *Psychological Review,* 1968, Vol. 75, 522-536.

Norman, D. A. *Memory and attention.* New York: Wiley, 1969.

Norman, D. A. (Ed.) *Models of human memory.* New York: Academic Press, 1970.

Peterson, L. R. Concurrent verbal activity. *Psychological Review,* 1969, Vol. 76, 376-386.

Peterson, L. R., & Peterson, M. J. Short-term retention of individual verbal items. *Journal of Experimental Psychology,* 1959, Vol. 58, 193-198.

Posner, M. I. Components of skilled performance. *Science,* 1966, Vol. 152, 1712-1718.

Posner, M. I. Abstraction and the process of recognition. In G. Bower & J. T. Spence (Eds.), *Advances in learning and motivation.* Vol. 3. New York: Academic Press, 1969.

Posner, M. I., Boies, S. J., Eichelman, W. H., & Taylor, R. L. Retention of visual and name codes of single letters. *Journal of Experimental Psychology Monographs,* 1969, Vol. 79, 1-16.

Posner, M. I., Lewis, J. L., & Conrad, C. Component processes in reading: a performance analysis. In preparation.

Quillian, M. R. Semantic memory. In M. Minsky (Ed.), *Semantic information processing.* Cambridge, Massachusetts: MIT Press, 1968.

Reitman, W. R. What does it take to remember. In D. A. Norman (Ed.), *Models of human memory.* New York: Academic Press, 1970.

Scoville, W. B. Amnesia after bilateral mesial temporal-lobe excision: introduction to case H. M. *Neuropsychologia,* 1968, Vol. 6, 211-213.

Shiffrin, R. M. Memory search. In D. A. Norman (Ed.), *Models of human memory.* New York: Academic Press, 1970.

Sidman, M., Stoddard, L. T., & Mohr, J. P. Some additional quantitative observations of immediate memory in a patient with bilateral hippocampal lesions. *Neuropsychologia,* 1968, Vol. 6, 245-254.

Spence, J. T., & Bower, G. H. (Eds.) *The psychology of learning and motivation.* Vol. 4. New York: Academic Press, 1970.

Spence, K. W., & Spence, J. T. (Eds.) *The psychology of learning and motivation.* Vol. 1. New York: Academic Press, 1967.

Spence, K. W., & Spence, J. T. (Eds.) *The psychology of learning and motivation.* Vol. 2. New York: Academic Press, 1968.

Sternberg, S. High speed scanning in human memory. *Science,* 1966, Vol. 153, 652-654.

Sternberg, S. Two operations in character recognition: some evidence from reaction-time measurements. *Perception & Psychophysics,* 1967, Vol. 2, 45-53.

Talland, G. A. *Deranged memory.* New York: Academic Press, 1965.

Talland, G. A. *Disorders of memory and learning.* Middlesex, England: Penguin, 1968.

Talland, G. A., & Waugh, N. C. (Eds.) *The pathology of memory.* New York: Academic Press, 1969.

Teuber, H. -L., Milner, B., & Vaughan, H. G., Jr. Persistent anterograde amnesia after stab wound of the basal brain. *Neuropsychologia,* 1968, Vol. 6, 267-282.

Warrington, E. K., & Weiskrantz, L. An analysis of short-term and long-term memory deficits in man. In J. A. Deutsch (Ed.), *Physiological basis of memory.* New York: Academic Press, 1972.

Wickelgren, W. A. Sparing of short-term memory in an amnesic patient: implications for strength theory of memory. *Neuropsychologia,* 1968, Vol. 6, 235-244.

Wickelgren, W. A. Multitrace strength theory. In D. A. Norman (Ed.), *Models of human memory.* New York: Academic Press, 1970.

Woodworth, R. S., & Schlosberg, H. *Experimental psychology.* New York: Holt, 1954.

AUTHOR INDEX

Numbers in italics refer to the pages on which the complete references are listed.

SUBJECT INDEX

431

Motor horn cells, 138
Motor learning, 3
Motor neuron, 137, 139, 158
Multicistronic, 35
Multipolar cell, 129
Muscles, 130
Myasthenia gravis, 61
Myelination, 48
Myograms, 138

N

Narcosis, 114
Negative adaptation, 130
Negative feedback, 209
Negative (cathodal) pulse, 197
Negative reinforcement, 6
Neocortex, 47
Neomycin, 52
Nerve impulse, 129, 133
Nerve-muscle preparation, 221
Neural refractory periods, 236
Neural transmitters, 60
Neuromuscular junction, 92, 146, 220
Neuromuscular synapse, 132
Neuron, 3, 156, 198
Neuronal plasticity, 32
Neuronal refractory periods, 238, 240
Nicotine, 86, 99
Nonspecific thalamic nuclei, 157
Nonspecific thalamus, 162
Noradrenergic transmitter, 246
Norepinephrine, 91
Nucleic acids, 2, 3, 30
Nucleoli, 33
Nucleophosphoprotein, 33
Nucleoproteins, 83, 90
Nucleus, 90

O

Occipital cortex, 144
Occipital lesions, 388
Olfactory bulbs, 187
Olfactory discrimination, 6
Olfactory memory, 4
Olfactory stimuli, 3
Oligochaetes, 134

Operant behavior, 119
Operant conditioning, 10, 125, 150, 156
Optic chiasma, 290
Optic lobes of locust, 141
Orbicularis oculi muscle, 160
Orbital frontal deficit, 316
Organelles, 41
Orienting response, 140
Overtraining effect, 7
Overtraining situation, 8

P

^{32}P. 44
Pacemaker neurons, 154
Paired-pulse technique, 219, 222, 226, 242
Pancreas, 34
Paramecium, 131
Paraphernalia, 159
Parietal area, 161
Parietal cortex, 161
Parietal lobe, 387
Partial reinforcement schedules, 194, 202
Passive avoidance, 92
Passive avoidance learning, 93
Pattern discrimination, 8
Pelvic splanchnics, 190
Pentylenetetrazol, 86, 89, 97
Peptides, 5, 16, 17, 37, 40, 42
Perikaryon, 28, 34
pH, 36
Photoreceptor, 130, 135
Physostigmine, 63, 64, 70, 92, 120
Picrotoxin, 86, 99, 100, 139
Pigeons, 212
Placing reflex, 277
Planarians, 2, 8-11, 12
Plasticity, 136, 137, 151, 157, 164
Polarization, 52
Pole climbing task, 90
Polyacrylamide, 36
Polychaetes, 134
Polynucleotides, 40
Polysaccharides, 36
Polysomes, 34, 49
Polysynaptic reflexes, 130
Pons, 156
Pontine reticular formation, 162
Ponto-bulbar reticular formation, 162